G. T. Krishnamurthy · S. Krishnamurthy

Nuclear Hepatology

A Textbook of Hepatobiliary Diseases

Springer
Berlin
Heidelberg
New York
Barcelona
Hong Kong
London
Milan
Paris
Singapore
Tokyo

Gerbail T. Krishnamurthy
Shakuntala Krishnamurthy

Nuclear Hepatology

A Textbook of Hepatobiliary Diseases

With 152 Figures in 246 Separate Illustrations, 10 in Color and 72 Tables

Springer

G.T. Krishnamurthy, S. Krishnamurthy
Department of Nuclear Medicine, Tuality Community Hospital, Tuality HEALTHCARE, Hillsboro, Oregon, USA

G.T. Krishnamurthy, MBBS, MS, FACP, FACNP
Formerly, Chief, Nuclear Medicine Service, Veterans Affairs Medical Center
Portland, Oregon, USA
Program Director, Nuclear Medicine Residency, Oregon Health Sciences University
Portland, Oregon, USA
Professor of Radiology, Pathology, and Adjunct Professor of Medicine
Oregon Health Sciences University, Portland, Oregon, USA
Clinical Professor of Radiology, University of Arizona, Tucson, Arizona, USA
Associate Professor of Medicine, University of California, Los Angeles, California, USA

S. Krishnamurthy, BSc, MBBS
Clinical Assistant Professor of Radiology, Oregon Health Sciences University, Portland, Oregon, USA

ISBN 3-540-65917-X Springer-Verlag Berlin Heidelberg New York

Library of Congress Cataloging-in-Publication Data
Krishnamurthy, Gerbail, 1937–
Nuclear hepatology: a textbook of hepatobiliary diseases / Gerbail Krishnamurthy, Shakuntala Krisnamurthy.
p. ; cm.
Includes bibliographical references and index.
ISBN 354065917X (alk. paper)
1. Liver--Radionuclide imaging. 2. Biliary tract--Radionuclide imaging. I. Krishnamurthy, Shakuntala, 1942– II. Title.
[DNLM: 1. Liver Diseases--radionuclide imaging. 2. Biliary Tract Diseases--physiopathology. 3. Biliary Tract Diseases--radionuclide imaging. 4. Liver Diseases--physiopathology. 5. Radiopharmaceuticals--diagnostic use. WI 700 K92n 2000]
RC847.5.I42 K75 2000
616.3'607575--dc21 00-021831

Springer-Verlag is a company in the BertelsmannSpringer publishing group.

Printed in Germany

Cover-Design: Erich Kirchner, Heidelberg
Typesetting: Verlagsservice Teichmann, Mauer

SPIN: 107 111 82 21/3135 – 5 4 3 2 1 0 – Printed on acid-free paper

Dedicated with love and affection
to our children Anil and Kalpana,
who provided us a constant source of inspiration
throughout the conception
and completion of this textbook

Preface

Recent advances in technology have greatly impacted upon the practice of nuclear medicine in general, and the approach to hepatobiliary diseases in particular. Emphasis is now placed more on non-invasive functional imaging with quantification, a feature unique to nuclear medicine and not available from any other competing diagnostic imaging modality. By providing a measure of severity of disease, quantification aids not only in timing of therapy but also for testing whether or not the chosen therapy has achieved the intended goals and objectives. This is the first textbook of its kind in the new millennium on nuclear hepatology to fully integrate quantitative physiology with morphology in the diagnosis of hepatobiliary diseases.

The conception of nuclear hepatology occurred in the late 1940s with the introduction of radiocolloids, whose rate of clearance from blood was used as a measure of hepatic blood flow. Radiocolloid imaging of the liver, introduced first in the mid 1950s, was the most popular nuclear medicine imaging procedure in the 1970s and early 1980s, accounting for nearly 50% of the total workload in many nuclear medicine departments. Nuclear medicine shifted its focus during the mid 1980s from morphology alone to imaging of morphology integrated with quantitative physiology. Introduction of functional imaging radiopharmaceuticals, sophisticated gamma cameras, and powerful online computers with rapid data processing software all made it possible to quantify function as an integral part of imaging. Clarification of the function of the sphincter of Oddi through manometric studies, and availability of cholecystokinin for clinical studies, provided the ingredients necessary for integration of basic physiology and morphology with pathophysiology in the diagnosis of various hepatobiliary diseases.

As the only two authors, we have avoided unnecessary repetitions. Anatomy, histology (Chap. 1), and physiology (Chap. 2) of the hepatobiliary system are covered in sufficient detail necessary for image interpretation. Pharmacokinetics and clinical application of both morphology and physiology imaging agents (Chap. 3) are described, and for obvious reasons the physiology imaging agents are described in much greater detail than the morphology imaging agents. Imaging of morphology (Chap. 4) emphasizes its complementary role with ultrasound, CT, and MRI studies. Data acquisition and method of quantification of various physiological parameters are described (Chap. 5) with sufficient detail for easy adaptation. The reciprocal relationship between the function of the gallbladder and sphincter of Oddi, and the action of hormones (cholecystokinin) and drugs (opioids) on them in both health and disease (Chap. 6), are discussed in depth.

The minimum expectation by a referring physician from an imaging procedure is to be able to differentiate intrahepatic from extrahepatic cholestasis, which is essential for designing an appropriate management strategy. To highlight this importance, the differential diagnostic parameters of intrahepatic (Chap. 7) and extrahepatic (Chap. 8) cholestasis are described separately. Diseases of the gallbladder (Chap. 9) with or without accompanying morphological changes and their identification with quantitative functional parameters are presented. Functional imaging with quantification provides a sound basis for the diagnosis of biliary dyskinesia (Chap. 10), especially in the separation of sphincter of Oddi spasm from cystic duct syndrome. Diagnosis of hepatobiliary diseases in the newborn and children (Chap. 11) and evaluation of liver function before and after transplantation (Chap. 12) are presented in detail. The role of nuclear hepatology studies in the separation of native from donor liver function in the case of auxiliary liver transplantation is described.

The ability to radiolabel bile in vivo with technetium-99m, to acquire data directly from the liver, and to quantify function totally under basal conditions without needing sedation or indwelling catheters, offers a unique opportunity to study most liver diseases associated with bile formation and flow. We have emphasized mostly those diagnostic imaging procedures that are clinically well established and also have pointed out yet unharnessed areas where there is great potential for further progress. Emphasis is placed on developing newer or modifying current techniques in the identification of end-stage liver disease and also in the evaluation of transplant related complications. This textbook is intended to serve as a ready reference as well as a clinical and procedural guide in meeting the needs of practitioners of nuclear medicine, radiology, internal medicine, pediatrics, gastroenterology, hepatology, primary care, general surgery, and liver transplant surgery and others who take care of patients with hepatobiliary diseases.

We have made sincere efforts to give due credit to all those authors whose innovative work has made it possible for us to write this textbook. Our understanding of the role of quantitative hepatobiliary imaging and its clinical application were made possible largely through the voluntary participation of many of our patients in clinical research studies over several years and we acknowledge their contribution in completing this book. We are indebted to Dr. Paul H. Brown, Associate Professor of Radiology, Oregon Health Sciences University, Portland, and Mrs. Judy Hays, Assistant Librarian, Tuality Community Hospital, Hillsboro, Oregon, for reviewing several chapters and for checking references for accuracy and completion, respectively.

Portland

GERBAIL T. KRISHNAMURTHY
SHAKUNTALA KRISHNAMURTHY

Contents

Morphology and Microstructure of the Hepatobiliary System

1.1 Morphology

Embryology

The liver and biliary system develop from an endodermal bud which sprouts during the 5th week of intrauterine life when the embryo is about 3 mm in length [1]. The bud arises along the ventral surface at the junction of the foregut with the midgut, and soon differentiates into a cranial (pars hepatica) branch and a caudal (pars cystica) branch. The ventral pancreas sprouts near the caudal bud and the dorsal pancreas arises on the opposite side at the foregut-midgut junction (Fig. 1.1.1). When the embryo is about 5 mm in length, the cranial and caudal branches grow further connected by a common stalk which later becomes the common bile duct. By the time the embryo is about 7 mm in length, the cranial branch (pars hepatica) divides into two cellular columns which later become the physiologic right and left hepatic lobes [2]. The gallbladder develops from the caudal branch (pars cystica) and continues its connection with the common stalk through a channel which later becomes the cystic duct. Canalization takes place to form a patent biliary tree (gallbladder, cystic duct, right and left hepatic duct, common hepatic duct and the common bile duct). When the embryo is about 10 mm in length, the gut begins to make a 90° clockwise rotation and completes it by the time it is 12 mm in length, which brings the ventral pancreas in close contact with the dorsal pancreas, facilitating their fusion into a single pancreas, before birth [3]. This rotation also brings the common bile duct posterior to the duodenum. Many congenital abnormalities around this region are secondary to malrotation at this junction. The liver begins bile secretion by the 12th intrauterine week, thus completing the formation of the hepatobiliary system, the most complex metabolic factory in the human body. In adults, the liver weighs about 1500–1800 g and forms about 1/50 of the body weight. In children, however, it forms a relatively much larger fraction (1/20) of the total body weight.

Liver Lobes and Surfaces

Most of the liver is situated in the upper quadrant of the abdomen underneath the right hemidiaphragm, with the superior border situated at the level of the right fifth intercostal space. Liver consists of five surfaces: anterior, posterior, right lateral, superior, and inferior. The anterior, right lateral, and posterior surfaces are smooth and superior and inferior surfaces are rough with grooves and fissures for entry and exit of the vascular and biliary structures. The liver can be divided into right and left lobes on

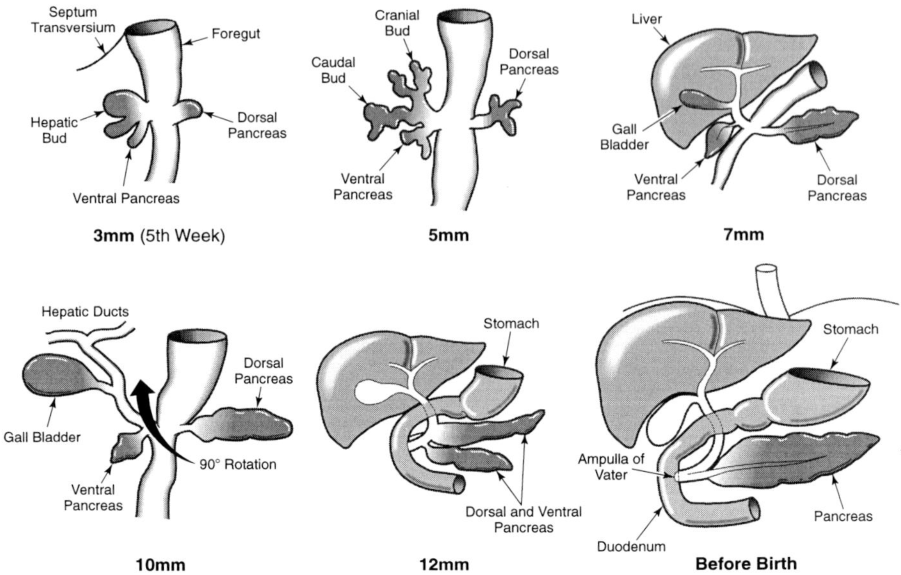

Fig. 1.1.1. Embryology of the hepatobiliary system. The hepatic bud arises from the endoderm of the primitive foregut at its junction with the midgut when the embryo is about 3 mm in length. The hepatic bud divides into cranial (pars hepatica) and caudal (pars cystica) branches when the embryo reaches 5 mm size. The ventral pancreas arises from the pars cystica, which later gives rise to the biliary system. After a 90° clockwise rotation (10-mm embryo), the ventral pancreas fuses with the dorsal pancreas. This rotation brings the common bile duct posterior to the duodenum (12 mm). The common bile duct opens through the ampulla of Vater into the duodenum at the posteromedial wall at an elevation called the papilla

the basis of either anatomic or physiologic markers (Fig. 1.1.2). Anatomically, the liver is divided into right and left lobes on the basis of the line of attachment of the falciform ligament. The anatomic division serves no useful purpose in the management of liver disease and hence has been given less importance in recent years. The physiologic division, on the other hand, has gained more popularity recently as it follows embryologic development and delineates functional lobes and segments whose line of demarcation is used for liver resection during transplant or tumor surgery. The physiologic division into right and left lobes is indicated by a deep fissure called the plane of Sérégé-Cantlie that passes from the gallbladder fossa in front to the inferior vena cava in the back [3].

The falciform ligament, the marker of the anatomic right and left lobes, lies to the left of the deep fissure (Sérégé-Cantlie) that divides the liver into physiologic right and left lobes. The caudate lobe situated posteriorly, and the quadrate lobe situated anteriorly, both form part of the anatomic right lobe, but both of these structures belong to the physiologic left lobe (Fig. 1.1.2). The anatomic right lobe is six times larger than the anatomic left lobe, whereas the physiologic right lobe is almost the same size as the physiologic left lobe. It is important, therefore, to be very specific while describing lobes of the liver, whether one is referring to the anatomic or to the physiologic division. Throughout this book we will follow the physiologic division unless mentioned otherwise.

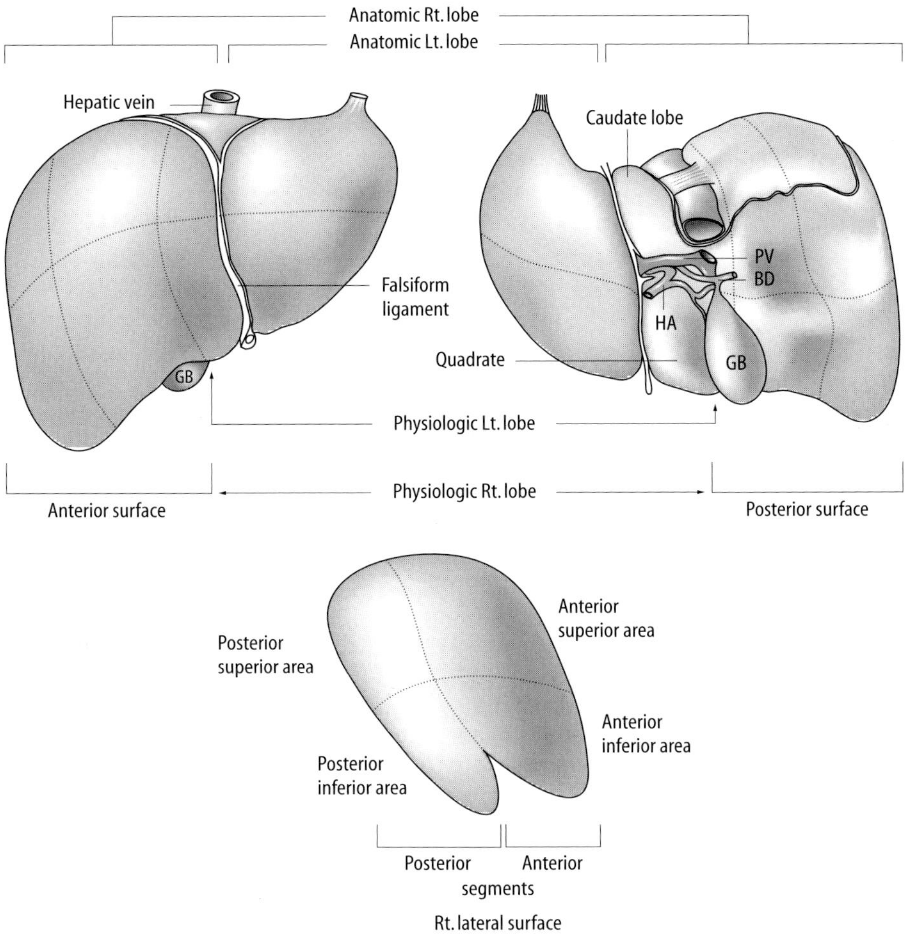

Fig. 1.1.2. Surfaces, segments, and lobes of the liver. The anatomic left lobe (divided by the falciform ligament) is much smaller than the anatomic right lobe, but the physiologic left lobe is almost as large as the physiologic right lobe. The quadrate lobe, which forms a part of the anatomic right lobe, becomes a part of the physiologic left lobe. Liver consists of three lobes (including the caudate lobe), four segments, and eight areas. *HA*, hepatic artery; *BD*, bile duct; *PV*, portal vein; *GB*, gallbladder

Segments and Areas

The liver is divided into lobes, segments, and areas. The division can be made on the basis of either the vascular structures [3–5] or the bile ducts [6]. As the vessels (hepatic artery and portal vein) and bile ducts travel together to every lobe, segment, and area of the liver, there is usually no difference as to which structure is chosen as the reference point for the division. Areas are either named by numbers or given a directional nomenclature, similar to the division of the lungs into lobes and segments. Couinaud [4] and Bismuth [7] gave numbers, whereas Healey and Schroy [6] preferred directional nomenclature. The imaging technology (nuclear medicine, CT, MRI, and ultrasound) has chosen numerical segments for the division [8–14]. Table 1.1.1 shows names and numbers adopted by different authors. The directional nomenclature used by Healey and Schroy [6] is much easier to remember whereas the numbers require memorization. Recent authors in general seem to prefer the numbers proposed by Couinaud and Bismuth [14].

Table 1.1.1. Nomenclature for hepatic lobes, segments, and areas as adopted by different authors

Liver lobe	Hjortsjo [3]	Healey and Schroy [6]	Couinaud [4]	Bismuth [7]
Caudate lobe	Dorsal segment	Lobus caudatus	I	I
Left lobe	Dorsolateral segment	Lateral superior area	II	II
	Ventrolateral segment	Lateral inferior area	III	III
	Central segment	Medial superior area	IV	IVa
	Dorsoventral segment	Medial inferior area	IV	IVb
Right lobe	Ventrocaudal segment	Anterior-inferior area	V	V
	Dorsocaudal + intermediocaudal	Posterior-inferior area	VI	VI
	Dorsocranial + intermediocaudal	Posterior-superior area	VII	VII
	Ventrocranial	Anterior-superior area	VIII	VIII

The middle hepatic vein passes in between the right and left lobes. The right lobe is divided into anterior and posterior segments by the fissure of the right hepatic vein which runs almost in the middle of the right lobe. The left lobe is divided into medial and lateral segments by the left hepatic vein in the middle. The right and left branches of the portal vein divide the liver segments into superior and inferior areas. The liver, therefore, consists of two large lobes, four segments, and eight areas (Fig. 1.1.3). The caudate lobe (#I) despite being very small in size is considered as a separate lobe mainly because of its unique vasculature.

Blood Vessels, Bile Ducts, Lymphatics, and Nerves

Hepatic Artery

After arising from the celiac axis, the hepatic artery runs between the two layers of the hepatogastric ligament (lesser omentum) and enters the liver at the hilum. It is situated anterior to the portal vein and onto the left side of the common bile duct (Fig. 1.1.3). In 90% of patients, the hepatic artery divides into right and left branches before entering the hilum of the liver. In the remaining 10%, the hepatic artery divides into three terminal branches, the third branch entering the quadrate lobe (area IV) directly. The hepatic artery supplies about 400 ml arterial blood/min at 100 mmHg systolic pressure, and accounts for 25% of the total liver blood flow [15].

The cystic artery to the gallbladder usually arises from the right hepatic artery in the triangle of Calot, which is bordered by the inferior liver surface above, common hepatic duct to the left, and the cystic duct to the right. Often the cystic artery may arise from the main hepatic artery, left hepatic artery or the gastroduodenal artery. Soon after its origin, the cystic artery enters the gallbladder at its neck and divides immediately into a superficial branch and a deep branch, both of which were first identified by Vesalius in 1564 [3]. The superficial branch supplies blood mostly to the free inferior wall covered by the peritoneum and the deep branch supplies blood to the superior wall, which lies in direct contact with the inferior liver surface.

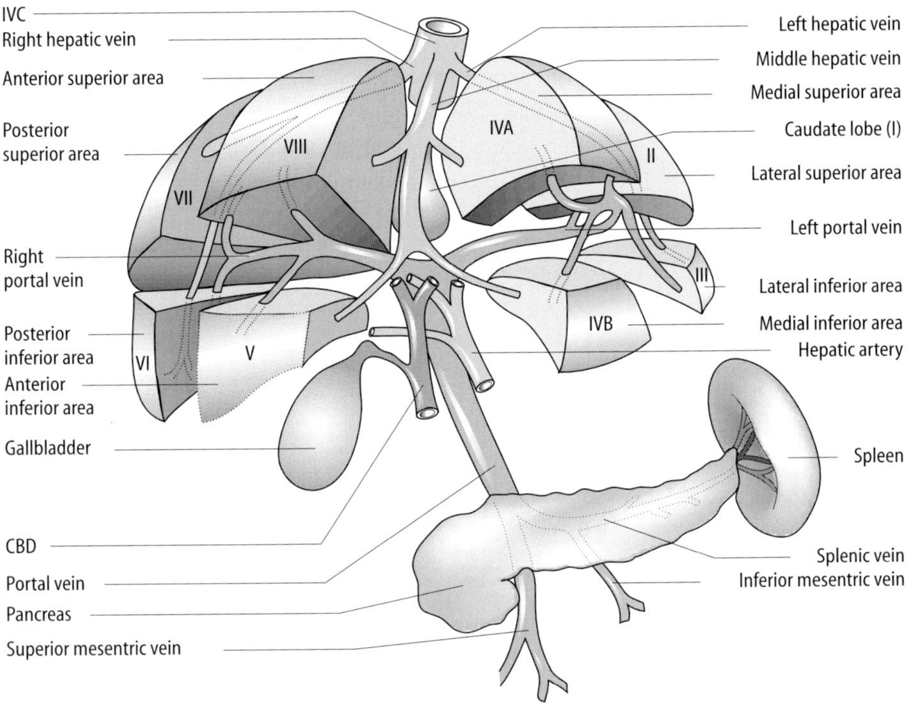

Fig. 1.1.3. Hepatic and portal venous system. The left hepatic vein, carrying blood from the lateral segment of the left lobe, joins the middle hepatic vein, carrying blood from the medial segment of the left lobe and anterior segment of the right lobe, to form a single venous trunk before joining the inferior vena cava. The right hepatic vein carries blood mostly from the posterior segment of the right lobe and joins the inferior vena cava separately. The portal vein is formed by the union of the superior mesenteric and splenic veins. It divides into right and left portal branches, which travel in opposite directions at 180° and enter the parenchyma in the middle dividing liver into superior and inferior areas. *CBD*, common bile duct; *IVC*, inferior vena cava

Portal Vein

The portal vein is formed by the union of the splenic and superior mesenteric veins and measures about 5.5–8 cm in length and enters the liver at the porta hepatis (Fig. 1.1.3). It divides at a 180° angle into right and left portal vein branches, which enter the parenchyma in the middle, dividing the liver into superior and inferior areas. The right portal vein gives off anterior and posterior segmental branches and the left portal vein gives off medial and lateral segmental branches. Segmental veins give off at least one branch to each area of the liver. Two small veins, one each from right and left portal vein branches, enter the caudate lobe. The portal vein supplies about 1200 ml blood/min (75% of the total liver blood supply) at 7–10 mmHg systolic pressure [15].

Hepatic Veins

There are three distinctly separate hepatic veins: right, middle, and left. They interdigitate and overlap with the portal venous system and divide the liver into four segments.

The left hepatic vein drains blood mostly from the superior and inferior area of the lateral segment of the left lobe. Small tributaries are also received from the medial segment of the left lobe (Fig. 1.1.3). The middle hepatic vein runs along the gallbladder fossa-inferior vena cava plane (Sérégé-Cantlie) and divides the liver into physiologic right and left lobes. It receives blood from the superior and inferior areas of the medial segment of the left lobe, and the superior and inferior areas of the anterior segment of the right lobe. The middle and left hepatic veins unite to form a single trunk before joining the inferior vena cava. The right hepatic vein is the largest of the three veins and drains blood mostly from the superior and inferior areas of the posterior segment of the right lobe. Small tributaries are also received from the anterior segment of the right lobe. The right hepatic vein joins the inferior vena cava directly as a separate branch. The venous blood from the caudate lobe also drains directly into the inferior vena cava. Because of this separate venous pathway directly into the inferior vena cava, the caudate lobe often maintains normal function during thrombosis of the hepatic veins (Budd-Chiari syndrome). The patients with Budd-Chiari syndrome demonstrate a normal pattern of ^{99m}Tc-sulfur colloid uptake by the caudate lobe, whereas the rest of the liver parenchyma shows a marked reduction or no radiocolloid uptake at all.

Bile Ducts

The biliary tree consists of a network of progressively increasing in size ductal system originating at the hepatocytes as the bile canaliculus (Fig. 1.1.4). Bile canaliculi from the adjoining hepatocytes unite to form the cholangioles (<20 μm), which in turn combine to form the interlobular ducts (20–100 μm) and later the area ducts (100–400 μm). Ducts from each area unite to form the segmental ducts (400–800 μm). The segments are positioned anterior and posterior in the right lobe, and medial and lateral in the left lobe [16]. The anterior segmental duct unites with the posterior segmental duct (72%) to form the right hepatic duct (Fig. 1.1.5). The right

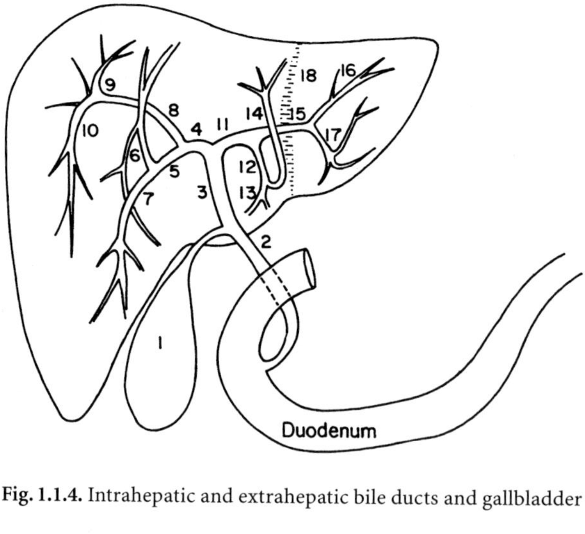

1-Gallbladder
2-Common Bile Duct
3-Common Hepatic Duct
4-Right Hepatic Duct
5-Anterior Segment Duct
6-Anterior Superior Area Duct
7-Anterior Inferior Area Duct
8-Posterior Segment Duct
9-Posterior Superior Area Duct
10-Posterior Inferior Area Duct
11-Left Hepatic Duct
12-Medial Segment Duct
13-Medial Inferior Area Duct
14-Medial Superior Area Duct
15-Lateral Segment Duct
16-Lateral Superior Area Duct
17-Lateral Inferior Area Duct
18-Falciform Ligament

Fig. 1.1.4. Intrahepatic and extrahepatic bile ducts and gallbladder posterior segmental duct unites with the left hepatic duct directly in 22%, and in the remaining 6% of people the right anterior segmental duct joins the left hepatic duct directly [6].

In the left lobe, the medial segmental duct usually unites with the lateral segmental duct (62%) to form the left hepatic duct. The left medial segmental duct joins the left inferior area duct in 25% of cases. Other variations are less frequent (Fig. 1.1.6). It is rare for either the left medial or the left lateral segmental duct to join the right hepatic duct directly. The medial segmental duct drains bile from the anatomic quadrate lobe and the lateral segmental duct drains bile from the entire anatomic left lobe. In a ^{99m}Tc-HIDA (hepatic iminodiacetic acid) study, the medial segmental duct and the lateral segmental duct appear as separate trunks in an anterior view image. Anterior and posterior segmental ducts of the right hepatic lobe become superimposed in the

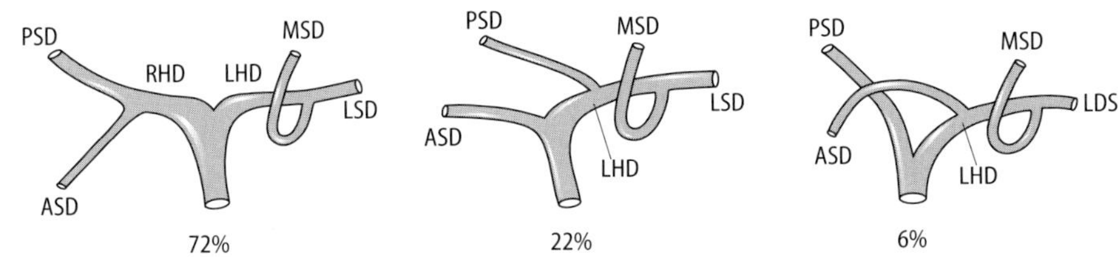

Fig. 1.1.5. Variations in bile drainage from the right lobe. The anterior segmental duct (*ASD*) usually joins with the posterior segmental duct (*PSD*), forming the right hepatic duct (*RHD*) in 72%. Sometimes either *PSD* (22%) or *ASD* (6%) may join the left hepatic duct directly. Both *RHD* and *LHD* unite to form the common hepatic duct

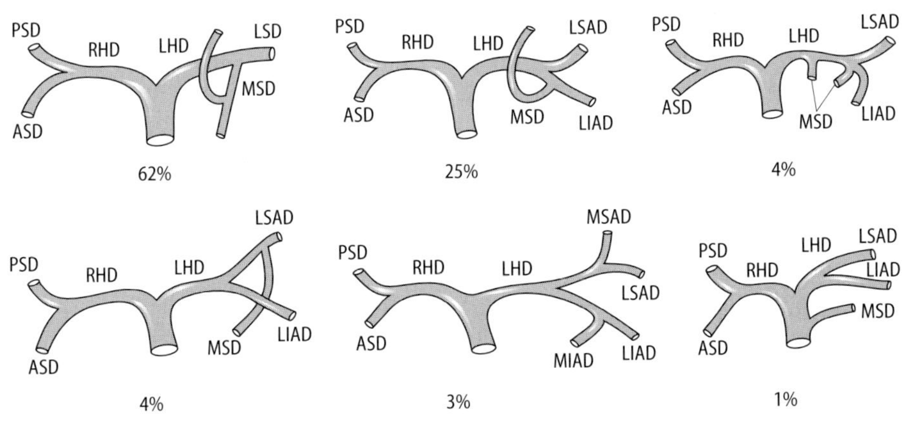

Fig. 1.1.6. Variations in drainage of bile from the left lobe. The medial segmental duct (*MSD*) usually unites with the lateral segmental duct (*LSD*) in 62%, forming the left hepatic duct (*LHD*), which later unites with the right hepatic duct (*RHD*), forming the common hepatic duct. In the remaining 38% of patients the main difference in bile drainage pertains to variations in area ducts joining with each other. It is rare for either the left medial or the left lateral segmental duct from the left lobe to join directly with the right hepatic duct (*RHD*). *LSAD* = lateral superior area duct; *LIAD* = lateral inferior area duct; *MIAD* = medial inferior area duct; *MSAD* = medial superior area duct; *PSD* = posterior segmental duct; *ASD* = anterior segmental duct

anterior view image. A right lateral view, therefore, is necessary to separate the right anterior segmental duct from the right posterior segmental duct (Fig. 1.1.2). There is profuse arterial arborization and a generous blood supply to both intrahepatic and extrahepatic bile ducts.

Based upon its pattern of bile drainage, the caudate lobe is divided anatomically into three parts: (1) caudate process, (2) right caudate lobe, and (3) left caudate lobe. Bile from the caudate process drains mostly into the right posterior segmental duct and less often into the left hepatic duct. Bile from the right caudate lobe enters either the right posterior segmental duct or the left hepatic duct with equal frequency. Bile from the left caudate lobe enters the left hepatic duct [6].

Lymphatics

The lymph vessels from the liver parenchyma generally follow the course of the blood vessels and bile ducts and join with the gallbladder lymph vessels at the porta hepatis, and later divide into two main lymph channels; one channel follows the course of the common bile duct and the other follows the course of the hepatic artery. Both channels pass through several lymph nodes. The lymph channel following the course of the hepatic artery drains lymph primarily into nodes around the celiac axis and the other channel, which follows the course of the common bile duct, drains lymph into lymph nodes around the pancreas [3]. The lymph from the liver parenchyma and bile ducts ultimately reaches the cisterna chyli (Fig. 1.1.7). The location of the liver lymph nodes is highly variable with the exception of one node situated at the junction of the gallbladder neck with the cystic duct (node of Mascagni). Enlargement of the node of Mascagni during generalized lymphadenopathy may cause cystic duct obstruction and block bile entry into the gallbladder, mimicking findings of an acute cholecystitis. Small lymph vessels around the central vein accompany the hepatic veins and inferior vena cava and drain lymph directly into the thoracic duct [17].

Nerves

The hepatobiliary system is supplied by both somatic and autonomic nervous systems. The somatic nerve supply comes from the lower thoracic intercostal nerves (T7–11) and the right phrenic nerve (C3, 4). The lower thoracic intercostal nerves supply the parietal peritoneum. The right phrenic nerve supplies the diaphragm and the peritoneum covering the liver and the gallbladder. The pain due to distension of the liver capsule, gallbladder wall, or bile ducts is transmitted through these nerves (Fig. 1.1.7).

The autonomic nerve supply is by both sympathetic and parasympathetic nervous systems. The parasympathetic nerve fibers travel via the vagus which arises from the medulla and traverses down, one on each side of the neck and mediastinum to reach the abdomen. Due to clockwise rotation of the gut during early intrauterine life (Fig. 1.1.1), the left vagus nerve becomes the anterior and the right vagus the posterior trunk. Both of these nerve trunks were first identified and correctly described by Vesalius in 1543 [18]. The anterior trunk (left vagus) enters the anterior gastric plexus at the gastroesophageal junction. A branch from the anterior gastric plexus, the anterior hepatic nerve, enters the porta hepatis and bifurcates; one branch supplies the intrahepatic and proximal extrahepatic bile ducts and blood vessels and the other

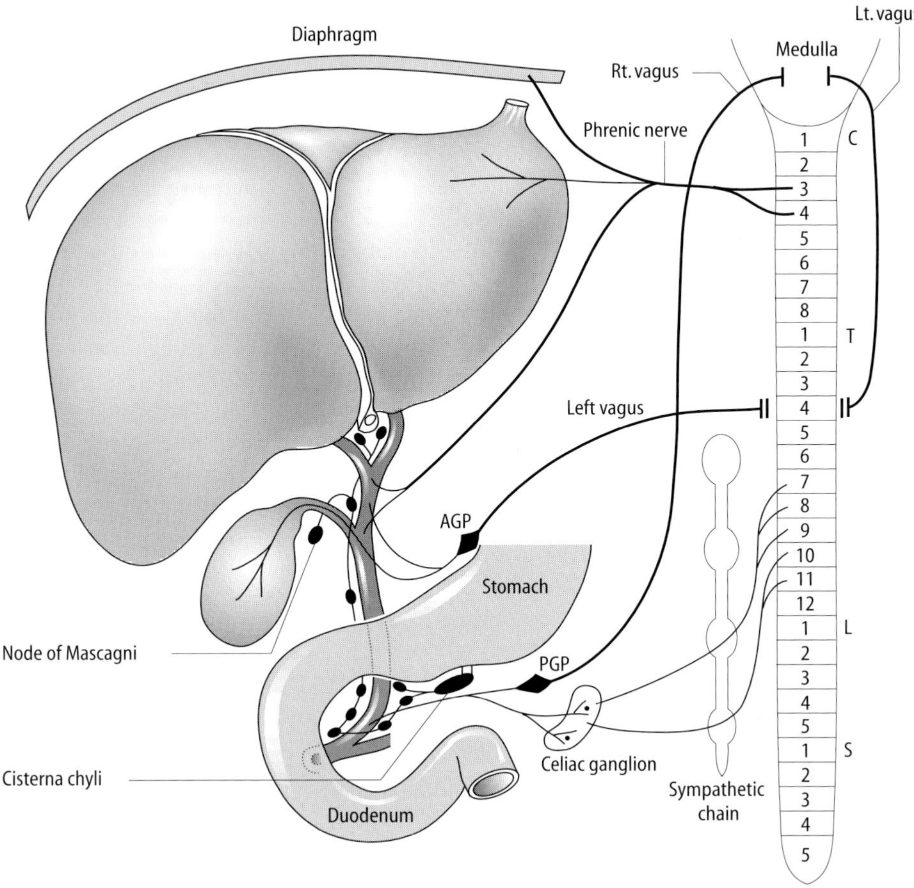

Fig. 1.1.7. Nerve supply and lymphatic drainage of the hepatobiliary system. The vagus (parasympathetic) nerve from the medulla descends along each side of the neck and mediastinum and enters the abdomen. The left vagus gives off branches to the anterior gastric plexus (*AGP*), from where the vagal branches reach the liver and gallbladder and intrahepatic ducts. The right vagus gives off branches to the posterior gastric plexus (*PGP*), from where the vagal branches are given off mainly to the common bile duct and the sphincter of Oddi. The phrenic nerve from cervical 3–4 supplies the liver capsule and the peritoneum covering the liver and gallbladder. Sympathetic nerve fibers reach the biliary system via the splanchnic nerves (T7–11) after passing through the celiac ganglion. The lymph from the gallbladder is drained to a node near the neck (node of Mascagni) and then to the nodes along the common bile duct, which also receive lymph from the lower half of the liver. The liver and gallbladder lymph vessels enter the peripancreatic lymph nodes and ultimately drain lymph into the cisterna chyli

branch supplies the gallbladder. The posterior vagal trunk (right vagus) passes behind the stomach and enters the posterior gastric plexus. A few of its branches enter the celiac ganglion. From the posterior gastric plexus the nerve fibers enter the distal common bile duct and the sphincter of Oddi (Fig. 1.1.7).

The parasympathetic nerve supply to the gallbladder comes primarily from the anterior trunk (left vagus). The distal common bile duct and the sphincter of Oddi receive their parasympathetic nerve supply primarily from the posterior trunk (right vagus). The parasympathetic motor function of the gallbladder, therefore, is controlled mainly through the anterior trunk (left vagus) and that of the sphincter of Oddi mainly through the posterior trunk (right vagus). An injury or section of the anterior trunk (left vagus) alone during vagotomy, therefore, has the same effect as complete vagotomy (cutting of both vagi) as far as the motor function of the gallbladder is concerned. Parasympathetic ablation enhances muscular relaxation and increases bile stasis within the gallbladder promoting cholelithiasis [19–21]. Stimulation of the parasympathetic system, on the other hand, increases the tonicity of the gallbladder and promotes complete bile emptying.

The hepatobiliary system receives the sympathetic nerve supply via the greater (T7–9) and lesser splanchnic nerves (T10, 11). The axons from preganglionic sympathetic nerve cells in the lateral horn of the thoracic T7–11 segments travel via the greater and lesser splanchnic nerves and enter the celiac ganglion. The postganglionic sympathetic fibers from the celiac ganglion enter the liver, gallbladder, common bile duct, and sphincter of Oddi. Sympathetic nerve stimulation relaxes the gallbladder wall. The hepatic artery and its branches are supplied by sympathetic nerves that control the vascular tone. The pain sensation of the hepatobiliary system is carried to the central nervous system via both the splanchnic nerves and the branches of the right phrenic nerve (Fig. 1.1.7).

Biliary Apparatus

Intrahepatic Ducts

The hepatobiliary system is analogous to a tree. The hepatocytes represent the leaves, the canaliculi the stalk, and the area and segmental ducts the branches of the tree. The common hepatic duct and the common bile duct represent the trunk and the sphincter of Oddi the roots of the tree. The gallbladder is akin to a fruit [22]. Bile canaliculi from the hepatocytes join to form the cholangioles, which in turn unite to form the interlobular bile ducts and then into larger area ducts. Ducts from each area unite to form the segmental ducts. The anterior and posterior segmental ducts unite to form the right hepatic duct, and the medial and lateral segmental ducts unite to form the left hepatic duct (Fig. 1.1.4).

Extrahepatic Ducts

The right and left hepatic ducts leave the liver parenchyma and proceed inferiorly for a distance of 0.5–1.5 cm before joining to form the common hepatic duct [6]. The common hepatic duct is 2–7 cm in length and joins with the cystic duct to form the common bile duct.

Gallbladder

The gallbladder lies along the inferior liver border in a groove between the right lobe and the quadrate lobe (medial segment of the left lobe). It consists of a fundus, body, and neck (Fig. 1.1.8). The gallbladder measures about 7–10 cm in length, 3–5 cm in width, and 40–50 ml in volume [23]. The superior one-third of the wall is in direct contact with the liver and hence lacks the peritoneal covering. The rest of the gallblad-

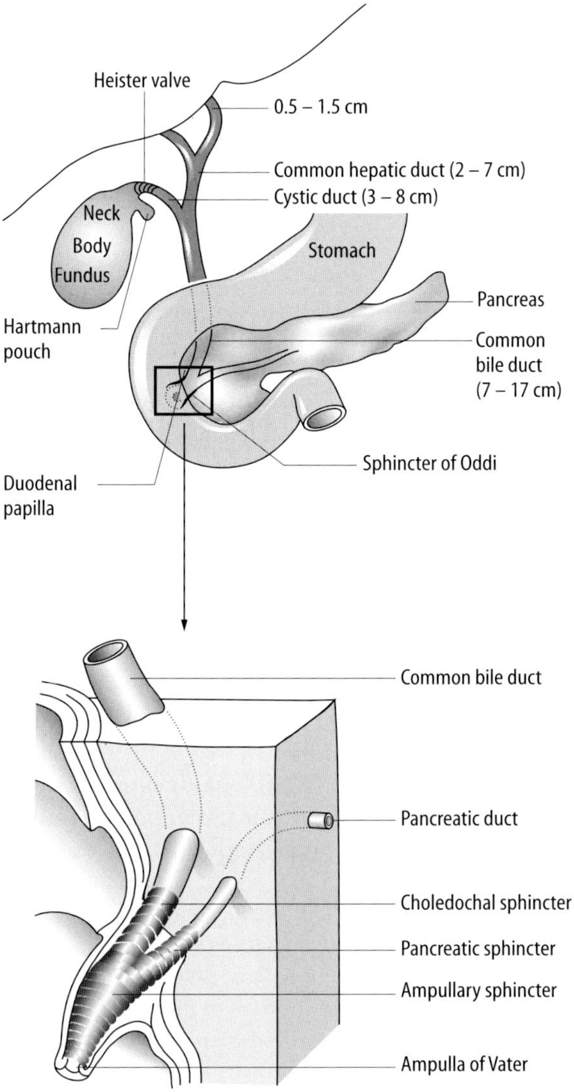

Fig. 1.1.8. Extrahepatic biliary tract. The distal one-third of both right and left hepatic ducts, and the entire common hepatic and common bile ducts, are extrahepatic in location. The gallbladder consists of a fundus, body, neck, and cystic duct. The mucous membrane in the neck and cystic duct is thrown into folds which acts as a valve (Heister's valve) for bile entry and exit. A pouch near the neck (Hartmann's pouch) often lodges gallstones. The sphincter of Oddi (enlarged) at the distal end of the common bile duct consists of three separate sphincters. The distal common bile duct is surrounded by the choledochal sphincter (sphincter of Boyden). The distal pancreatic duct (duct of Wirsung) is surrounded by a separate pancreatic sphincter. The common channel formed by the union of two ducts is surrounded by the ampullary sphincter. The common channel (ampulla of Vater) opens into the duodenum at an elevation called the papilla. The name sphincter of Oddi refers to all three sphincters

der wall is covered with the visceral peritoneum. The gallbladder is a pear shaped organ with the extension of the fundus below the inferior liver margin. The position of the fundus on the body surface corresponds to the point of intersection of the lateral margin of the right rectus muscle with the right costal margin. A line drawn between the left anterior superior iliac spine and the umbilicus points to the position of the fundus when it is extended upwards to meet with the right costal margin. A pouch like structure (Hartmann's pouch) at the neck often lodges gallstones, initiating cystic duct obstruction and subsequent acute cholecystitis. The mucous membrane is thrown into folds in the neck and cystic duct and acts as a valve (Heister's valve) for bile entry and exit into and out of the gallbladder, respectively. The cystic duct measures about 3–8 cm in length and less than 3 mm in diameter and joins the common hepatic duct at a 45° angle (in 80%) to form the common bile duct. Sometimes, the cystic duct may directly join the right hepatic or the left hepatic duct. There are many variations in the way the cystic duct joins with the common hepatic duct, right hepatic, or left hepatic duct [24]. The artery to the gallbladder (cystic artery) arises usually from the right hepatic artery (72%) or from its accessory branches (13%) and less often directly from the hepatic artery (6%) or the gastroduodenal artery.

The gallbladder is supplied by both the sympathetic and parasympathetic nervous systems, which control its tone, contraction, and relaxation. The gallbladder lymph, after passing through a node at the neck (node of Mascagni), enters the hepatic plexus and ultimately reaches the cisterna chyli (Fig. 1.1.7). The gallbladder is absent in 1:1600 live births and in about 8% of cases it is entirely intrahepatic in location [25]. The C loop of the duodenum and the hepatic flexure of the colon are in close proximity to the gallbladder.

Common Bile Duct

The common bile duct is formed by the union of the common hepatic duct with the cystic duct. It varies in length from 7 to 17 cm and the lumen is less than 8 mm in diameter (Fig. 1.1.8). The common bile duct is divided into: supraduodenal, retroduodenal, intrapancreatic, and intraduodenal segments. The supraduodenal segment is the longest and measures 2–4 cm in length. The retroduodenal and intrapancreatic segments each measure about 2.5–3 cm in length. The intraduodenal segment is the narrowest part of the common bile duct. The retroduodenal segment lies behind the duodenal bulb and may be non-visualized in a ^{99m}Tc-HIDA study if there is fluid collection in the duodenum. The common bile duct enters the posteromedial wall of the second part of the duodenum and unites with the pancreatic duct (duct of Wirsung), forming a common channel, the ampulla of Vater, which finally enters the duodenal lumen at an elevation called the "papilla." The papilla lies about 8–10 cm away from the pylorus of the stomach. The common bile duct joins with the pancreatic duct, forming a common channel of 10–12 mm length in 86% of cases. The two ducts join together at the ampulla just before opening into the duodenum in 6% of cases, and in the remaining 8% both ducts open separately into the duodenum [3].

References

1. Linder HH, Green RB. Embryology and surgical anatomy of the extra hepatic biliary tract. Surg Clin N Amer 1964;44:1273–1285
2. Netter FH. CIBA collection of medical illustration, Volume lll, Digestive system, part lll. Liver, biliary tract, and pancreas. CIBA, Summit NJ, 1964
3. Hess W. Surgery of the biliary passages and the pancreas. D Von Nostrand Company Inc, Princeton, NJ, 1965
4. Couinaud C. Le foie etudes anatomiques et chirurgicales, Masson, Paris, 1957
5. Reifferscheid M. Chirurgie der leber. Georg Thieme Verlag, Stuttgart, 1957
6. Haley JE, Schroy PC. Anatomy of the biliary ducts within the human liver. Analysis of the prevailing pattern of branchings and the major variations of the biliary ducts. Arch Surg 1953;66:599–616
7. Bismuth H. Surgical anatomy and anatomical surgery of the liver. World J Surg 1982;6:3–9

8. Goldsmith MA, Woodburn RT. Surgical anatomy pertaining to liver resection. Surg Gynecol Obstet 1957;141:429–437
9. Sugarbaker PH. En bloc resection of hepatic segments 4B, 5 and 6 by transverse hepatectomy. Surg Gynecol Obstet 1990;170:250–252
10. Sugarbaker PH, Nelson RC, Murray DR, Chezmar JL, Barnardino MF. A segmental approach to computerized tomographic portography for hepatic resection. Surg Gynecol Obstet 1990;171:189–195
11. Nelson RC, Chezmar JL, Sugarbaker PH, Murray DR, Bernardino MF. Pre-operative localization of focal liver lesions to specific liver segments: utility of CT during arterial portography. Radiology 1991;181:443–448
12. Laforture M, Madore F, Patriquin H, Breton G. Segmental anatomy of the liver: a sonographic approach to the Couinaud nomenclature. Radiology 1991;181:443–448
13. Soyer P. Segmental anatomy of the liver: utility of a nomenclature accepted world wide. AJR. Amer J Roentgenol 1993;161:572–573
14. Dodd GD lll, An American's guide to Couinaud's numbering system. AJR. Amer J Roentgenol 1993;161:574–575
15. Sherlock S, Dooley J. Diseases of the liver and biliary system. 10th edition, Blackwell Science, Malden, MA, 1997
16. Roberts SK, Ludwig J, LaRusso NF. The pathology of biliary epithelia. Gastroenterology 1997;112:269–279
17. Jones AL. The architecture of bile secretion. A morphological perspective of physiology. Dig Dis Sci 1980;25;609–629
18. Holle F. Historical outline. In: Holle F, Anderson S. eds. Vagotomy: latest advances. Springer-Verlag, New York, 1974
19. LaRusso D, Misciagno G, Noviello MR, Torantino S. Cholelithiasis after billroth ll gastric resection. Surgery 1988;103:579–583
20. Griffiths JMT, Holmes G. Cholecystitis following gastric surgery. Lancet 1994;2:780–782
21. Turunen M, Antila L. Gallbladder disease following gastrectomy. Acta Chir Scand 1964;127:134–137
22. Krishnamurthy S, Krishnamurthy GT. Evolution of nuclear hepatology as a clinical subspeciality. J Nucl Med Technol. 1995;23 (suppl): 35S–45S
23. Gunnarson E, Investigation of the distension capacity of the human gallbladder. Acta Radiol (Stockh) 1961;56:161–165
24. Goor DA, Ebert PA. Anomalies of the biliary tree. Report of a repair of an accessory bile duct and review of the literature. Arch Surg 1972;104:302–309
25. Boyden EA. The accessory gallbladder – an embryological and comparative study of aberrant biliary vesicles in man and domestic mammals. Am J Anat 1926;38:177–231

1.2 Microstructure

The liver is the largest organ in the body and consists of an intricate structure to carry out both the complex exocrine (bile secretion) and endocrine (protein synthesis) functions efficiently. The organ shape and structure are well maintained despite the paucity of connective tissue.

A lobule was viewed as the basic microarchitecture of the liver for well over a century [1]. A lobule consists of a tributary of the hepatic vein at the center and portal triad (consisting of the terminal branch of the hepatic artery, portal vein, and bile duct) at the periphery, and the space in between is occupied by hepatocytes and cells of the sinusoidal space. A new concept, an acinus, as being the basic liver microscopic unit was proposed first in 1958 and is now well accepted because it explains the function and regeneration of the liver much better than the lobule model [2]. An acinus is diamond shaped with a central vein (hepatic vein) at one corner and a portal triad at the other two corners. The liver consists of the polygonal cells (hepatocytes), sinusoidal cells, canalicular cells, and other supporting cells (Fig. 1.2.1). An adult liver consists of well over 250 billion cells of which 60% are hepatocytes [3]. In the rat, the hepatocytes constitute 78% of the liver by volume. The peripheral polygonal cells in zone 1, which receive blood through the portal vein and hepatic artery, are able to sustain ischemia much better than the cells in zone 3, which lie closer to the central vein [4].

Vascular Compartment

This compartment is situated between two single-layer plates of hepatocytes and consists of two spaces: (1) the sinusoidal space and (2) the perisinusoidal space of Disse (Fig. 1.2.1). The sinusoidal space is much larger of the two and accounts for two-thirds of the vascular compartment. Four types of cells are found in the vascular space: (1) endothelial cell (sinusoidal lining cell), (2) Kupffer cell, (3) lipocyte (Ito cell or fat storing cell), and (4) pit cell [5]. These four cells together constitute the functional unit of the hepatic sinusoid (Table 1.2.1).

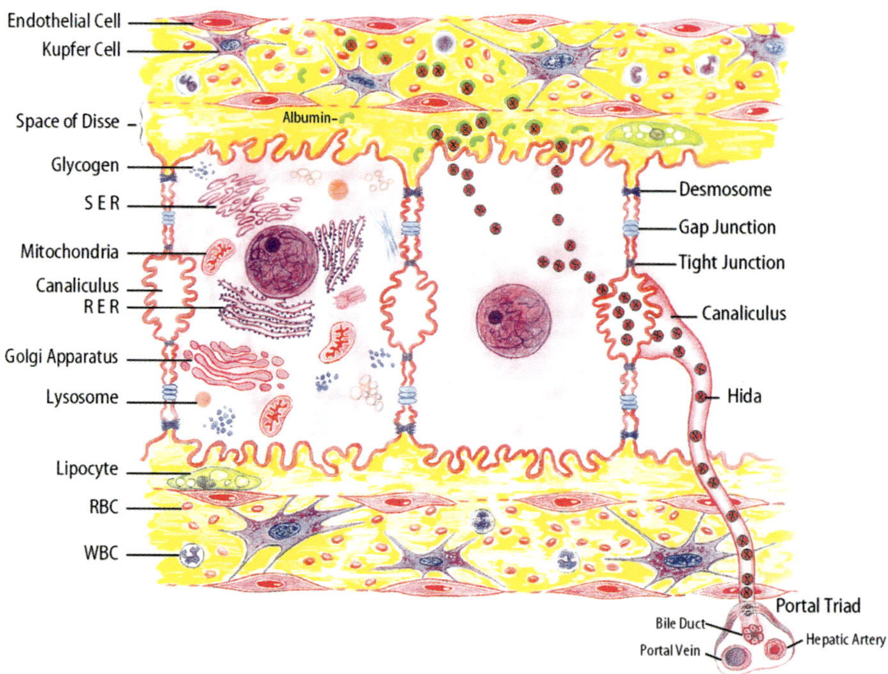

Fig. 1.2.1. Microstructure of the liver. The vascular space is divided into two compartments by the endothelial cells: (1) sinusoidal space and (2) perisinusoidal space of Disse. Kupffer cells are located in the sinusoidal space and lipocytes (Ito cells) in the perisinusoidal space of Disse. The basolateral border of the hepatocyte faces the space of Disse. Canaliculi are invagination of the lateral wall of two adjacent hepatocytes. Canaliculi join to form the canal of Hering, which turn unite to form the interlobular ducts. The portal triad consists of a branch of the bile duct, hepatic artery, and portal vein. Substrates move from the basolateral border to the canaliculi after passing through the hepatocyte. *SER*, smooth endoplasmic reticulum; *RER*, rough endoplasmic reticulum [25]

Table 1.2.1. Function of various cells of the liver

Hepatocyte	Endothelial cell	Kupffer cell	Lipocyte	Canalicular cell
Bile secretion	Plasma filtration	Phagocytosis of colloids, bacteria, endotoxin, tumor cells.	Storage of fats, vitamin A, and retinoid	Bile transit
Phosphorylation	Endocytosis			Water secretion
Heme synthesis	Removal of collagen, Fc fragment of IgG, C3b complement.	Receptor for Fc fraction, C3b complement	Collagen secretion	Electrolyte transfer
Protein synthesis				
Beta oxidation		Secretion of TNFa, collagenase, interleukins, arachidonic acid.		
Glycogenesis				
Bilirubin conjugation		Erythroblastosis		
Drug detoxification		Storage of iron, ferritin, hemosiderin, immune complex.		
Lipoprotein synthesis				
Storage of ferritin, vitamin B_{12}		Produce endogenous pyrogen		

Endothelial Cells

These are flat cells lining the vascular space and consist of numerous fenestrae in between [6]. The fenestrae (holes) vary in size from 0.1 to 3 μm in diameter and selectively allow certain plasma constituents to pass through from the sinusoidal space to the perisinusoidal space of Disse (Fig. 1.2.1). The microvilli of the hepatocytes in the perisinusoidal space of Disse are often seen through these fenestrae when viewed with a scanning electron microscope. The number of fenestrae decreases and the hole diameter increases in patients with alcoholic liver disease and cirrhosis [7–9]. The main function of the fenestrae is to act as a selective filter, allowing only those constituents that need to enter the perisinusoidal space of Disse and excluding others from the entrance. Red blood cells and leukocytes are excluded, whereas the electrolytes, plasma proteins (albumin), vitamins and other essential nutrients are allowed free entry into the perisinusoidal space of Disse.

Kupffer Cells

Kupffer described two types of cells, one in 1876 [10] and the other in 1899 [11]. It was first thought that the cell described in 1876 was the reticuloendothelial cell bearing his name (Kupffer cell). However, in 1951, Ito showed that this cell is the fat storing (lipocyte, Ito cell) cell situated in the perisinusoidal space of Disse [12]. The cell described by Kupffer in 1899 is now recognized as the Kupffer cell. The Kupffer cells are highly specialized macrophages distributed irregularly within the sinusoidal space. There is no direct connection between two adjacent Kupffer cells. Their surface is irregular with folds and ruffles. They are highly mobile scavenger cells often found within the space of Disse or may lie free within the sinusoidal space, unattached to the endothelial cell. The cytoplasm is rich in lysosomes, Golgi apparatus, and rough endoplasmic reticulum (Fig. 1.2.1). The Kupffer cells proliferate locally to maintain their population but at times of greater need they increase their number by calling in reinforcements from the bone marrow.

Lipocyte or Ito Cells

These cells, the "Sternzellen of Von Kupffer," first described in 1876, are the resting fibroblasts in the perisinusoidal space of Disse that are now organized as the fat storing cells [12, 13]. For many years it was thought that these cells did not have any specific function in humans. Lipocytes are rich in vitamin A and are the storage site for retinoids. They become activated during liver injury and play a dominant role in repair and fibrosis [14]. The activation of lipocytes and resultant fibrosis leads to collagen deposition in the subendothelial space of Disse. Other accompanying effects include a reduction in the number of fenestrae, and a loss of microvilli along the perisinusoidal surface of the hepatocytes, both of which result in a decrease in the delivery of organic anions (including HIDA) into the perisinusoidal space of Disse.

Pit Cells

These cells are found within the sinusoidal space. They are highly mobile killer lymphocytes and contain organelles necessary for removal of tumor cells and virus infected hepatocytes.

Hepatocytes

The hepatocyte is the largest cell in the liver and varies in size from 13 to 30 μm with an average diameter of 25 μm. Each milligram of liver tissue consists of 202,000 cells, of which 60% are hepatocytes and the rest are sinusoidal and other supporting cells. There are about 250 billion hepatocytes in an adult liver [15]. A hepatocyte is polyhedral, multifaceted (as many as eight surfaces) and measures about 11,000 μm^3 in volume. Because of their relatively larger size, hepatocytes account for 78% of the liver by volume. Sinusoidal cells account for 6% and the extracellular space occupies the remaining 16% of the liver volume. On the basis of function, the hepatocyte plasma membrane is divided into three domains: (1) basolateral domain, (2) contact or contiguous domain, and (3) canalicular domain.

The basolateral domain faces the perisinusoidal space of Disse and accounts for 70% of the wall surface. It consists of 30–50 microvilli, which increases the absorptive surface by six times [16]. The microvilli extend along the paracellular space until the two adjacent hepatocytes come in close contact at the point of the desmosome. This surface is bathed in plasma filtered through the fenestrae of the sieve plate of the endothelial cells, and allows metabolic exchange between the plasma and the hepatocyte. Organic anions, including ^{99m}Tc-HIDA, enter the hepatocyte along this domain.

The contact domain accounts for 15% of the surface and is placed between two adjacent hepatocytes. The tight junction situated near the canaliculus prevents plasma constituents from entering the canalicular space directly from the space of Disse. The gap junction can be located anywhere along the lateral border and provides direct communication between adjacent hepatocytes on a selective basis.

The canalicular domain accounts for the remaining 15% of the cell surface and is situated at the center of two adjacent hepatocytes. It represents a specialized part of the hepatocyte. The canalicular wall consists of microvilli, which increase the functional surface.

Hepatocyte contains a nucleus and a nucleolus which are rich in deoxyribonucleic acid. The smooth endoplasmic reticulum (SER) are tubular structures containing microsomes and carry out bilirubin conjugation and detoxification of drugs and other organic anions. SER are steroid sensitive and participate in enzyme induction when phenobarbital is administered. The rough endoplasmic reticulum (RER) contains ribosomes and is responsible for protein synthesis including albumin. Lysosomes are cytoplasmic particles close to bile canaliculi and contain hydrolytic enzymes including acid phosphatase. Lysosomes perform a scavenger function and remove from blood excess material including ferritin, bile pigments, and metals such as copper. The Golgi apparatus consists of particulates and vesicles and lies close to bile canaliculus. The lysosomes and Golgi apparatus together perform the tasks of storage, entrapment, and final excretion into bile of various non-essential body constituents. The mitochondria, which participate in oxidative phosphorylation, heme synthesis, and citric acid cycle, are scattered throughout the cell. The hepatocytes and cells in the sinusoidal and canalicular space are supported by a cytoskeleton consisting of microtubules and microfilaments. The cells of the sinusoidal and perisinusoidal space of Disse are supported by collagen, laminin, protoglycan fibronectin, and heparan sulfate [15, 16].

Bile Canaliculus

Bile canaliculi are a simple convoluted border of the hepatocyte. The microvilli are convolutions, which increase surface area for bile secretion (Fig. 1.2.1). A canaliculus varies from 0.1 to 1 μm in diameter. At the periphery of a hepatic lobule several bile canaliculi join to form the canal of Hering, which acts as a transitional zone between intralobular and interlobular ductal systems. The interlobular ducts unite to form area ducts which drain bile from an area of the liver. Area ducts unite to form the segmental ducts which in turn unite to form the lobar ducts. The cells lining the ducts (cholangioles) are cuboidal in shape and contain apical microvilli which project into the duct lumen [17].

Gallbladder and Cystic Duct

The gallbladder wall consists of three layers: (1) serosal layer, (2) fibromuscular layer, and (3) mucosal layer. The serosal layer is the peritoneum which covers about two-thirds of the gallbladder wall with the exception of the superior one-third, which is in direct contact with the liver. The fibromuscular layer consists mostly of elastic fibrous tissue. The muscular layer is irregular and consists of longitudinal and circular muscle fibers which are well developed around the fundus and the infundibulum, and scanty over the body and neck of the gallbladder. The mucosa consists of a single layer of cells with three different cell types: columnar cells, pencil cells, and basal cells. The mucosal layer is thrown into folds, which increases the surface area of the gallbladder. The columnar cells have microvilli, 0.7–0.8 μm in length, along the luminal surface. The intercellular space between two adjacent columnar cells is narrow at the luminal end but is widely open towards the fibromuscular layer [18]. Water and electrolytes are continuously absorbed from the lumen, through these intercellular spaces, making room for entry of fresh hepatic bile into the gallbladder during fasting [19]. The wall is impermeable to bile acids, bilirubin, radiocontrast agents, and other organic anions including ^{99m}Tc-HIDA. The neck contains mucus secreting cells. Pencil cells which are long and narrow are found mainly in the body and extend from the basement membrane to the lumen. Basal cells are small and are concentrated more towards the fibromuscular layer.

The water absorbed from the gallbladder lumen through the lateral intercellular spaces enters the gallbladder venous blood through several small veins which drain into the hepatic or portal veins directly. There is no one single large cystic vein. The venous blood from the free wall of the gallbladder drains into venous radicles which eventually enter the portal venous system.

The cystic duct, common hepatic duct, and common bile duct possess a mucosa, submucosa, and muscularis. The mucosal cells are a continuation of the gallbladder mucosal cells and contain the columnar cells with a ciliated border. The walls of the common hepatic duct and common bile duct are composed of a thick layer of connective tissue interspersed with a few muscle cells. This structural configuration is well suited for the bile ducts to participate in bile concentration and discharge.

Sphincter of Oddi

For well over a century, the study of this small segment of the biliary tract has fascinated anatomists, physiologists, and microscopists [20]. More recently, it has gotten the attention of gastroenterologists, hepatologists, and electron microscopists. For many years it was believed that the sphincter was a mere extension of the smooth muscle from the duodenal wall. Boyden's detailed work in 1937 clearly established it as a true sphincter, separate from the duodenal wall musculature [21]. The common bile duct enters the posteromedial wall of the second part of the duodenum tangentially and traverses for about 2 cm before joining the pancreatic duct (duct of Wirsung) to form a common channel, the ampulla of Vater. The common channel travels for 10–15 mm before entering the duodenal lumen at an elevation, the papilla, which is about 7–10 cm from the pylorus of the stomach (Fig. 1.1.8). The circular and longitudinal muscle fibers form a sphincter called the sphincter choledochus (sphincter of Boyden) at the distal end of the common bile duct before it joins the pancreatic duct. The sphincter is about 10–15 mm in length and mostly intramuscular. The contractions of this sphincter prevent reflux of pancreatic secretions into the common bile duct. The distal pancreatic duct (duct of Wirsung) is also surrounded by a distinct sphincter called the pancreatic sphincter whose contractions prevent reflux of bile into the pancreatic duct. The pancreatic sphincter is absent in about 20% of subjects [22]. The common channel formed by union of the common bile duct and the pancreatic duct is called the ampulla of Vater and is surrounded by a weak sphincter called the sphincter of Ampulla (pylorus of Westphal). The name "sphincter of Oddi" commonly refers to the function of all three sphincters situated at the distal end of the common bile duct and the pancreatic duct. Variations of the common bile duct length, its union with the pancreatic duct, and its opening into the duodenum are frequent and are related to embryologic development [23]. The common bile duct opens through the ampulla of Vater into the lumen of the second part of the duodenum in 82% of cases. The opening is lower than usual in 5%, opens at an angle in 7%, or opens into the transverse duodenum (third part) in the remaining 6% of patients [24].

References

1. Kiernan P. The anatomy and physiology of the liver. Philosophical Tr Roy Soc, London 1883;133:711–715
2. Rapapport AM. The structural and functional unit in the human liver (liver acinus). Anat Rec 1958;130:673–689
3. McMinn RMH. Anatomy of the liver and biliary tree. In: S Marlow, S Sherlock (eds) Surgery of the gallbladder and bile ducts. pp 1–18. Butterworth & Co Ltd, Boston, 1981
4. Bloulin A, Bolender RP, Weibel ER. Distribution of organelles and membranes between hepatocytes and non-hepatocytes in the rat liver parenchyma. A stereological study. J Cell Biol 1977;72:441–455
5. Gendrault J, Montecino-Rodriguez, Cinqualbre J. Structure of the normal human liver sinusoid after perfusion fixation. In: Knook DL, Wisse E (eds) Liver sinusoidal cells. Elsevier Biomedical Press, Amsterdam, 1982, pp 93–100
6. Wisse E. An electron microscopic study of the fenestral endothelial lining of rat liver sinusoid. J Ultrastructure Research 1970;31:125–150
7. Toner PG, Carr KE. Ultrastructure of the liver and biliary apparatus. In: Marlow S, Sherlock S. Eds, Surgery of the gallbladder and bile ducts. Butterworth & Co Ltd, Boston, 1981, pp 19–65
8. Wisse E, DeZanger RB, Charles K, Van Der Smissen P, McCuskey RS. The liver sieve: considerations concerning the structure and function of endothelial fenestrae, the sinusoidal wall and the space of Disse. Hepatology 1985;5:683–692
9. Horn T, Christoffersen P, Henrikseen JH. Alcoholic liver injury: defenestration in non-cirrhotic livers. A scanning microscopic study. Hepatology 1987;7:77–82
10. Kupffer C Von. Uberdie sternzallen der leber. Arch Mikr Anat 1876;12:353–357
11. Kupffer C Von. Uber die sogenanten sternzellen der sangetheier leber. Arch Mikr Anat 1899;54:254–260
12. Ito T. Cytological studies on stellate cells of Kupffer and fat storing cells in the capillaries of the human liver. Acta Anat Nippon 1951;26:42 (abstract)
13. Wake W. The sternzellen of Von Kupffer – After 106 years. In: Knook DL, Wisse E (eds) Sinusoidal liver cells. Elsevier Biomedical Press, Amsterdam, 1982, pp 1–12
14. Friedman SL. The cellular basis of hepatic fibrosis. Mechanism and treatment strategies. N Engl J Med 1993;328:1828–1835
15. Sherlock S, Dooley J. Diseases of the liver and biliary system. 10th edition, Blackwell Science, Malden, MA, 1997
16. Feldman G. The cytoskeleton of the hepatocyte. J Hepatology. 1989;8:380–384
17. Jones AL, Schmucker DL, Reston RH, Murakami T. The architecture of bile secretion. A morphological perspective of physiology. Dig Dis Sci 1980;25:609–629
18. Eveff RD, Higgins JA, Brown AC. The fine structure of normal mucosa in human gallbladder. Gastroenterology 1964;47:49–60
19. Tormey JM, Diamond JM. Studies on the structural basis of water transport across epithelial membranes. Federation Proceedings 1966;25:692–707
20. Oddi R. D'une disposition a sphincter del'ouverture du canal cholique. Arch Ital Biol 1887:8:317–322
21. Boyden EA. The sphincter of Oddi in man and certain representative mammals. Surgery 1937;1:25–37
22. Boyden EA. The anatomy of the choledochoduodenal junction in man. Surg Gynecol Obstet 1957;104: 641–652
23. Linder HH. Embryology and anatomy of the biliary tree. In: Way LW, Pelligrini CA (Eds) Surgery of the gallbladder and bile ducts. WB Saunders Co, Philadelphia, 1987. pp 3–22
24. Linder HH, Pena VA, Ruggieri RA. A clinical and anatomical study of anomalous termination of the common bile duct into the duodenum. Ann Surg 1976;184:626–632
25. Krishnamurthy S, Krishnamurthy GT. Evolution of nuclear hepatology as a clinical subspeciality. J Nucl Med Technol 1995;23 (suppl):35S–45S

Liver and Spleen Function

Liver is the largest organ and carries out the most complex biologic functions in the body. It secretes bile, synthesizes proteins, metabolizes nutrients, hormones, and drugs and detoxifies noxious endogenous and exogenous substrates. To accomplish all of these functions, the liver is located centrally in the body with well designed architecture and is supplied with a generous amount of blood. Secretion of bile is one of many important liver functions. Bile promotes digestion and absorption of essential nutrients and also serves as a vehicle to get rid off biologic waste products from the body. The biliary tree is designed not only for continuous bile secretion but also for periodic bile storage and discharge at the time when food enters the small intestine. Spleen carries out many functions whose importance has been recognized only recently. This chapter will discuss various functions of these two organs.

2.1 Liver Function

The liver secretes about 600–800 ml of bile per day, 25–33 ml/h or 0.42–55 ml/min [1]. Under normal hydration, the osmolality of the hepatic bile is similar to that of plasma and ranges between 290 and 320 mosmol/l. Bile secretion is independent of hepatic perfusion pressure; thus it differs from that of urine formation, which is very much dependent upon the glomerular filtration pressure in the kidneys [2, 3]. Bile promotes the dual function of absorption of essential nutrients from the intestinal lumen into the blood stream and discharge of biologic waste products from the blood into intestinal lumen. The hepatic bile is composed of 98% water and 2% solutes, which include bile acids, phospholipids, cholesterol, conjugated bilirubin, electrolytes, and proteins (Table 2.1.1). Bile formation takes place in three steps: (1) uptake of solutes and solvents by the hepatocyte from the blood stream, (2) intracellular transit of these substances through the hepatocyte, and (3) secretion by the hepatocyte into bile canaliculi. All three domains of the hepatocyte plasma membrane participate in the uptake and excretion [4]. The uptake from the blood in the space of Disse takes place along the basolateral domain and bile secretion occurs at the canalicular domain. The lateral domain, the wall facing two adjacent hepatocytes, plays a major role in water and solute transport and regulation of the total volume of bile secreted per day.

Table 2.1.1. Composition of human hepatic and gallbladder bile

Substrate concentration	Hepatic bile	Gallbladder bile
Water (g/dl)	98	92
Na^+ (mEq/l)	150	130
K^+ (mEq/l)	5	10
Ca^{2+} (mEq/l)	5	23
Cl^- (mEq/l)	100	25
HCO_3^- (mEq/l)	28	10
Bile salts (g/dl)	1	6
Bilirubin (g/dl)	0.05	0.3
Cholesterol (g/dl)	0.1	0.6
Fatty acids (g/dl)	0.12	0.8
Lecithin (g/dl)	0.04	0.3

Hepatocyte Uptake

Of the several different available pathways for hepatocyte uptake (Fig. 2.1.1), three appear to play a major role: (1) the cotransport pathway, involving sodium taurocholate (NTCP) and a Na^+ bicarbonate pathway, (2) the sodium-independent organic anion transporting polypeptide pathway (OATP), including ^{99m}Tc-HIDA, and (3) the Na^+/K^+ ATPase pump, bile acid-amino acid, and Na^+-H^+ exchanger [5]. The Na^+/K^+ pump is dependent upon ATPase, which is heavily concentrated along the basolateral border of the hepatocyte [6]. The Na^+-K^+ ATPase pump enables net movement of three Na^+ ions out of the hepatocyte for every two K^+ ions moving into the hepatocyte from the space of Disse. The net effect of these electrolyte exchange is a higher concentration of K^+ inside than outside and a higher concentration of Na^+ outside than inside the hepatocyte. Due to this ion imbalance, the inside of the hepatocyte carries a higher negative charge (–35 mV) than its outside environment [7].

Bile acid uptake occurs via a sodium taurocholate cotransporter (NTCP) pathway facilitated by a 48- and 49-kDa protein present along the basolateral domain. Bile acids also make use of a 54-kDa multispecific carrier protein to a minor extent. The potassium channel promotes sodium-dependent bile salt uptake. Organic anions (bilirubin, indocyanine green, Bromsulphalein and also ^{99m}Tc-HIDA) make use of a non-sodium-dependent, carrier protein called sinusoidal multispecific organic anion transporter (OATP) present along the basolateral border. Sodium$^+$/H^- exchange and Na^+/HCO_3^- cotransport systems help to maintain the constancy of intracellular pH.

Transport Through the Hepatocyte

Bile acids are transported through the hepatocyte via a 33-kDa cytosolic protein, 3α-hydroxysteroid dehydrogenase. Organic anions (including ^{99m}Tc-HIDA) are transported through the hepatocyte by as yet ill defined mechanisms.

Secretion into Bile Canaliculi

The quantity of solute transported across the canalicular membrane is the rate limiting step in the volume of bile normally secreted per day. Canalicular membrane contains several ATP dependent and independent transport pumps to enable secretion of solutes from the hepatocyte into canaliculi [8]. These pumps include ATP dependent multidrug-resistance-1 p-glycoprotein (MDR1), phospholipid transporter multidrug-

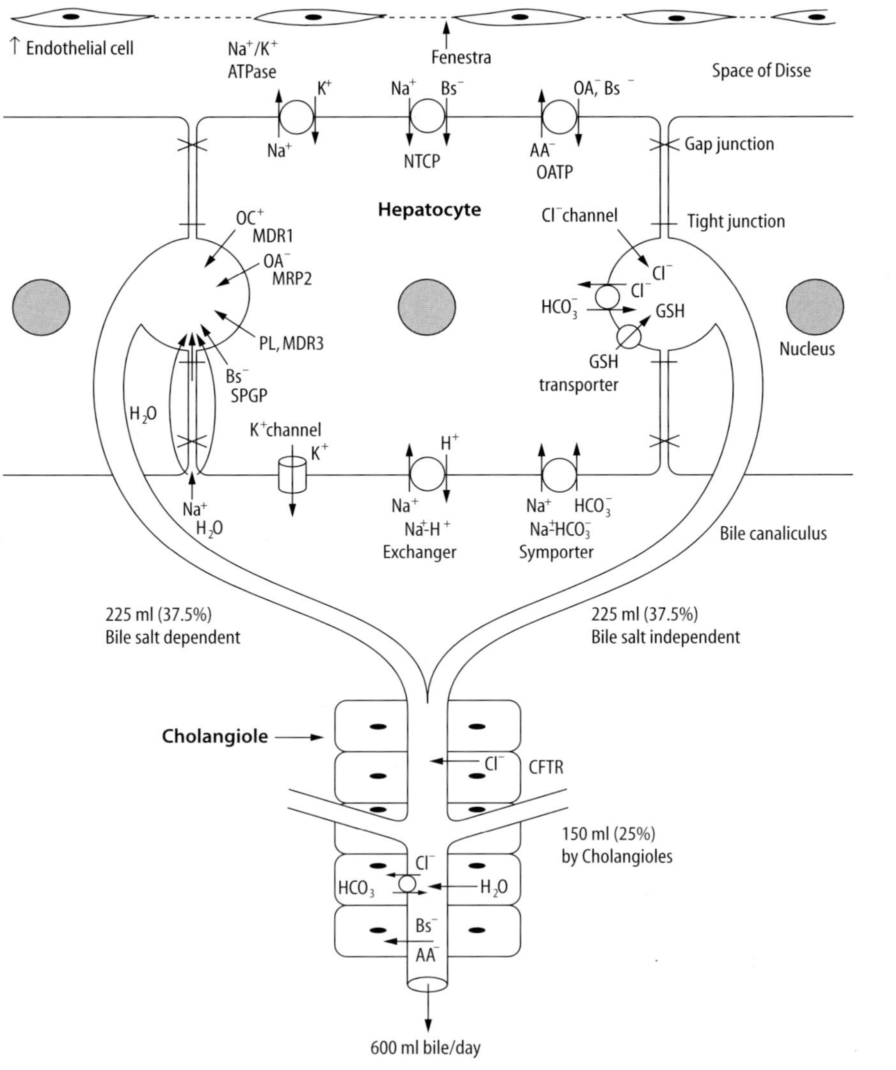

Fig. 2.1.1. Mechanism of bile secretion. The uptake of solutes from the space of Disse occurs along the basolateral domain of the hepatocyte by many different pathways. Organic anions (*OA*$^-$) and bile salts (*BS*$^-$) are exchanged for amino acids (*AA*$^-$) through the organic anion transport pump (*OATP*). Sodium dependent bile salt uptake occurs via the sodium taurocholate pump (*NTCP*). Sodium/potassium exchange occurs through Na^+/K^+ ATPase and sodium-hydrogen exchange via their exchanger protein. Sodium is also cotransported with bicarbonates through their symporter. After intracellular transit, solute secretion into bile takes place along the canalicular domain. Organic anions are secreted through the multispecific organic anion transporter (*MRP2*), organic cations (OC^+) through multidrug-resistant-1 p-glycoprotein (*MDR1*), and phospholipids (*PL*) through MDR3. Chloride channel, glutathione (*GSH*) transporter, chloride (Cl^-)/bicarbonate (HCO_3^-) exchange, and canalicular bile salt export pump (*BSEP* or *SPGP*) also participate. Cholangioles reabsorb BS^-, AA^-, and glucose, exchange Cl^- for HCO_3^-, and secrete chloride into the lumen through cystic fibrosis transmembrane regulator (*CFTR*). Water enters the canalicular bile by three different routes: (1) transcellular, (2) paracellular, and (3) a combination of paracellular and transcellular

resistance-3 p-glycoprotein (MDR3), canalicular multispecific organic anion transporter (MRP2), and canalicular bile salt export pump (BSEP or SGPG). The ATP independent transport systems include a chloride channel, a chloride-bicarbonate anion exchanger and a glutathione (GSH) transporter (Fig. 2.1.1). Bile salts are secreted into the canaliculi also by a sodium independent mechanism, facilitated by a 100-kDa polypeptide. Other organic anions such as bilirubin, BSP, indocyanine green, and glutathione (^{99m}Tc-HIDA) are secreted by an ATP dependent carrier protein MRP2. The secretion of organic cations (e.g., cancer chemotherapy agents, cyclosporin A, calcium channel blockers and other drugs) is mediated by MDR1, a 170-gene product [9]. After passing through the tight junction (leaky tight junction), sodium and other cations enter the canaliculi through the space between the lateral domain of two adjacent hepatocytes, and the water then simply follows the electrolytes.

Of the daily total bile of 600 ml, 450 ml (75%) is secreted by the hepatocyte and 150 ml (25%) is added by the cells lining the canaliculi (cholangioles or cholangiocytes). Of a total of 450 ml hepatocellular bile, 225 ml (50%) is bile salt dependent and the remaining 225 (50%) ml is bile salt independent. Figure 2.1.1 summarizes the mechanisms and associated carrier proteins that play a part in transport substances from blood into the hepatocyte and finally into bile canaliculi. Movement of sodium in and out of the hepatocyte is an important step in the uptake and excretion of solutes by the hepatocyte. Bilirubin transport from blood into the hepatocyte and then into the canaliculi is mediated by a saturable process and it competes with other organic anions [10].

Protein Secretion

Liver is the main source of plasma proteins, albumin and globulins. Serum albumin synthesized entirely by the hepatocytes accounts for 60% of plasma proteins, is composed of 585 amino acids, and does not contain any carbohydrate moiety. In addition to maintaining the osmotic pressure, albumin functions as a carrier protein for drugs, metals, vitamins, amino acids, steroid, fatty acids, and ^{99m}Tc-HIDA. Other proteins secreted by hepatocytes include α_1-antitrypsin, a_1-fetoprotein, α_2-macroglobulin, antithrombin III, ceruloplasmin, C-reactive protein, fibrinogen, haptoglobin, hemopexin, and transferrin (Table 2.1.2). Most of these proteins are composed of a carbohydrate moiety and hence are called glycoprotein [11].

Table 2.1.2. Plasma proteins secreted by hepatocytes [11]

Protein	Molecular weight (kDa)	Function	Ligand binding	Plasma conc. (mg/dl)
Albumin	66	Osmotic pressure		4500–5000
		Carrier protein	Hormones, amino acids, fatty acids, vitamins	
α_1-Antitrypsin	54	Trypsin and general protease inhibitor	Present in serum and tissue secretions	1.3–1.4
α-Fetoprotein	72	Osmotic regulation	Hormones, amino acids	Undetectable in adults
		Carrier protein		Present in fetal blood
Antithrombin III	65	Regulation of coagulation	Binding to protease	15–60
Ceruloplasmin	134	Copper transport	Six copper atoms per mol	15–60
C-reactive protein	105	Tissue inflammation	Complement C1q	Increased inflammation
Fibrinogen	340	Fibrin precursor during hemostasis	–	200–450
Transferrin	80	Iron transport	Two iron atoms per mol	3–6.5
Haptoglobin	100	Transport of hemoglobin	Hemoglobin	40–180
Prothrombin	72	Hemostasis	Calcium chelation	10.0

Bile Flow

Water is the major component of the hepatic bile and it enters the canaliculi mainly through three routes: (1) passing directly through the hepatocyte (transcellular), (2) passing through the tight junction (leaky tight junction!) between two lateral domains of adjacent hepatocytes (paracellular), and (3) by a combination of transcellular and paracellular pathways (first through the hepatocyte into the paracellular space and then through the tight junction into the canaliculi). The hepatic bile is relatively more dilute (contains less bile salts, bilirubin, chloride, and bicarbonate per liter) than the gallbladder bile (Table 2.1.1).

Bile Storage and Concentration by the Gallbladder

A major portion of the bile secreted by the liver during fasting enters the gallbladder and a minor fraction enters the duodenum directly, depending upon the tonus of the sphincter of Oddi (Fig. 2.1.2). During a period of 10 h in the night, the liver produces about 250 ml bile (25 ml/h or 0.42 ml/min), of which 175 ml (70%) enters the gallbladder (17.5 ml/h or 0.3 ml/min). Since the gallbladder can usually fill to its maximum capacity of 50 ml during a period of 6 h, it must absorb at least 0.3 ml water/min to be

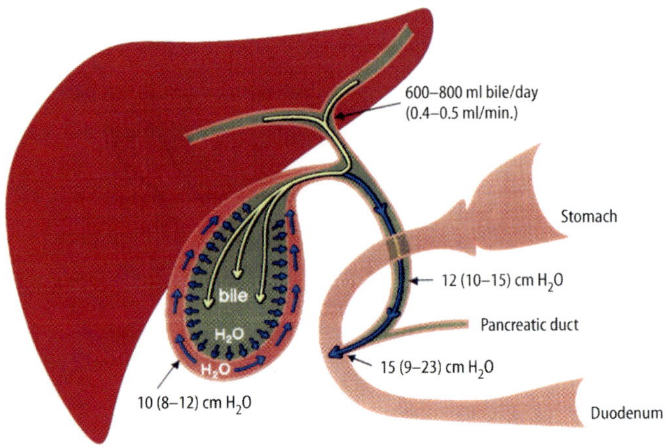

Fig. 2.1.2. Bile entry mechanism into the gallbladder. A higher mean (range) pressure at the sphincter of Oddi (15 cm H_2O) than the gallbladder, and absorption of water through the wall during fasting, facilitate constant hepatic bile entry into the gallbladder

able to accommodate the constant inflow of fresh hepatic bile during fasting. This is accomplished primarily by absorption of water and electrolytes through the gallbladder wall. As much as 90% of water can be absorbed through the gallbladder wall during a 6-h period. Dietschy demonstrated that 100 ml hepatic bile placed inside the gallbladder reduces to less than 10 ml in 6 h mainly through absorption of water (Fig. 2.1.3). As a consequence of this selective water absorption, the concentration of solutes increases in the gallbladder bile [12,13]. This process of selective absorption of water resulting in a higher concentration of bile salts, bilirubin, cholesterol, fatty acids, and lecithin in the gallbladder bile than hepatic bile is called the concentration function of the gallbladder [14,15]. A normal gallbladder can sequester all of 3–6 g total body bile salts within it after an overnight fast.

The volume of hepatic bile that enters the gallbladder during fasting is controlled by two mechanisms, the tonus of the sphincter of Oddi and absorption of water through the gallbladder wall (Fig. 2.1.2). Under basal conditions, the mean pressure in the sphincter of Oddi is 15 cm water, the common bile duct 12 cm water, and the gallbladder 10 cm water. By choosing the path of least resistance, the hepatic bile enters the gallbladder. The tonus of the sphincter of Oddi is dependent upon the frequency and amplitude of phasic waves contractions. The phasic wave frequency ranges from 1 to 13/min with an average of 6 contractions/min [16]. High frequency contractions (>8/min) are relatively rare (14%). Sphincter of Oddi phasic wave contractions occur in conjunction with phase III of the migrating motor complex, which begins in the stomach and traverses through the duodenum and jejunum [17].

The second mechanism that promotes hepatic bile entry into the gallbladder is the rate of absorption of water through the gallbladder wall. During fasting, the lateral intercellular channels between the columnar epithelial cells are widely opened allowing the passage of sodium and water from the gallbladder lumen into the interstitial spaces first and then the hepatic venous blood (Fig. 2.1.4). These lateral intercellular

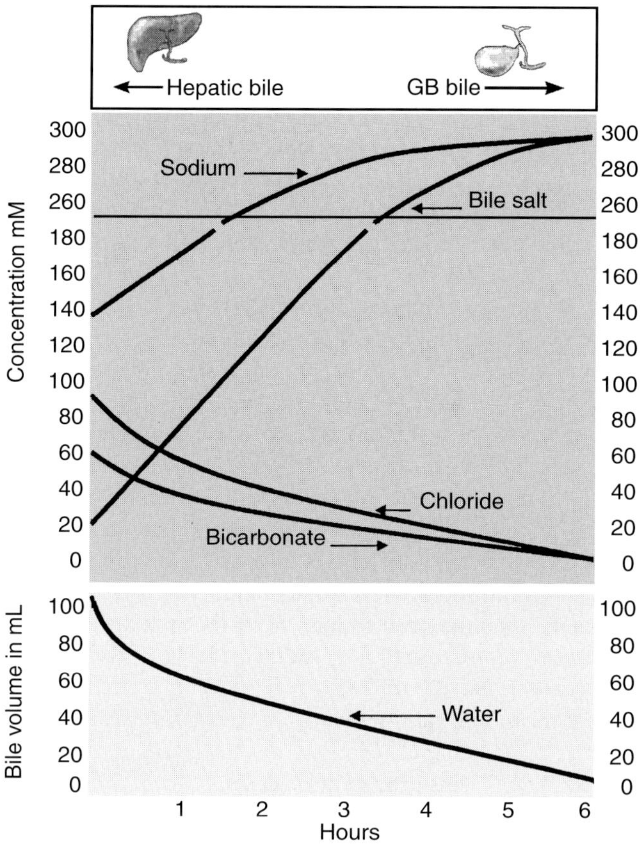

Fig. 2.1.3. Mechanism of bile concentration. Mainly through different rates of absorption, gallbladder (rabbit) increases the concentration of sodium and bile salts and decreases the concentration of chloride and bicarbonate in its bile, when compared to hepatic bile. Gallbladder bile volume decreases by 90% to achieve these concentrations [14]

spaces collapse when the gallbladder wall contracts following ingestion of a meal, or injection of cholecystokinin, or upon injection of ouabain, which is known to inhibit water transport across most epithelial membranes [14]. Spontaneous gallbladder emptying and refilling plays a minor role in making room for the fresh hepatic bile. In about 250 normal subjects monitored continuously for 2 h with ^{99m}Tc-HIDA by the authors, spontaneous gallbladder emptying to the extent of 5–10% was noticed in less than 5% of subjects. The bile that enters the duodenum during fasting normally moves antegrade towards the jejunum. Normally during fasting there is no bile reflux from the duodenum into the stomach.

Gallbladder Emptying

Emptying of the gallbladder is under both hormonal and nervous control, hormonal control playing the major role. Nervous control is exerted through both the sympathetic and parasympathetic systems as shown in Chap. 1, Fig. 1.1.7. The cholinergic parasympathetic nerve fibers to the gallbladder come primarily from the anterior gastric plexus (left vagus). Gallbladder emptying in response to sham feeding is mediated through these cholinergic nerve fibers and can be blocked with atropine or after vagotomy [18]. The parasympathetic cholinergic nerve fibers to the sphincter of Oddi come mainly from the posterior gastric plexus (right vagus). Sympathetic postganglionic nerve fibers reach the gallbladder and the sphincter of Oddi from the celiac ganglion. Sympathetic nerve stimulation relaxes the gallbladder wall and promotes hepatic bile entry.

The hormone induced contraction and emptying of the gallbladder occurs mainly through endogenous release of cholecystokinin (CCK), demonstrated first in 1928 by Ivy and Oldberg [19]. Cholecystokinin, a linear 33 or 39 amino acid polypeptide, is produced from a large precursor protein with 114 amino acids. Most of the biologic function of the hormone is confined to the last four carboxy-terminal amino acids. A much shorter cholecystokinin with only eight carboxy-terminal amino acids (CCK-8) carries most of the biologic function of the parent molecule with 33 amino acids [20]. The contraction and emptying of the gallbladder begins within 2–3 min after an intravenous administration of CCK-8, but it may take as long as 10–20 min to begin emptying following a meal [21]. This time delay in gallbladder emptying after a meal is due to a combination of time taken for the meal to pass from the stomach into the

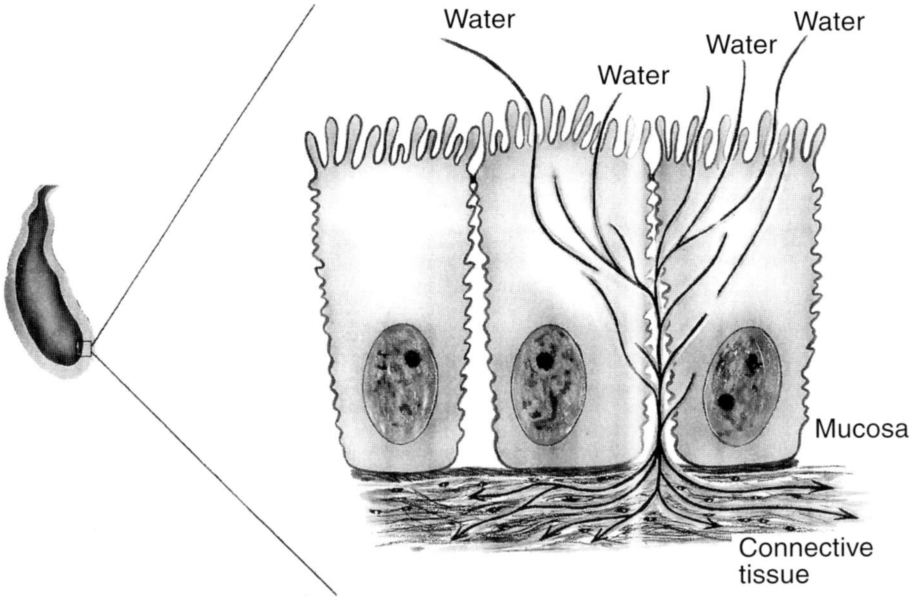

Fig. 2.1.4. Absorption of water through the gallbladder epithelium. Lateral intercellular channels between the columnar epithelial cells are widely open during fasting allowing free passage of water from the lumen into the connective space. Water absorption creates space for constant entry of hepatic bile into the gallbladder during fasting [14]

duodenum and the time taken for the CCK secreting cells in the duodenal mucosa to release enough hormone into the blood stream. Cerulein, motilin, and other gastrointestinal hormones with an identical carboxy-terminal tetrapeptide also induce gallbladder contraction and emptying [22].

References

1. Fitz JG. Cellular mechanism of bile secretion. In: Zakim D, Boyer TD, eds. Hepatology. A textbook of liver disease. Philadelphia, WB Saunders Co. 1996: pp 362–376
2. Boyer JL, Klatskin G. Canalicular bile flow and bile secretory pressure. Evidence for a non-bile salt dependent fraction in the isolated perfused rat liver. Gastroenterology 1970;59:853–859
3. Brauer RW, Leong SF, Holloway RJ. Mechanism of secretion. Effect of perfusion pressure and temperature on bile flow and bile secretion pressure. Am J Physiology 1954;177:103–106
4. Jones AL, Schmucker DL, Renston RH, Murakami T. The architecture of bile secretion. A morphological perspective of physiology. Dig Dis Sci 1980;25:609–629
5. Sherlock S, Dooley J. Cholestasis. Diseases of the liver and biliary system, 10th edition, Blackwell Science, Malden, MA. 1997, pp 217–237
6. Sellinger M, Barrett C, Malle P, Gordon ER, Boyer JL. Cryptic Na^+, K^+-ATPase activity in the rat liver canalicular plasma membranes: evidence for its basolateral origin. Hepatology 1990;11:223–229
7. Meier PJ. Molecular mechanisms of hepatic bile salt transport from sinusoidal blood into bile. Am J Physiol 269:G801–G812, 1995
8. Trauner M, Meier PJ, Boyer JL. Molecular pathogenesis of cholestasis. N Engl J Med 1998:339:1217–1227
9. Kamimato Y, Gatmaitan Z, Hsu J, Arias IM. The function of Gp 170, the multidrug resistance gene product, in rat liver canalicular membrane vesicles. J Biol Chem 1989;264:11693–11698
10. Goresky CA. Initial distribution and rate of sulfobromophthalein in the liver. Am J Physiology 1964;207:13–16
11. Donohue TM Jr., Tuma DJ, Sorrell MF. Plasma proteins metabolism. In: Zakim D, Boyer TD. Hepatology. A text book of liver disease, 3rd edition. Philadelphia, WB Saunders Co., 1996;130–148
12. Krishnamurthy GT, Bobba VR, McConnel D, Turner F, Mesgarzadeh M, Kingston E. Quantitative biliary dynamics: Introduction of a new noninvasive scintigraphic technique. J Nucl Med 1983;24;217–223
13. Vlahcevic ZR, Heuman DM, Hylemon PB. Physiology and pathology of enterohepatic circulation of bile acids. In: Zakin D, Boyer TD (eds.). Hepatology. A textbook of liver disease. 1996. Philadelphia, W.B. Saunders Co. pp 376-417
14. Wheeler HO. Concentrating function of the gallbladder Am J Med 1971;51:588–595
15. Krishnamurthy S, Krishnamurthy GT. Evolution of nuclear hepatology as a clinical subspeciality. J Nucl Med Technol 1995;23:35S-45S (supplement)
16. Thune A, Scicchitano J, Roberts-Thompson I, Toouli J. Reproducibility of endoscopic sphincter of Oddi manometry. Dig Dis Sci 1991;36:1401–1405
17. Lee SK, Kim MH, Seo DW, Yoo BM, Lee MH, Myung SJ, Min YI. Frequency of phasic wave contraction is variable during long-term sphincter of Oddi manometry. Am J Gastroenterol 1996;91:2395–2398
18. Fisher RS, Rock E, Malmud LS. Gallbladder emptying response to sham feeding in humans. Gastroenterology 1986;90:1854–1857
19. Ivy AC, Oldberg E. A hormone mechanism of gallbladder contraction and evacuation. Am J Physiology 1928;86:599–613
20. Mutt V. Cholecystokinin: isolation, structure, and function. In: Jerzy Glass GB. ed. Gastrointestinal hormones. New York, Raven Press, 1980, pp 169–221
21. Bobba VR, Krishnamurthy GT, Kingston E, Turner FE, Brown PH, Langrell K. Gallbladder dynamics induced by a fatty meal in normal subjects and patients with gallstones: Concise communication . J Nucl Med 1984;25:21–24
22. Bloom SR, Adrian TE, Mitchenere P, et al. Motilin induced gallbladder contraction. A new mechanism. Gastroenterology 1981;80:1113

2.2 Spleen Function

The spleen is composed mostly of reticuloendothelial cells and lymphoid tissue. It carries out the following important biologic functions:

1. Hemopoiesis
2. Destruction of senescent red blood cells, leukocytes, and platelets
3. Culling and pitting
4. Phagocytosis
5. Reservoir function
6. Immunologic function

The spleen is usually seen during radionuclide imaging with radiocolloids and radiolabeled red blood cells, leukocytes, monoclonal antibodies, or peptides (somatostatin). As the spleen does not concentrate ^{99m}Tc-GSA or ^{99m}Tc-HIDA, it is not seen during functional liver or hepatobiliary imaging, respectively.

A normal spleen weighs between 80 and 200 g with an average of 150 g [1]. In the posterior view of a radiocolloid scan, the spleen normally measures 10.5 cm along the oblique axis. The spleen has to enlarge more than 2.5 times its normal size before it is palpable in the left upper quadrant, during a routine physical examination. Most of the palpable spleens are enlarged but not all non-palpable spleens are normal in size.

During the first 6 months of intrauterine life, the spleen functions as a major hematopoietic organ, and this function normally disappears by birth. In thalassemia and myeloid metaplasia, the spleen is capable of resuming its intrauterine function in adult life to produce red blood cells. The normal function in adults is destruction of senescent red blood cells, leukocytes, and platelets. Excessive destruction of blood cells by the spleen results in anemia, leukopenia, or thrombocytopenia [2]. The volume of red blood cells in the body and their destruction by the spleen are measured by labeling the cells with chromium-51 [3]. During labeling, hexavalent chromium-51 (Na_2CrO_4) crosses the red cell membrane and attaches to hemoglobin after reduction into a trivalent form [4]. The physical half-life of chromium-51 is 27 days. Random labeling, elution of chromium-51, and death of senescent red cells, all account for the mean red blood cell (RBC) survival half-time of 35 days (normal life span of RBCs is 120 days). Chromium-51 released after RBC death is taken up by the reticuloendothelial cells and it does not label other red blood cells in blood, and hence serves as an ideal marker for RBC survival studies.

The selective removal of abnormal red cells by the spleen is called culling, and removal of intraerythrocytic inclusions without destroying the RBCs is called pitting. Howell-Jolly bodies, the remnant of the RBC nucleus, are removed from the RBCs by the spleen. The appearance of Howell-Jolly bodies in the peripheral blood, therefore, is an indication of either splenectomy or a non-functioning spleen [5]. Hypersplenism is documented by showing increased spleen/liver and increased spleen/precordial count ratios in association with decreased RBC survival time. Return of splenic function after splenectomy is attributed to autotransplantation (due to spillage) of the splenic tissue on the peritoneal surface or an accessory spleen [6]. Imaging of the spleen with radiocolloids, a popular modality in the 1970 and 1980s, has been largely replaced today by computerized tomography and ultrasound. Radiocolloid spleen imaging is now obtained occasionally to clarify an abnormality that has already been detected with other diagnostic methods or to document splenomegaly in the diagnosis of polycythemia rubra vera [7].

The spleen capsule has a thin muscle layer whose contraction squeezes out the sequestered RBCs, WBCs, and platelets into the peripheral circulation. Injection of epinephrine induces smooth muscle contraction with a subsequent rise in peripheral cell count. The spleen offers a protective role for the lung tissue and pulmonary hypertension is shown to develop after splenectomy in some patients [8]. The immunologic function of the spleen is carried out by the lymphocytes and reticuloendothelial cells (phagocytosis). The spleen produces antibodies against many microorganisms, especially polysaccharide encapsulated bacteria such as pneumococci. Overwhelming infection sometimes follows after splenectomy in children. Human splenic autotransplantation produces significant antipneumococcal antibody in response to administration of pneumococcal vaccine [9].

References

1. Mattsson O. Scintigraphic spleen volume calculation. Acta Radiol [Diagn] (Stockh) 1982;23:471–477
2. Spencer RP, Pearson HA. The spleen as a hematological organ. Semin Nucl Med 1975;5:95–102
3. Gray SJ, Sterling K. The tagging of red blood cells and plasma proteins with radioactive chromium. J Clin Invest 1950;29:818
4. Pollycove M, Tono M. Blood volume. In: Sandler MP, Patton JH, Coleman RE, Gottschalk A, Wackers FJTh, Hopper PB. Diagnostic Nuclear Medicine, 3rd edition, Williams and Wilkins, Baltimore, 1996, pp 827–834
5. Crosby WH, Normal functions of the spleen relative to red blood cells. A review. Blood 1959;14:399–408
6. Pearson HA, Johnston D, Smith KA, Touloukian RJ. The born-again spleen. Return of splenic function after splenectomy for trauma. New Eng J Med 1978;298:1389–1392
7. Spencer RP. Spleen imaging. In: Sandler MP, Patton JH, Coleman RE, Gottschalk A, Wackers FJTh, Hopper PB. Diagnostic Nuclear Medicine, 3rd edition, Williams and Wilkins, Baltimore, 1996, pp 865–874
8. Hoeper MM, Niedermeyer J, Hoffmeyer F, Flemming P, Fabel H. Pulmonary hypertension after splenectomy? Ann Intern Med 1999;130:506–509
9. Leemans R, Manson W, Snijder JAM, Smit JW, Klasen HJ, The TH, Timens W. Immune response capacity after human splenic autotransplantation. Restoration of response to individual pneumococcal vaccine subtypes. Ann Surg 1999;229:279–285

Imaging Agents

Historical Evolution

The conception of nuclear hepatology took place in the late 1940s with the introduction of radiocolloids, whose rate of clearance from the circulation was used as an indicator of liver function [1]. The birth of nuclear hepatology occurred in 1954 with the successful imaging of the liver morphology with gold-198 colloid using an automated rectilinear scanner developed by Cassen [2, 3]. Morphology imaging with radiocolloid was supplanted by liver physiology imaging with the introduction of ^{131}I-rose bengal in 1955 by Taplin et al. [4]. Imaging of morphology gained clinical popularity after the introduction of technetium-99m colloid in 1965 [5] and a rapid leap in imaging of physiology occurred with the introduction of ^{99m}Tc-HIDA (hepatic iminodiacetic acid) agents in 1976 [6].

3.1 Morphology and Physiology Imaging Agents

The liver carries out the most complex biologic function through the hepatocytes, Kupffer cells, endothelial cells, fat cells (Ito cells), blood vessels, and biliary epithelial cells. Liver imaging agents can be classified broadly into two groups: (1) those that identify pathology mainly through detection of changes in liver morphology and (2) those that identify pathology by identifying changes in liver physiology (Table 3.1.1). A wide variety of imaging agents now available enable the study of specific cell function (Table 3.1.2). Radiocolloids are the most common agents for imaging morphology and ^{99m}Tc-HIDA compounds are the preferred agents for physiology. Since liver morphology imaging is now carried out mostly with CT or ultrasound, imaging of physiology is currently the most common diagnostic procedure in nuclear hepatology. Both groups of agents are described below.

Radiocolloids

Radiocolloids are small particles, 5 µm to 1 µ in size, that are removed from circulation by the reticuloendothelial cells of the liver, spleen, and bone marrow. They carry a negative charge of –30 mV and do not pass through the dialysis membrane permeable to ions. However, they readily pass through an ion-exchange column and show no movement on paper chromatography [7]. Although gold-198 is no longer used for imaging, a thorough understanding of its pharmacokinetic provides a sound basis for understanding the biokinetics of the ^{99m}Tc-S colloid and is described briefly below.

Table 3.1.1. Classification of liver imaging agents

1. Morphology imaging agents	Radiocolloids (^{198}Au, ^{99m}Tc-S-colloid) ^{67}Ga-citrate
2. Physiology imaging agents	These agents can be further divided into four subgroups based on specific function
°a) Hepatobiliary agents	^{99m}Tc-HIDA, ^{99m}Tc-PG, ^{131}I-rose bengal, etc.
°b) Blood pool agents	^{99m}Tc-RBC, ^{99m}Tc-albumin
°c) Receptor specific agents	^{99m}Tc-GSA, ^{111}In-octreotide, ^{111}In-monoclonal antibody, ^{99m}Tc-monoclonal antibodies
°d) Miscellaneous agents	^{111}In-WBC, ^{99m}Tc-WBC (HMPAO), and other agents that are developed primarily for imaging of other organs but pass through the liver during their elimination enabling imaging of the hepatobiliary system, e.g., ^{99m}Tc-Sestamibi, ^{99m}Tc-Tetrofosmin, ^{99m}Tc-HMPAO

Table 3.1.2. Cell, mechanism of uptake, disposition, and dose of radiolabeled agents for imaging of the liver and spleen

Agent	Uptake by	Mechanism of uptake	Excretion into bile	Dose (mCi)
^{99m}Tc-S-colloid	Kupffer cell	Phagocytosis	No	2–5
^{99m}Tc-GSA	Hepatocyte	ASGP receptor	No	2–8
^{99m}Tc-HIDA	Hepatocyte	RME	Yes	2–8
^{99m}Tc-RBC	Hemangioma	Blood pool	No	10–20
^{99m}Tc-HMPAO-WBC	Infection	Chemotaxis	No	10–20
^{111}In-WBC (oxine)	Infection	Chemotaxis	No	0.5–1.0
^{111}In-Octreotide	Somatostatin-receptor	Receptor-ligand interaction	No	3–8
^{111}In-MOAB	TAG-72	Antigen-antibody interaction	No	2–5
^{67}Ga-citrate	Hepatocyte	Unknown	No	2–10

ASGP, asialoglycoprotein, GSA, galactosyl human serum albumin, HIDA, hepatic iminodiacetic acid, RME, receptor mediated endocytosis

Gold-198 Colloid

Gold-198 (^{198}Au) colloid is one of the smallest radiocolloid particles known to nuclear medicine. The particles vary in size from 5 to 50 μm with an average size of 30 μm and clear from blood with a $T_{1/2}$ of 3 min. Gold-198 has a physical half-life of 2.7 days, decays by beta minus emission, and emits a monoenergetic gamma photon of 411 keV for imaging. The adult dose ranges from 100 to 150 μCi in 25 μg to 2.5 mg gold. The three organs which concentrate ^{198}Au colloid include liver, spleen, and bone marrow; with the smallest particles preferentially taken up by the bone marrow and the largest particles by the spleen [9]. The percentage dose localized in each organ depends upon its function and size, and the size and electrochemical character of the radiocolloid particles. Normally the liver weighs about 1500–1800 g, the spleen 150–200 g, and the bone marrow ~1500 g (Table 3.1.3). Normally, about 90% of a ^{198}Au colloid dose is taken up by the liver, 7% by reticuloendothelial (RE) cells of the bone marrow, and 3% by the spleen [10]. In moderate hepatocellular disease, the liver mass increases (2400 g) due to fatty infiltration, and the mass of the spleen increases (250 g) due to portal hypertension. In advanced cirrhosis, the liver actually shrinks in size (1400 g) due to fibrosis, whereas the spleen continues to increase in size (400 g) due to the increase in portal hypertension. The mass of reticuloendothelial cells in the bone marrow does not change. In moderate liver disease, the uptake by the liver decreases to 70%. In advanced cirrhosis when the liver shrinks in size, the radiocolloid uptake may fall below 35%. As the uptake of radiocolloid by the liver decreases, the uptake by the spleen and bone marrow increases, in direct proportion to the degree of portal hypertension.

Table 3.1.3. Liver, spleen, and bone marrow mass in normal subjects and patients with liver disease [10]

Clinical status	Mass of organ (g) Liver	Spleen	Bone marrow
Normal	1807	174	1500
Early to intermediate liver disease	2400	250	1500
Intermediate to advanced liver disease	1400	400	1500

Technetium-99m-Sulfur Colloid

Technetium-99m-sulfur colloid particles are much larger and with a wider variation in size than ^{198}Au colloid particles, the average size being about 300 μm (Table 3.1.4). The usual dose for planar imaging in adults is 2–5 mCi. Liver perfusion and single photon emission computed tomography (SPECT) studies require a much larger dose, in the range of 5–10 mCi. Technetium-99m has a physical half-life of 6 h and emits a gamma photon of 140 keV energy, which makes it ideal for imaging. Intravenously injected particles clear from blood with a $T_{1/2}$ of 2.5 min.

Table 3.1.4. Characteristics of ^{99m}Tc-S-colloid

Parameter	
Half-life (h)	6.03
Blood clearance ($T_{1/2}$, min)	2.5
Particle size range (μm)	100–1000
Particle mean size (μm)	300
Decay constant (/h)	0.1149
Mean disintegration (%)	87
G-rad/μCi/h	0.0369
Adult dose (mCi)	2–8
Dose to liver from a study (rads)	0.68–2.72

Normally, about 85% of the injected dose of ^{99m}Tc-S-colloid is taken up by the liver, 7% by the spleen, 5% by the bone marrow, and the remaining 3% by other organs such as the lungs or stomach [11]. In moderate parenchymal liver disease, the radiocolloid uptake by the liver decreases and the uptake by the spleen and bone marrow increases. In severe parenchymal liver disease (cirrhosis) when the liver shrinks in size, ~30% of the dose is taken up by the liver, and as much as 30% by the spleen, 25% by the red marrow, and the remaining 13% of the dose is taken up by other organs including the lungs, kidney, and stomach (Table 3.1.5). As most liver morphology imaging is currently obtained with CT, or ultrasound, radiocolloid imaging is chosen primarily for delineating the functional characteristics of the lesion that has already been detected with one of the other imaging modalities. Radiocolloid spleen imaging is often obtained for accurate measurement of spleen size in the diagnosis of polycythemia rubra vera and other myeloproliferative disorders. Technetium-99m-S-colloid preparations are also used in the measurement of gastric emptying time, evaluation of shunt (LeVeen) patency, and for the detection of acute GI bleeding, gastroesophageal reflux, or pulmonary aspiration of gastric contents, etc.

Table 3.1.5. Relative distribution of 99mTc-sulfur-colloid (% injected dose) in normal subjects and patients with liver disease [11]

Clinical status	Liver	Spleen	Marrow	Other
Normal	85	7	5	3
Mild to moderate liver disease	67	13	12	8
Moderate to severe liver disease	32	30	25	13

The radiocolloid dose is used within 6 h of its preparation, and the particles are shaken vigorously just prior to injection to prevent settlement at the bottom of the vial. As free ^{99m}Tc-pertechnetate appears in the breast milk, mothers are instructed not to feed their infants with breast milk for the next 24 h, and to use formula milk instead. The breast milk expressed prior to radiocolloid injection and stored is preferable to formula milk. The usual pediatric dose is 15–75 μCi/kg (0.56–2.78 MBq/kg). For bone marrow imaging in pediatrics, the dose is 30–150 μCi/kg (1.1–5.6 MBq/kg). The minimum dose per study is 600 μCi (22.2 MBq). For gastroesophageal reflux and pulmonary aspiration studies, ^{99m}Tc-S-colloid dose is given orally mixed with a liquid or a semisolid meal.

Mechanism of Radiocolloid Uptake

Metchnikoff in 1884 first observed a process where highly mobile polymorphonuclear leukocytes ingested (phagocytosis) foreign particles, microorganisms, and cellular debris, removing them from the circulation. Similar phenomena were observed in the cells lining the liver sinusoids [12]. Kupffer in 1899 described the nature of these cells in the hepatic sinusoids which today bear his name as Kupffer cells [13]. Aschoff in 1924 introduced the concept of the reticuloendothelial system consisting of the mesenchymal cells distributed throughout the body [14]. Radiocolloid uptake is seen primarily by three organs in the body: liver, spleen, and bone marrow. Lung and other organ uptake normally is not high enough to be seen on the images.

The uptake of radiocolloids by the RE system cells is dependent upon various factors including particle size, charge, dose, chemical composition, and other factors. The maximum phagocytic capacity in humans is 1.07 mg/min/kg body weight [15]. The RE system acts as a biologic filter by removing effete cells and foreign material from blood and thus restricting the general toxic effect on the body. The filtering mechanism becomes more and more efficient in the spleen as the particle size increases. The smallest particles are removed preferentially by the bone marrow, medium size particles by the liver, and the largest particles by the spleen. As the ^{198}Au colloid particles are the smallest (30 μm), most of them are taken up by the liver and bone marrow and very few particles by the spleen, explaining why the spleen is usually not visualized well in the scans obtained with gold-198.

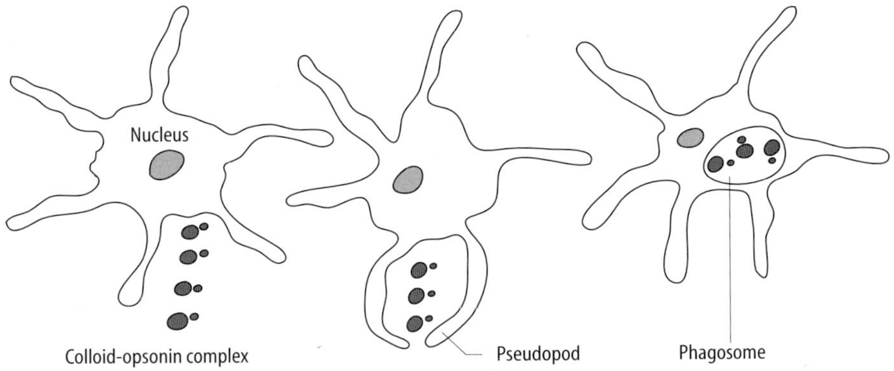

Fig. 3.1.1. Mechanism of radiocolloid uptake. After intravenous injection, radiocolloid comes in contact with plasma proteins, forming a radiocolloid-opsonin complex. The complex is encircled by pseudopodes of the Kupffer cells in the liver and reticuloendothelial (*RE*) cells in the spleen and bone marrow. After complete engulfment, the radiocolloid forms a phagosome within the cytosol

Upon intravenous injection, radiocolloid particles are coated by plasma opsonins, making them susceptible to phagocytosis. A radiocolloid-opsonin complex attaches to the RE cell membrane and initiates phagocytosis (Fig. 3.1.1). The cytoplasm of the RE cell flows around the opsonized radiocolloid particles as pseudopods, encircles the particle, and ultimately incorporates into the cytoplasm, forming a phagosome [16, 17]. The ultimate fate of the radiocolloid in the phagosome depends upon its nature. The phagosome is either destroyed and its contents stored in the cytosol or it is destroyed, digested, and its contents released back into the circulation. Gold-198 radiocolloids are stored intracellularly whereas the ^{99m}Tc-S-colloids are digested and released into the circulation [18].

Dosimetry of Radiocolloids

The liver is the critical organ for radiocolloids and receives 39 rads/mCi ^{198}Au and 0.34 rad/mCi ^{99m}Tc-S-colloid (Table 3.1.6). From one imaging study, the liver receive 5.8 rads from ^{198}Au (200-μCi dose) and 0. 68 rads from ^{99m}Tc-S-colloid (2-mCi dose). Radiation to the liver decreases as the severity of liver disease increases. The total body receives 1.4 rads/mCi with ^{198}Au and 0.019 rads/mCi with ^{99m}Tc-S-colloid. The introduction of ^{99m}Tc-sulfur-colloid in 1965 was a major breakthrough that revolutionized liver morphology imaging in the late 1970s and through the early 1980s.

Table 3.1.6. Absorbed dose (rads/mCi) from ^{99m}Tc-sulfur-colloid in normal subjects and patients with liver disease [11]

Organ	Normal	Moderate disease	Severe disease
Liver	0.34	0.21	0.16
Spleen	0.21	0.28	0.42
Red marrow	0.02	0.04	0.07
Ovaries	0.005	0.008	0.012
Testes	0.001	0.002	0.003
Total body	0.019	0.019	0.019

Technetium-99m-HIDA Agents

Functional imaging in nuclear hepatology took a quantum leap with the introduction of ^{99m}Tc-HIDA agents by Loberg et al. in 1976 [6]. Hepatobiliary diseases are quite common and they often present clinically with dramatic suddenness requiring immediate diagnosis and therapy (acute cholecystitis). ^{99m}Tc-HIDA agents fulfill the requirement for rapid diagnosis.

Labeling

Technetium-99m-HIDA agents are lidocaine analogues. Lidocaine has been used in clinical practice for many years and its pharmacokinetics are well understood. Liver is the primary site of uptake and metabolism of lidocaine, indocyanine green and other organic variations [19–21]. Lidocaine ($C_{14}H_{22}N_2O$) has a molecular weight of 270.80 and clears from blood in a biexponential fashion; the fast component has a $T_{1/2}$ of 7 min, and the slow component a $T_{1/2}$ of 108 min. Lidocaine shows a high first pass extraction by the liver. About 90% of extracted lidocaine is metabolized into monoethylglycylxylidine and the remaining 10% is excreted in urine unchanged. Age does not affect the biokinetic behavior of lidocaine.

Based upon its wide clinical application in cardiology and with the knowledge that lidocaine is metabolized primarily in the liver, it was hypothesized that technetium-99m-labeled lidocaine or its analogues could find a potential imaging application in either cardiology or hepatology. Since technetium-99m could not be attached to lidocaine directly, iminodiacetic acid (IDA) was chosen as a bifunctional chelate to carry the ligand (lidocaine) at one end and the radiotracer (^{99m}Tc) at the other end [6]. Each molecule of labeled ^{99m}Tc-HIDA complex, therefore, consists of two molecules each of the ligand and the chelate and an atom of technetium-99m in the middle (Fig. 3.1.2). When ^{99m}Tc-HIDA was injected into mice and gamma camera imaging began, the investigators were startled not to find any myocardial uptake but were immensely pleased to see radioactivity first in the hepatocytes and later throughout the biliary system [22]. For the lack of any other better terminology, the investigators settled on a new name, **h**epatic **i**mino**d**iacetic **a**cid, or HIDA. Thus the major portion of the name (HIDA) reflects the chelate (IDA) more than it does the ligand (lidocaine), which provides the most critical functional information.

Radiolabeling with technetium-99m does not affect the blood clearance or the hepatic uptake of lidocaine but it alters the intrahepatic transit. Unlike lidocaine,

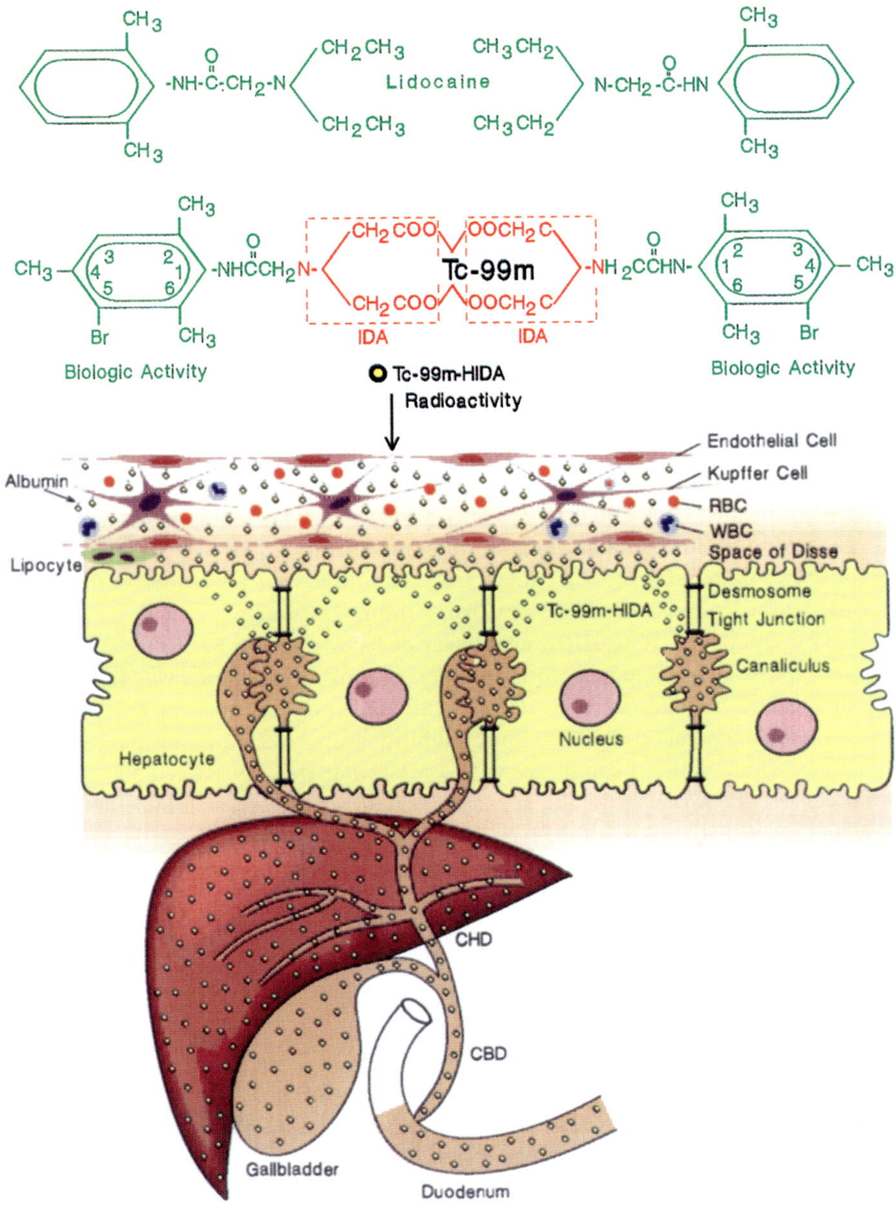

Fig. 3.1.2. Molecular structure and hepatobiliary transit of ^{99m}Tc-HIDA. Lidocaine (*green*) is the ligand with the biologic function, technetium-99m (*black*) is the radiotracer, and iminodiacetic acid (*IDA*) is the chelate (*red*) that binds them together. A radiolabeled whole complex consists an atom of ^{99m}Tc, two molecules of lidocaine, and two molecules of IDA. Albumin delivers the radiotracer to the space of Disse where the dissociation takes place. ^{99m}Tc-HIDA is taken up by the hepatocyte and secreted into bile canaliculi in free form, where it mixes with the hepatic bile and serves as an ideal in vivo radio tracer for imaging of the entire hepatobiliary tree [27]

^{99m}Tc-HIDA is not metabolized during its transit through the hepatocyte. It is secreted as native ^{99m}Tc-HIDA into the bile canaliculi. This feature is readily demonstrated by reinjection of radiolabeled gallbladder bile intravenously into the same animal where the exact kinetics of the original injection are reproduced. Lidocaine forms a dimer with technetium-99m which increases the molecular weight from 270.8 for lidocaine to 833 for ^{99m}Tc-HIDA complex (Fig. 3.1.2). An increase in molecular weight enhances hepatocyte uptake and excretion. Labeling with technetium-99m imparts hepatic specificity. Lidocaine labeled with carbon-14 or tin-113m, on the other hand, does not show hepatic uptake and excretion; instead it is excreted mostly through urine [6].

Structure-Function Relationship

The basic configuration of all ^{99m}Tc-HIDA agents is very similar (Fig. 3.1.3). The bifunctional chelate, IDA, attaches to a molecule of lidocaine at one end and to an atom of technetium-99m at the other end. Technetium-99m is the radiotracer and the biologic function resides with lidocaine. The biokinetic behavior of the labeled complex can be altered by making substitutions in the benzene ring at positions 2, 4, 6 (ortho), 4 (para), or 5 (meta) with a methyl, ethyl, isopropyl, or isobutyl group. A halogen is attached in the meta position (mebrofenin). More than 30 new compounds were created by making various substitutions at different positions [23–25]. Six of the compounds have undergone critical clinical trials and three have been approved for routine use by the United States Food and Drug Administration.

Hepatic uptake of ^{99m}Tc-HIDA agents varies from a low of 82.5% to 98.1% [26]. Hepatic uptake of ^{99m}Tc-disofenin is 89% and that of mebrofenin 98% (Table 3.1.7). The uptake and excretion of ^{99m}Tc-HIDA agents are dependent upon various factors of which molecular structure, weight, lipid solubility, and protein binding are important parameters. Radiolabeled complexes with a molecular weight between 300 and 1000 are preferentially taken up by the hepatocytes and rapidly secreted into the bile. An isopropyl substitution at the 2 and 6 positions (disofenin) makes it a better agent than

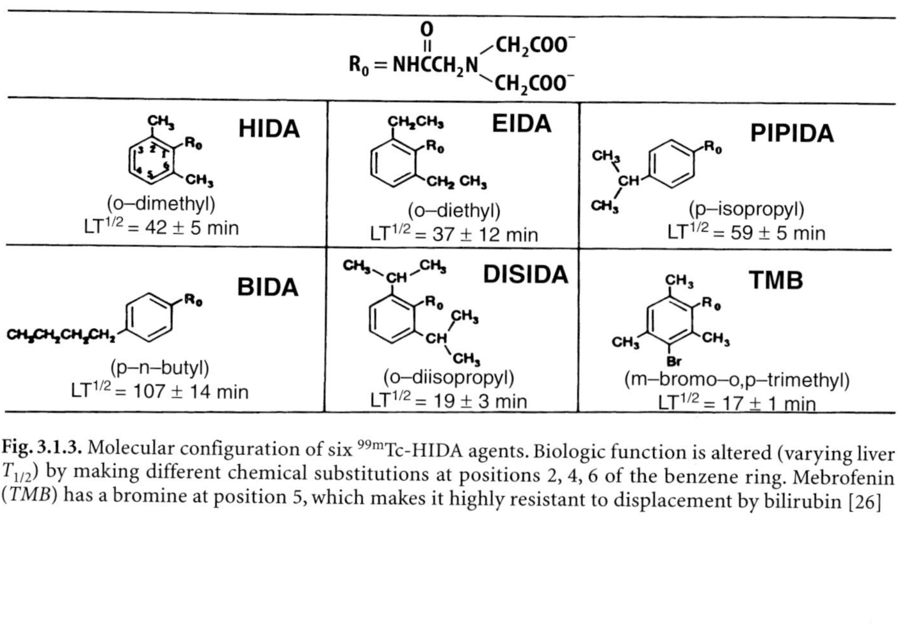

Fig. 3.1.3. Molecular configuration of six ^{99m}Tc-HIDA agents. Biologic function is altered (varying liver $T_{1/2}$) by making different chemical substitutions at positions 2, 4, 6 of the benzene ring. Mebrofenin (*TMB*) has a bromine at position 5, which makes it highly resistant to displacement by bilirubin [26]

a dimethyl or diethyl substitution at the same locations, or an isopropyl substitution at the para position (PIPIDA). A methyl substitution at positions 2, 4, 6 and a bromine atom at position 5 (mebrofenin) results in creating the best agent of all. ^{99m}Tc-Mebrofenin shows the highest liver uptake (98%) and resists strongly the displacement by a high bilirubin level. Both agents are secreted from the liver rapidly into bile with a mean excretion half-time of 17 min with mebrofenin and 19 min with disofenin. The dose not taken up by the liver is excreted through the kidneys. Urinary excretion of mebrofenin is 2% and disofenin 11% of the dose injected.

Table 3.1.7. Biokinetic features of Tc-99 m mebrofenin and Tc-99 m disofenin

Agent	Liver uptake (% dose)	Urine excretion (% dose)	Liver excretion ($T_{1/2}$, min)	Radiation (mrads) to Liver	Radiation (mrads) to Gallbladder
^{99m}Tc-Mebrofenin (Choletec)	98	2	17	70	410
^{99m}Tc-Disofenin (Hepatolite)	89	11	19	75	370

Biokinetics of ^{99m}Tc-HIDA Agents

Biokinetic behavior of ^{99m}Tc-HIDA agents can be divided into six functional phases: (1) blood transport, (2) uptake by the hepatocyte, (3) transit through the hepatocyte and secretion into bile canaliculi, (4) flow through the intrahepatic and extrahepatic ducts, (5) entry into the gallbladder, and (6) final discharge into the small intestine [26, 27].

Blood Transport. ^{99m}Tc-HIDA agents are transported in blood bound to serum albumin, forming an albumin-^{99m}Tc-HIDA complex [26]. Protein binding enhances hepatic delivery and hepatocyte uptake and decreases renal excretion. The agents clear from the blood at variable rates (Fig. 3.1.4). Hypoalbuminemia decreases hepatic delivery and increases renal excretion. The affinity of ^{99m}Tc-HIDA to bind with albumin is much lower than that of bromsulphalein and bilirubin [28]. A substitution at the para position improves both albumin binding and lipid solubility. Methyl substitution at the 2, 4, 6 positions and a bromine at the 5 position (mebrofenin) increases both hepatic delivery and hepatocyte uptake and markedly reduces renal excretion. A butyl substitution at the para position has a similar effect on the uptake [25]. Albumin bound ^{99m}Tc-HIDA leaves the sinusoidal space through the fenestrae of the endothelial cells and enters the perisinusoidal space of Disse, a space unique for liver capillaries. Disassociation between albumin-^{99m}Tc-HIDA takes place in the space of Disse very close to the basolateral border of the hepatocyte (Fig. 3.1.2). Only ^{99m}Tc-HIDA enters the hepatocyte, leaving albumin behind in the blood. This mechanism is common for most organic anions [28].

Hepatocyte Uptake. The mechanism of uptake of ^{99m}Tc-HIDA by the hepatocyte is similar to those of other organic anions [29, 30]. Liver concentrates three types of organic anions including bile acids, free fatty acids, and non-bile acid cholephils (bromsulphalein, bilirubin, rose bengal, indocyanine green and ^{99m}Tc-HIDA). Non-bile acid cholephils are taken up by the hepatocyte by a mechanism called receptor mediat-

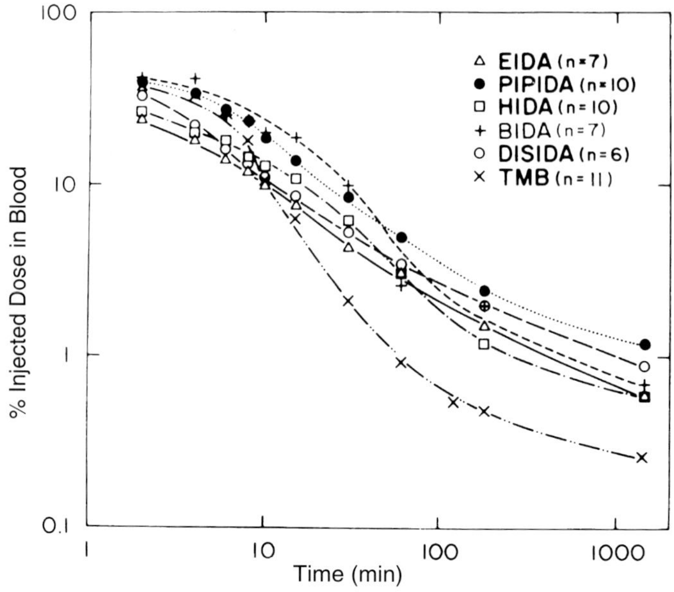

Fig. 3.1.4. Blood clearance of six ^{99m}Tc-HIDA agents. Note the fastest blood clearance with mebrofenin (*TMB*) [26]

ed endocytosis (RME). RME has been well documented for low density lipoprotein, IgA, insulin, transferrin, asialoglycoprotein and cholesterol [31]. It is believed that ^{99m}Tc-HIDA compounds follow the RME pathway taken by bilirubin and other organic anions. By subjecting cultured rat hepatocytes to different in vitro experimental conditions, Okuda et al. and Lan et al. have demonstrated three possible pathways for uptake of ^{99m}Tc-HIDA: (1) organic anion pathway probably through RME, (2) bile acid (bile salt) pathway, and (3) free fatty acid pathway [28, 32, 33].

Receptor Mediated Endocytosis. After dissociation from albumin in the space of Disse, ^{99m}Tc-HIDA attaches to its specific receptors through receptor protein (ligandin). These receptors are located along the basolateral border and along the walls of the coated pits, which are mere invaginations of the basolateral membrane into the hepatocyte cytosol [31, 34]. The ligand (^{99m}Tc-HIDA) and the receptor protein (ligandin) cluster in the coated pit (Fig. 3.1.5). This collection is one of the primary requirements for RME to progress. After separation from the surface membrane, the coated pit forms a coated vesicle, and ^{99m}Tc-HIDA becomes internalized within the hepatocyte. After losing the protein covering, the vesicle becomes an endosome. In the case of LDL, IgA, insulin, and transferrin, the protein coating the vesicle is clathrin. Cotransport through bile acids and free fatty acids occurs simultaneously with RME.

Despite sharing a common mechanism of uptake, there are a few differences in hepatocyte uptake between ^{99m}Tc-mebrofenin and ^{99m}Tc-disofenin. In cultured rat hepatocytes, bilirubin reduces the uptake of disofenin much more profoundly than

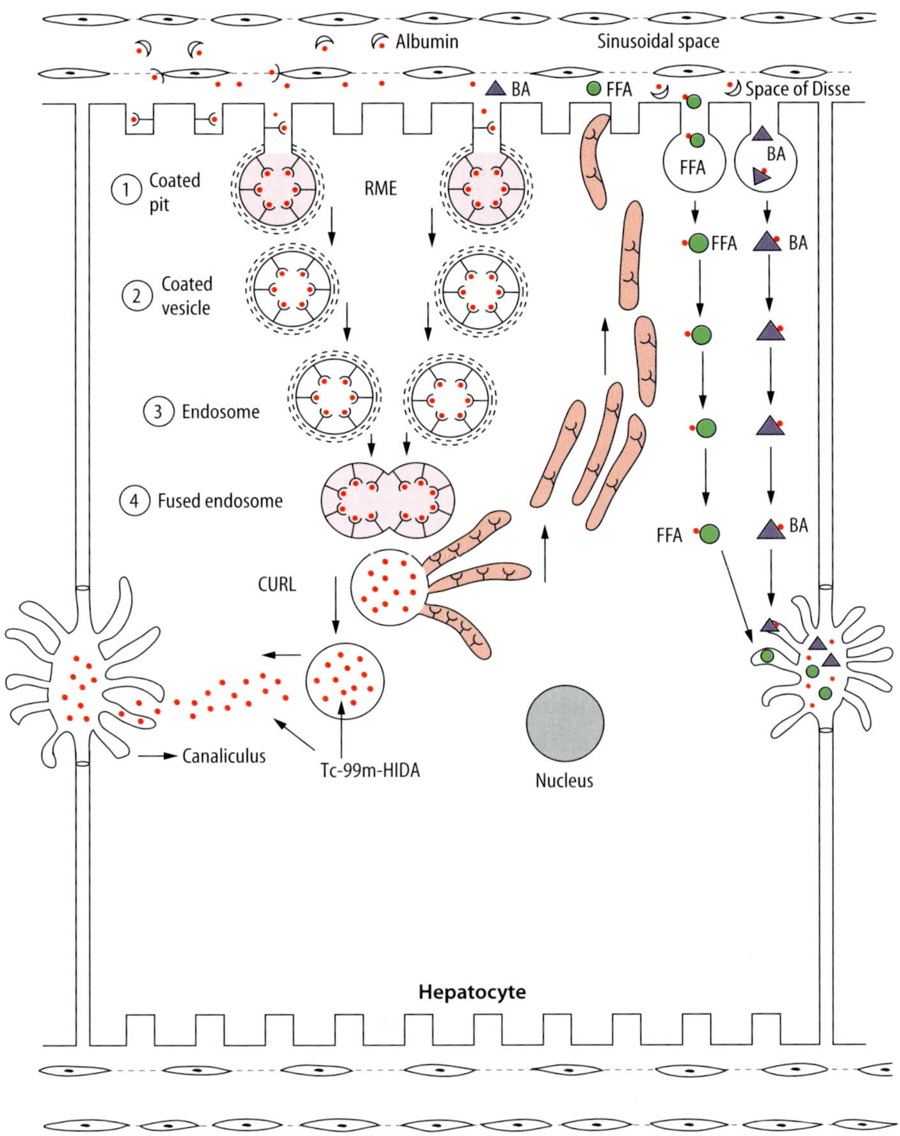

Fig. 3.1.5. Schematic representation of receptor mediated endocytosis for uptake and excretion of ^{99m}Tc-HIDA by the hepatocyte. Primary uptake occurs via receptor mediated endocytosis (*RME*). After detaching from albumin in the space of Disse, the radiotracer attaches to the ligandin receptors within the coated pits [1], which are invaginations of the basolateral border of the hepatocyte. A coated vesicle [2] is formed when it separates from the surface membrane. The coated vesicle rapidly loses its clathrin coat, forming an endosome [3]. Two endosomes combine together to form a fused endosome [4]. Hydrogen is pumped into fused intravesicular space, initiating uncoupling of receptor and ligand (*CURL*). Ligand enters the bile canaliculi and the receptor moves to the surface for recycling. ^{99m}Tc-HIDA in addition uses free fatty acid (*FFA*) and bile acid (*BA*) pathways for uptake and excretion in free form into bile canaliculi (modified from Steer [31])

that of mebrofenin. At 20 μM bilirubin in the culture medium, the hepatocyte uptake of ^{99m}Tc-disofenin decreases to 34% from a basal value of 100% without bilirubin in the culture medium. In contrast, the uptake of ^{99m}Tc-mebrofenin remains at 70% of the basal value under identical experimental conditions. Both disofenin and mebrofenin show a reduction in hepatocyte uptake when bile acids or free fatty acids are added to the culture medium, suggesting the existence of other uptake pathways. These results indicate that ^{99m}Tc-HIDA agents share a common pathway with organic anions (bilirubin), free fatty acid, and bile acids. Bromsulphalein (BSP) inhibits uptake by the hepatocyte of ^{99m}Tc-disofenin much more profoundly than ^{99m}Tc-mebrofenin (Table 3.1.8).

Table 3.1.8. Effect of 20 μM of various organic anions on the uptake (%) of ^{99m}Tc-disofenin and ^{99m}Tc-mebrofenin by cultured rat hepatocytes [32]

Agent	Basal uptake	BSP	Bilirubin	Tauro-cholate	Glyco-cholate	Cholate	Deoxy-cholate	Chenodeoxy-cholate
^{99m}Tc-Disofenin	100	59	34	61	59	66	42	42
^{99m}Tc-Mebrofenin	100	107	70	69	85	80	62	71

Transit Through the Hepatocyte and Secretion into Bile Canaliculi. Unlike bilirubin and other organic anions, ^{99m}Tc-HIDA agents are secreted into bile canaliculi in their native state, without undergoing any conjugation during their transit through the hepatocyte [6]. The mechanisms by which ^{99m}Tc-HIDA is transported through the hepatocyte and then secreted into the bile canalicular lumen are not clear. The general belief is that the mechanism is similar to those of non-cholephil organic anions, free fatty acids and bile acids. Vesicular transport and receptor-ligandin transport are thought to be involved. After losing the clathrin coat, the vesicle forms an endosome. Two endosomes together form a fused endosome. At this point, the ligand (^{99m}Tc-HIDA) and the receptor (ligandin) separate and start moving in two different directions. The ligand (^{99m}Tc-HIDA) enters the bile canaliculi and the ligandin moves to the hepatocyte surface for recycling [35]. Rough endoplasmic reticulum and the Golgi complex are known to synthesize the receptor. After entering the canaliculi, ^{99m}Tc-HIDA mixes thoroughly with the hepatic bile and from then on it serves as an ideal in vivo tracer for delineation of the entire hepatobiliary tree (Fig. 3.1.2). The curves generated over the liver provide a measure of the rapidity of uptake and excretion of ^{99m}Tc-HIDA (Fig. 3.1.6). The dose not taken up by the liver is excreted through urine (Fig. 3.1.7).

Currently ^{99m}Tc-disofenin and ^{99m}Tc-mebrofenin are the most popular agents (Fig. 3.1.8). ^{99m}Tc-mebrofenin, which has bromine at position 5 (meta), clears from the liver much more rapidly than ^{99m}Tc-disofenin (Fig. 3.1.9).

Flow Through Intrahepatic and Extrahepatic Ducts. The hepatic bile is radiolabeled instantly, as soon as ^{99m}Tc-HIDA secreted by the hepatocyte enters the bile canaliculi. In vivo bile radiolabeling under total basal conditions allows delineation of the entire intrahepatic and extrahepatic bile ducts. Of the 600 ml total bile produced per day, 450 ml is secreted by the hepatocytes and 150 ml by canalicular cells [36]. The bile within the ducts is radiolabeled as the hepatic bile passes through the ducts.

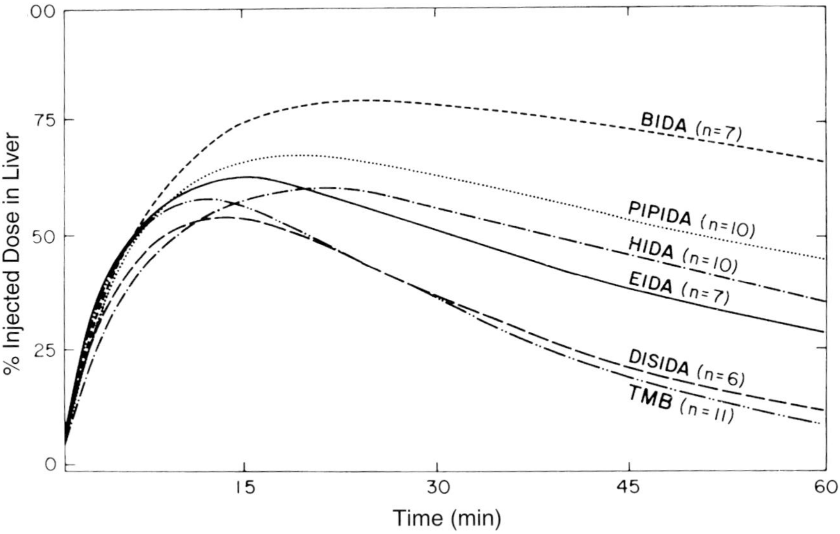

Fig. 3.1.6. Hepatic uptake and excretion of six ^{99m}Tc-HIDA agents. Fastest uptake and excretion is noted with disofenin (*DISIDA*) and mebrofenin (*TMB*)

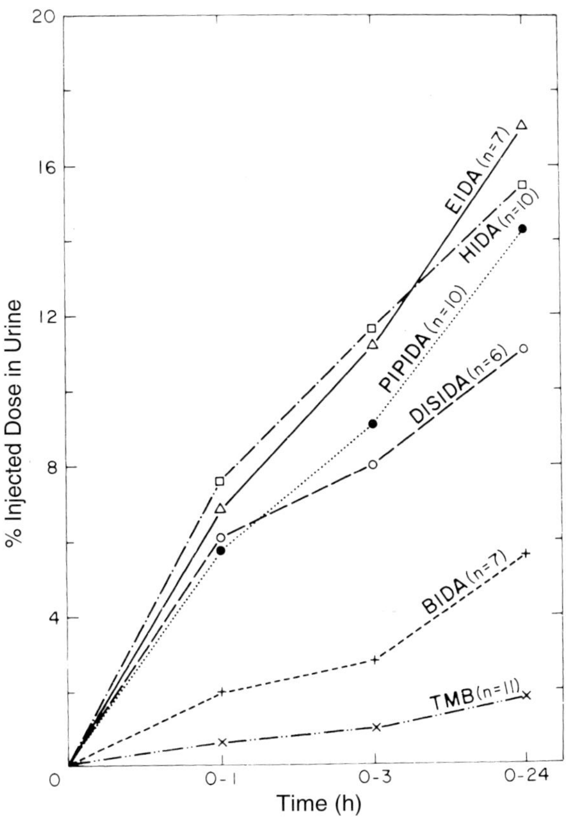

Fig. 3.1.7. Urinary excretion of six ^{99m}Tc-HIDA agents. Less than 2% of the injected dose of mebrofenin (*TMB*) is excreted in 24-h urine. Other agents show increasing amounts of urinary excretion [26]

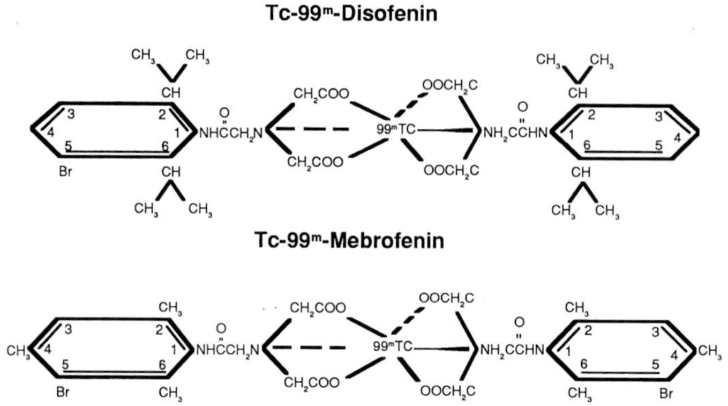

Fig. 3.1.8. Molecular structure of ^{99m}Tc-disofenin and ^{99m}Tc-mebrofenin. An atom of bromine at position 5, and three methyl groups at positions 2, 4, 6 in mebrofenin change its biologic behavior from that of disofenin with an isopropyl group at positions 2 and 6

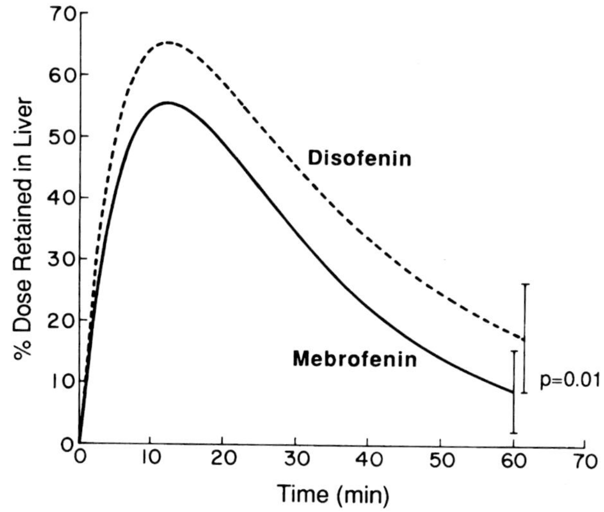

Fig. 3.1.9. Hepatic uptake and excretion of ^{99m}Tc-disofenin and ^{99m}Tc-mebrofenin. The uptake and excretion by the liver of ^{99m}Tc-mebrofenin are significantly faster when compared with ^{99m}Tc-disofenin [38]

Gallbladder Storage. About 70% of the hepatic bile secreted during fasting hours enters the gallbladder (0.3 ml/min) and the rest enters the duodenum directly [37]. A fully filled normal gallbladder can accommodate up to 50 ml bile. It would, therefore, take approximately 180 min (6 h) for a completely emptied gallbladder to refill to its full capacity. The ability to accommodate a constant inflow (0.3 ml bile/min) of hepatic bile during fasting is made possible by the absorption of an equal volume of water through the gallbladder wall (about 0.3 ml/min). The gallbladder wall absorbs water, chloride, and bicarbonates at a much faster rate than sodium, bile salts, and cholesterol from hepatic bile. By this selective absorption, the gallbladder can sequester all of the total body bile salts within it during 10–12 h of fasting. This selective process of solute concentration is called the concentration function of the gallbladder.

There is a rapid rise in ^{99m}Tc-HIDA counts when radiolabeled hepatic bile enters the gallbladder. Accumulation of a very high specific activity bile in a relatively small volume (50 ml) accounts for the gallbladder being the critical organ in a ^{99m}Tc-HIDA study [38], receiving about 908 mrads/mCi. The upper large intestine, lower large intestine, and small intestine receive decreasing doses (Table 3.1.9). Radiation to the gastrointestinal tract decreases in liver failure when kidneys become the preferential route of excretion for ^{99m}Tc-HIDA.

Table 3.1.9. Radiation absorbed dose (mrads/mCi) to various organs from ^{99m}Tc-HIDA in normal subjects and patients with increasing severity of liver disease [38]

Organ	Bilirubin level				
	Normal	Patients with increasing serum bilirubin level			
	<1 mg/dl	<1 mg/dl	1–5 mg/dl	5–10 mg/dl	>10 mg/dl
Gallbladder	908	728	617	309	101
Upper colon	302	235	198	100	36
Lower colon	199	154	131	68	27
Small intestine	189	147	125	65	25
Liver	76	91	90	47	18
Ovaries	62	50	43	25	13
Kidneys	43	58	67	105	132
Urinary bladder	35	46	53	87	111
Bone marrow	24	21	19	13	9
Spleen	9	8	7	5	3
Testes	4	4	4	4	5
Total body	16	15	14	9	6

Final Discharge into the Duodenum. When the food leaves the stomach and enters the duodenum, it stimulates cholecystokinin (CCK) secreting cells in the mucosa of the duodenum and jejunum to release endogenous CCK into circulation. It usually takes about 6–26 min (mean 16 min) after a meal for serum CCK levels to rise above the threshold to induce contraction and emptying of the gallbladder [39]. Once the gallbladder contraction is initiated, bile emptying is maintained for 1–2 h postmeal. In addition to initiating gallbladder contraction and emptying, CCK stimulates water secretion by cholangiocytes lining the bile ducts, and hastens bile flow by directly stimulating smooth muscle of the bile ducts [40]. CCK also increases intestinal peristalsis and facilitates movement of bile emptied from the gallbladder antegrade towards the jejunum and ileum. By inducing contraction of the pylorus of the stomach it prevents duodenogastric bile reflux. Highly concentrated gallbladder bile is discharged into the duodenum upon the arrival of food into the small intestine, where bile salts facilitate digestion and absorption of nutrients into the blood stream.

Other ^{99m}Tc-Labeled Hepatobiliary Agents

Some of the ^{99m}Tc-labeled potential hepatobiliary agents have not been approved by the United States Food and Drug Administration for routine clinical use. Some are approved in other countries. These agents include ^{99m}Tc-labeled penicillamine [41, 42], dihydrothiooctic acid [43], tetracycline [44], and pyridoxylidineglutamate [45]. ^{99m}Tc-Pyridoxylidineglutamate has been used extensively in Australia, Japan, and other Asian countries [46]. Some of the agents used for imaging of other organs pass through the liver and are secreted into bile and often they provide information about the hepatobiliary function (Fig. 3.1.10). Myocardial perfusion imaging agent, ^{99m}Tc-Sestamibi, is taken up by hepatocytes and secreted into bile and provides an opportunity to measure gallbladder ejection fraction with CCK in those rare patients where acalculous chronic cholecystitis (cystic duct syndrome) mimics an anginal type of pain.

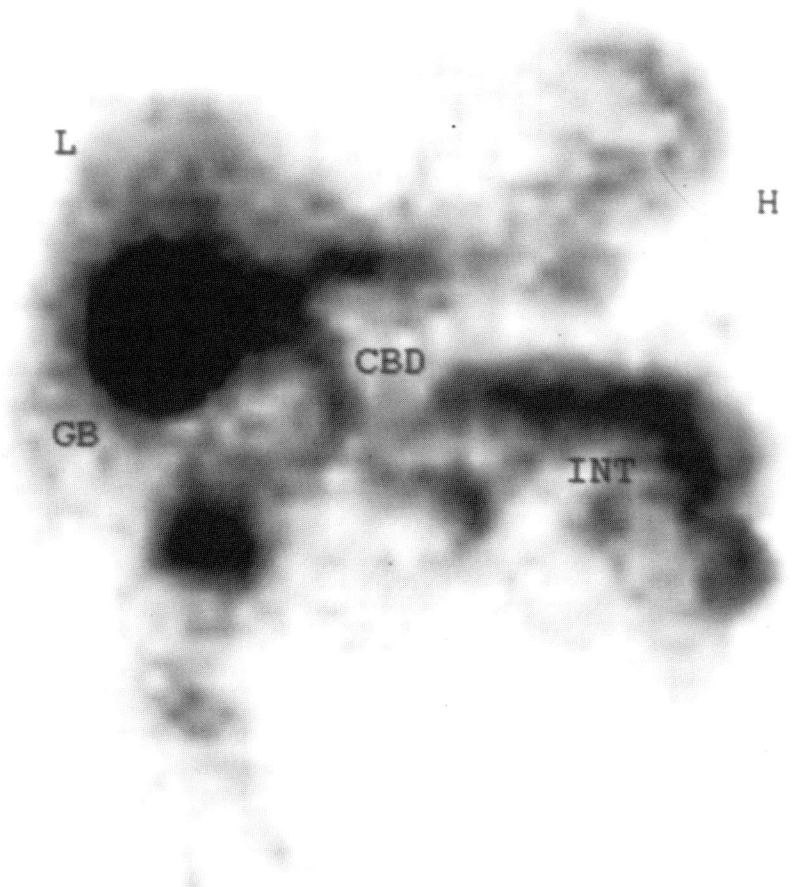

Fig. 3.1.10. Secretion of technetium-99m sestamibi into bile. Myocardial (*H*) perfusion imaging agent shows accumulation in the liver (*L*), bile ducts, and gallbladder (*GB*). *CBD*, common bile duct; *INT*, intestine

Technetium-99m-DTPA Galactosyl-Human Serum Albumin

The basolateral and lateral (not canalicular) border of the plasma membrane of the hepatocyte is rich in asialoglycoprotein (ASGP) receptors, which serve as the binding site for ^{99m}Tc-DTPA-galactosyl human serum albumin (^{99m}Tc-GSA). These receptors specific for the hepatocytes are not found in any other cells in the body [31]. After an intravenous injection, ^{99m}Tc-GSA circulates in the blood and is extracted by the hepatocyte plasma membrane and transferred to the lysosomes through receptor mediated endocytosis. Blood disappearance parallels the clearance of indocyanine green, considered a gold standard agent for hepatocyte function [47]. Studies in Japan have shown a great potential for the measurement of hepatic reserve prior to resection of the liver in patients with hepatocellular carcinoma, cholangiocarcinoma, cirrhosis, and metastatic disease. Rapid sequence SPECT imaging allows quantitative measurement of the functional reserve and enables the prediction of prognosis [48–50].

New SI Units for Measurement of Radiation

The international commission on radiation units and measurements recommended in 1974 that new SI (system international) units replace old CGS units for all scientific work after 1984. The old and new units of measurement and their relationship are shown in Tables 3.1.10, 3.1.11, and 3.1.12 [51].

Table 3.1.10. Old CGS and new SI units for measurement of radioactivity [51]

Old units (curies)	New SI units (becquerels)	Disintegrations per second (dps)
Megacurie (MCi)	37 PBq	$3.7+10^{16}$
Kilocurie (KCi)	37 TBq	$3.7+10^{13}$
Curie (Ci)	37 GBq	$3.7+10^{10}$
Millicurie (mCi)	37 MBq	$3.7+10^{7}$
Microcurie (μCi)	37 kBq	$3.7+10^{4}$
Nanocurie (nCi)	37 Bq	3.7+10
Picocurie (pCi)	37 mBq	$3.7+10^{-2}$

Table 3.1.11. Relationship between new becquerel and old curie units [51]

1 becquerel (Bq)	= 1 dis/s = $27.03+10^{-12}$ Ci	= 27.03 pCi
1 kilobecquerel (kBq)	= 10^3 Bq	= 27.03 nCi
1 megabecquerel (MBq)	= 10^6 Bq	= 27.03 μCi
1 gigabecquerel (GBq)	= 10^9 Bq	= 27.03 mCi

Table 3.1.12. Relationship between old and new SI units for measurement of radiation [51]

Parameter	Old unit	New SI unit	Conversion factor
Radioactivity	Curie (Ci) = $3.7+10^{10}$ dps	Becquerel (Bq) = 1 dps	1 Ci = $3.7+10^{10}$ Bq 1 Bq = $2.7+10^{-11}$ Ci
Radiation exposure	Roentgen (R) = $2.58+10^{-4}$ C/kg	Coulomb/kg (C/kg)	1 R = $2.58+10^{-4}$ C/kg 1 C/kg = $3.88+10^{3}$ R
Radiation absorbed dose	rad = 100 erg/g	Gray (Gy) = 1 J/kg	1 rad = 0.01 Gy 1 Gy = 100 rad
Radiation dose equivalent	rem = QF + rad	Sievert (Sv) = QF + Gy	1 rem = 0.01 Sv 1 Sv = 100 rem

References

1. Sheppard CW, Wells EB, Hahn PF, Goodell JBP. Studies of the distribution of intravenously administered colloidal sol of manganese dioxide and gold in human beings and dogs using radioactive isotopes. J Lab. & Clin Med 1947;32:274–277
2. Stirret LA, Yuhl ET, Cassen B. Clinical application of hepatic radioactive surveys . Am J Gastroenterology. 1954;21:310–317
3. Stirret LA, Yuhl ET, Libby RL. A new technique for diagnosis of carcinoma metastatic to the liver. Surg. Gynecol, Obstret. 1953;96:210–215
4. Taplin GV, Meredith OM Jr, Kade H. Radioactive (I-131 tagged) rose bengal uptake -excretion test for liver function using external gamma ray scintillation counting technique. J Lab & Clin Med 1955;45:665–678
5. Harper PV, Lathrop KA, Jimiriez F, Fink R, Gottschalk A. Technetium-99 m as a scanning agent. Radiology 1965;85:101–103
6. Loberg MD, Cooper M, Harvey E, Callery P, Faith W. Development of new radiopharmaceuticals based on N-substitution of iminodiacetic acid. J Nucl Med 1976;17:633–638
7. McAfee JG, Subramanian G. Radioactive agents for imaging. In: Freeman LM, Johnson (eds) Clinical radionuclide imaging Grune and Stratton Inc, Orlando 1984, Volume 1
8. Iya VK, Gopal GS, Chaudhuri SY, Colloidal gold. Preparation and particle size determination by electron microscope. Indian J Chem 1965;3:317–320
9. Dobson EL, Jones HB. The behavior of intravenously injected particulate material; Its rate of disappearance from blood as a measure of liver blood flow. Acta Med Scand (Suppl 144) 1952;273:1–50
10. MIRD: Dose estimates report number 4. Summary of current radiation dose estimates to humans with various liver conditions from Au-198 colloidal gold. J Nucl Med 1975;16:173–174
11. MIRD: Dose estimates report number 3. Summary of current radiation dose estimates to humans with various liver conditions from Tc-99 m sulfur colloid. J Nucl Med 1975;16:108A-108B
12. Metchnikoff E. In Immunite dans les maladies infectieuses. Paris Masson 1901
13. Kupffer C. Von. Uberdie sogenanuten sternzellen der saugentheirer leber. Arch Microsk Anat 1899;26:1
14. Ashoff I. Das reticulo-endotheliale system. Ergebn Inn Med Kinderheilk 1924;26:1
15. Iio M, Wagner Jr. H.N, Scheffel U, Jabbour B. Studies of the reticulo-endothelial system (RES) 1. Measurement of the phagocytic capacity of the RES in man and dog. J Clin Invest 1963;42:417–416
16. Saba TM. Physiology and physiopathology of the reticuloendothelial system. Arch Intern Med 1970;126:1031–1052
17. Stossel TP. How do phagocytes eat ? Ann Intern Med 1978;89:398–402
18. Kitani K, Taplin GV. Biliary excretion of 99 m Tc- albumin microaggregate degradation products (a method for measuring Kupffer cell digestive function) ? J Nucl Med 1972;13:260–265
19. Beckett AH, Boyes RN, Appleton PJ. The metabolism and excretion of lignocaine in man. J Pharm Pharmacology 1966;18:76–81 (suppl)
20. Rowland M, Thomson PD, Guichard A, Melmon KL. Disposition kinetics of lidocaine in normal subjects. Ann N Y Acad Sci 1971;179:383–398
21. Zito RA, Reid PR. Lidocaine kinetics predicted by indocyanin green clearance. New Engl J Med 1978;298:1160–1163
22. Ryan J, Cooper M, Loberg MD, et al. Technetium 99 m labeled N- (2,6 dimethylphenyl carbomoylmethyl) iminodiacetic acid (Tc-99m-HIDA). A new radiopharmaceutical for hepatobiliary imaging studies. J Nucl Med 1977;18:997–1004
23. Nunn AD, Loberg MD, Conley RA. A structure-distribution-relationship approach leading to the development of Tc-99 m mebrofenin: an improved cholescintigraphic agent. J Nucl Med 1983;24:423–430
24. Wistow BW, Subramanian G, Van Heertum RL, Henderson RW, Gagne GM, Hall RC, McAfee JG. An evaluation of Tc-99 m labeled hepatobiliary agents. J Nucl Med 1977;18:455–461
25. Subramanian G, McAfee JG, Henderson R, et al. A new bifunctional chelate for designing Tc-99 m labeled radiopharmaceuticals. In: Murry IP, Hoschl R. Eds. Proceedings of first Asia and Oceania congress of nuclear medicine, 1976. Sidney, Australia. Pink Panther Printers pp 144–149
26. Krishnamurthy S, Krishnamurthy GT. Technetium-99 m iminodiacetic acid organic anions: review of biokinetics and clinical application in hepatology. Hepatology 1989;9:139–153
27. Krishnamurthy S, Krishnamurthy GT. Evolution of nuclear hepatology as a clinical subspeciality. J Nucl Med Technol 1995;23:35S–45S (supplement)
28. Okada H, Nunes R, Vallabhajosula S, Strashun A, Goldsmith SJ, Berk PD. Studies of the hepatocellular uptake of the hepatobiliary scintiscanning agent Tc-99m-DISIDA. J Hepatol 1986;3:251–259

29. Berk PD, Stremmel W. Hepatocellular uptake of organic anions. In: H Popper, Schaffner F (eds). Progress in liver disease, vol 111 Grune and Stratton, New York 1988, pp 125–143
30. Chervu LR, Nunn AD, Loberg MD. Radiopharmaceuticals for hepatobiliary imaging. Semin Nucl Med 1982;12:5–17
31. Streer CJ. Receptor-mediated endocytosis: mechanisms, biologic function and molecular properties. In: Zakim D, Boyer TD (eds). Hepatology, a text book of liver disease. WB Saunders Co, Philadelphia, 1996 pp 149–214
32. Lan JA, Chervu LR, Johansen KL, Wolkoff AW. Uptake of Technetium-99 m Hepatobiliary agents by cultured rat hepatocyte. Gastroenterology 1988;95:1625–1631
33. Roy-Chowdhury J, Jansen PLM. Bilirubin metabolism and its disorders. In: Zakim D, Boyer TD. (eds). Hepatology, a text book of liver disease. WB Saunders Co Philadelphia 1996 pp 323–361
34. Goldstein JL, Anderson RG, Brown MS. Coated pits, coated vesicles, and receptor-mediated endocytosis. Nature 1979; 279:679–685
35. Pearse BM, Bretscher MS. Membrane recycling by coated vesicles. Ann Rev Biochem 1981;50:85–101
36. Sherlock S, Dooley J. Cholestasis. In: Sherlock S, Dooley J. Eds. Diseases of the liver and biliary system. Blackwell Scientific Publication, Boston. 1993 pp 214–235
37. Krishnamurthy GT, Bobba VR, McConnell D, Turner F, Mesgardeh M, Kingston E. Quantitative biliary dynamics: introduction of a new non-invasive scintigraphic technique. J Nucl Med 1983;24:217–223
38. Brown PH, Krishnamurthy GT, Bobba VR, Kingston E. Radiation dose calculation for Tc-99m-HIDA in health and disease. J Nucl Med 1981;22:177–183
39. Bobba VR, Krishnamurthy GT, Kingston E, Turner FE, Brown PH, Langrell K. Gallbladder dynamics induced by a fatty meal in normal subjects and patients with gallstones: concise communication. J Nucl Med 1984;25:21–24
40. Mutt V. Cholecystokinin: isolation, structure, and function. In: Jerzy Glass GB. Ed. Gastrointestinal hormones. Raven Press, New York, 1980.pp 169–221
41. Krishnamurthy GT, Tubis M, Endow JS, Blahd WH. Technetium-99m-penicillamine. A new agent for cholescintigraphy. J Nucl Med 1972;13:418 (Abstract)
42. Tubis M, Krishnamurthy GT, Endow JS, Blahd WH. 99 m Tc-penicillamine, a new cholescintigraphic agent. Comparison with oral cholecystography. J Nucl Med 1972;13;652–654
43. Tonkin AK, DeLand FH, Tc-99m-Dihydrothioctic acid. A new polygonal cell imaging agent. J Nucl Med 1974;15: 539- ??
44. Fliegel CP, Dewanjee MK, Holman LB, Davis MA, Treves S. 99mTc-Tetracycline as a kidney and gallbladder imaging agent. Radiology 1974;110:407–412
45. Baker RJ, Bellen JC, Ronai PM. Tc-99m-pyridoxylidineglutamate: a new hepatobiliary radiopharmaceutical. 1. Experimental aspects. J Nucl Med 1975;16:720–727
46. Ronai PM, Baker RJ, Bellen JC, Collins PJ, Lander H. Technetium-99m-pyridoxylidineglutamate: a new hepatobiliary radiopharmaceutical. ll. Clinical aspects. J Nucl Med 1975;16:728–737
47. Hwang E, Taki J, Shuke N, Nakajima K, Kinuya S, Konishi S, Michigishi T, Aburano T, Tonami N. Preoperative assessment of residual hepatic functional reserve using Tc-99m-DTPA-galactosyl human serum albumin dynamic SPECT. 1999;40:1644–1651
48. Sasaki N, Shiomi S, Iwata Y, Nishiguchi S, Kuroki T, Kawabe J, Ochi H. Clinical usefulness of scintigraphy with Tc-99m-galactosyl human serum albumin for prognosis of cirrhosis of the liver 1999;40:1652–1656
49. UetakeM, Koizumi K, Yagawa A, Nogata H, Tezuka T, Kono H, Ozawa T, Kusano T, Miyabukuro M, Hosaka M. Use of Tc-99 m DTPA galactosyl human serum albumin to predict postoperative residual liver function. Clin Nucl Med 1999;24:428–434
50. Akaki S, Mitsumori A, Kanazawa S, Togami I, Takeda Y, Hiraki Y. Lobar decrease in 99m-Tc-GSA accumulation in hilar cholangiocarcinoma. J Nucl Med 1999;40:394–398
51. Brown, PH. Mathematics and statistics. In Bernier DR, Christian PE, Langan JK (eds), Nuclear Medicine, Technology and techniques. Mosby, St Louis 4th edition 1997, pp 1–35

3.2 Radiolabeling of Red Blood Cells and Leukocytes

Radiolabeled red blood cells are used in nuclear medicine mainly for the assessment of vascular spaces, for measurement of left ventricular volume and ejection fraction, and for localization of bleeding sites. Radiolabeled leukocytes are used primarily for the detection and localization of abscesses and delineation of sites of diffuse or focal infection. Major applications in nuclear hepatology include differentiation of hemangiomas from other focal liver lesions with ^{99m}Tc-labeled red blood cells, and differentiation of abscesses from other cystic liver lesions with indium-111 oxine or ^{99m}Tc-hexamethyl propyleneamine oxime (HMPAO)-labeled leukocytes.

Red Blood Cell Labeling with ^{99m}Tc

Technetium-99m-labeled red blood cells (RBCs) are used for blood pool imaging in the separation of vascular malformation (hemangiomas) from other non-vascular liver lesions. Radiolabeling of RBCs with chromium-51 was first accomplished by Gray and Sterling in 1950 for the main purpose of measuring their survival in the diagnosis of hemolytic anemias [1]. Technetium-99m-labeled RBCs are used primarily for blood pool imaging, and survival studies cannot be carried out due to the short physical half-life of Tc-99m of only 6 h [2]. Three methods of RBC labeling are available: an in vivo method, in vitro method, and a combined in vivo and in vitro method. The in vivo method is technically simple but results in a slightly higher background radiation. The in vitro method, on the other hand, is technically more involved but gives excellent lesion to non-lesion contrast due to low background radiation.

In Vitro Method

About 1 ml patient blood is drawn into a heparinized syringe and added to the mixing vial containing 50 µg stannous chloride, 3.7 mg sodium citrate, 5.5 mg dextrose, and 0.11 mg sodium chloride (Ultratag Kit, Mallinckrodt, St. Louis, Mo.). Stannous (2^+) chloride readily crosses the red cell membrane and attaches to the heme component of the hemoglobin molecule, ready to do its job of reducing the valence of ^{99m}Tc-pertechnetate from 7^+ to 4^+. About 0.6 ml 0.1% sodium hypochlorite is added later as an oxidizing agent which converts all the excess stannous chloride (2^+) into the stannic (4^+) state in plasma but not inside the RBC due to its inability to cross the intact red cell membrane. About 20–30 mCi $^{99m}TcO_4$ (pertechnetate) is added to the reaction vial. ^{99m}Tc-pertechnetate readily crosses the red cell membrane and attaches to the globin molecule after it has been reduced from a valence of 7^+ to 4^+ by the waiting stannous (2^+) chloride on the heme fraction of hemoglobin molecule. Once ^{99m}Tc is reduced from the 7^+ to the 4^+ valence state, it does not come out of the hemoglobin molecule. The entry of ^{99m}Tc through the red cell membrane thus becomes one-way traffic. After 15–20 min of gentle incubation at room temperature, most of the ^{99m}Tc is trapped inside the RBC [2]. The in vitro method is a very efficient labeling technique and does not necessitate blood centrifugation to remove plasma, because 97% of technetium-99m is associated with the RBC and less than 3% remains in plasma. Hemoglobin contains 95% of the total red cell radioactivity, of which 77% is associated with globin and the rest with the heme fraction of the hemoglobin molecule [3].

In Vivo Method

Stannous chloride (10–20 μg/kg) from a commercial pyrophosphate kit is injected intravenously. Tin (2^+) enters the red cell membrane and attaches to hemoglobin to be ready to act as a reducing agent when ^{99m}Tc-pertechnetate enters the cell. About 30 min later, 20–30 mCi ^{99m}Tc-pertechnetate in saline is injected intravenously. ^{99m}Tc-pertechnetate crosses the red cell membrane, is reduced by stannous chloride and later binds firmly to hemoglobin.

Combined In Vivo and In Vitro Method

Pre-tinning is accomplished first by intravenous injection of cold stannous pyrophosphate made for bone scanning. Fifteen to 20 min later, about 3–4 ml patient blood is drawn into a 50-ml volume syringe and 20–30 mCi ^{99m}Tc-pertechnetate is added to the syringe, shaken gently for 10 min and reinjected through the same catheter. Because of the higher efficiency of labeling and lower background, the in vitro method may be preferred over the in vivo method in the detection of hepatic hemangiomas (blood pool) and gastrointestinal bleeding [4, 5].

Leukocyte Labeling

Leukocytes labeled with either indium-111 oxine or ^{99m}Tc-HMPAO are used in nuclear hepatology for the diagnosis of liver abscess, empyema, or acute cholecystitis [6, 7].

Indium-111 Oxine

About 50–60 ml patient blood is drawn into a heparinized syringe and 10 ml 0.9% sodium chloride containing 6% hetastarch is added to blood and mixed thoroughly [8]. The mixture is allowed to sediment for 40 min. After the sedimentation, leukocyte rich plasma is collected, diluted with saline in a ratio of 2:1, and centrifuged at 150 *g* for 10 min. The leukocyte rich pellet is washed twice with 10 ml saline, and centrifuged each time for 10 min at 150 *g* after washing. Washed cells are then resuspended in 4.5 ml saline. About 0.3–0.5 ml indium-111 oxine containing 0.4–0.5 mCi (14.8–18.5 MBq) indium-111 is added to the reaction vial and incubated gently for 15 min at room temperature. Indium-111 oxine penetrates the leukocyte membrane and, once inside the cell, indium-111 and oxine dissociate. Oxine diffuses out of the cell into the labeling medium, leaving indium-111 behind trapped inside the cell [6]. The suspension is then centrifuged for 8 min at 90 *g* and the supernatant is discarded and the pellet containing labeled leukocytes is resuspended in platelet-poor plasma. About 6 ml of the suspension containing 0.3–0.4 mCi indium-111 leukocytes is injected intravenously. Indium-111-labeled leukocytes clear from blood with a $T_{1/2}$ of 6 h, which is very close to the value of 7 h for cells labeled with the "gold standard" ^{32}P-di-isopropylfluorophosphate. After labeling, each leukocyte receives approximately 1480 rad (14.8 Gy) radiation from Auger electrons of 0.6–25.4 keV energy from indium-111. This amount of radiation from its own source does not affect its function [8].

The major advantage of ^{111}In-oxine-labeled leukocytes over ^{67}Ga-citrate or ^{99m}Tc-HMPAO WBCs for imaging abscesses is that the entire abdomen, with the exception of the liver and spleen, remains free of any secreted radioactivity into the bowel [9]. Abdominal infection is diagnosed by taking early images at 2–10 min and repeat images within 30–60 min after injection. Delayed images at 24 h may be needed in some patients. In the case of chest infection, the earliest images that will provide any useful information are taken at 3–4 h after injection. Due to the usual margination of leukocytes in the lungs, early chest images are usually not diagnostic [10].

^{99m}Tc-HMPAO

The blood separation step for leukocyte labeling with ^{99m}Tc-HMPAO remains identical to that of labeling with ^{111}In-oxine described above. After separation, leukocytes are resuspended in 20% plasma/ACD solution. About 20–25 mCi ^{99m}Tc-HMPAO is added to the reaction vial and incubated gently for 10 min at room temperature, washed with plasma, and resuspended in plasma and reinjected. The labeling yield is between 50% and 60% with 80% activity bound to granulocytes [11]. The labeled leukocytes clear from blood with a $T_{1/2}$ of 4 h, which is slightly shorter than for ^{111}In-labeled granulocytes. The main advantage of ^{99m}Tc-HMPAO is that a much larger dose can be given yet the total body and organ radiation dose is much less. The agent is easily available at all times of need at a very reasonable cost. The main disadvantage is that free ^{99m}Tc-HMPAO, not bound to leukocytes, is taken up by the hepatocytes and secreted into bile. Intestinal luminal activity interferes with the diagnosis in images taken beyond 30 min after injection. A negative scan rules out abdominal infection. More and more studies in recent years are being done with ^{99m}Tc-HMPHO [11]. Interference from secreted bile radioactivity is avoided by taking abdominal images early, within 10–20 min after injection. The absorbed radiation dose from labeled red blood cells and leukocytes is shown in Table 3.2.1.

Table 3.2.1. Radiation absorbed dose from ^{99m}Tc-labeled RBCs and WBCs and indium-111-labeled WBCs

Organ	^{99m}Tc-RBCs (rad/mCi; Gy/37 MBq)	^{99m}Tc-WBCs (HMPAO) (rad/mCi; Gy/37 MBq)	^{111}In-WBCs (rads/mCi; Gy/37 MBq)
Liver	0.07	0.15	5.0
Spleen	0.05	0.22	40.0
Lungs	0.06	–	–
Kidneys	0.05	–	–
Ovaries	–	0.03	0.4
Testes	–	0.19	0.02
Bone marrow	0.03	0.16	4.0
Whole body	0.02	0.03	–

References

1. Gray SJ, Sterling K. The tagging of red blood cells and plasma proteins with radioactive chromium. J Clin Invest 1950;29:1604–1610
2. Srivastava SC, Chervu LR. Radionuclide-labeled red blood cells: current status and future prospects. Semin Nucl Med 1984;14:68–82
3. Srivastava SC, Strau RF. Blood cell labeling with 99mTc: Progress and perspectives. Semin Nucl Med 1990;20:41–51
4. Front D, Isreal O, Groshar D, Weininger J. Technetium-99 m labeled red blood cell imaging. Semin Nucl Med 1984;14:226–250
5. Birnbaum BA, Weinreb JC, Megibow AT, Sanger JJ, Lubat E, Kanamuller H, Noz ME, Bosniak MA. Definitive diagnosis of hepatic hemangioma: MR imaging VS Tc-99m-labeled red blood cell SPECT. Radiology 1990;176:95–101
6. Thakur ML, Segal AW, Louis L, Welch MJ, Peters TJ. Indium-111-labeled cellular blood components: mechanism of labeling, and intracellular location in human neutrophills. J Nucl Med 1977;18:1022–1026
7. Lantto EH, LanttoTJ, Vorne M. Fast diagnosis of abdominal infections and inflammations with Technetium-99 m -HMPAO labeled leukocytes. J Nucl Med 1991;32:2029–2034
8. Datz FL. In-111-labeled leukocytes for the detection of infection: current status. Semin Nucl Med 1994;24:92–109
9. Leddin DJ, Paterson WG, DaCosta LR, Dinda PK, Depew WT, Markotich J, McKaigney JP, Groll A, Beck IT. In-111 labeled autologous leukocyte imaging and fecal excretion. Comparison with conventional methods of assessment of inflammatory bowel disease. Dig Dis Sci 1987;32:377--387
10. McAfee JG. Editorial: What is the best method for imaging focal infections ?. J Nucl Med 1989;31:413–416
11. Allan RA, Sladen GE, Bassingham S, Lazarus C, Clarke SE, Fogelman I. Comparison of simultaneous 99mTc-HMPAO and 111-In oxine labeled white cell scans in the assessment of inflammatory bowel disease. Eur J Nucl Med 1993;20:195–200

3.3 Gallium-67-Citrate

The tumor detection capability of ^{67}Ga-citrate was described first by Edwards and Hays in 1969 [1]. Very soon it was recognized that in addition to the detection of varieties of tumors (lymphomas, hepatomas, malignant melanoma, and squamous cell carcinomas), Ga-67 was also taken up in high concentration by infectious lesions and abscesses. Benign conditions such as pseudonodules of cirrhosis and other non-specific inflammations do not concentrate the agent [2]. This differential uptake by benign versus malignant lesions and the ability to detect infection led to widespread clinical application of ^{67}Ga-citrate imaging in the 1970s and 1980s, before CT and ultrasound became popular imaging techniques for the detection of focal hepatic lesions. Gallium-67 imaging is reemerging primarily for determining the therapeutic response to various chemotherapeutic agents in various malignancies.

Pharmacokinetics

Gallium-67 is produced in an accelerator by bombarding a zinc target with protons as represented by the equation [^{67}Zn (p, n) ^{67}Ga]. It has a physical half-life of 78.3 h and decays by electron capture to stable zinc. It has three principle gamma photons with mean energies of 93.7 keV (36%), 185 keV (20%), and 300 keV (16.0%). Upon intravenous injection, ^{67}Ga-citrate is transported in blood bound to plasma proteins, mainly transferrin and to a minor extent to lactoferrin and ferritin. Two different mechanisms are involved with reference to cellular uptake: normal soft tissues concentrate gallium-67 bound to transferrin, whereas tumors concentrate the fraction that is either free or bound loosely to other proteins [3]. In the hepatocytes, Ga-67 uptake is seen mostly in association with lysosomes and mitochondria and to a lesser extent in the cytosol. The nucleus concentrates less than 10% of the total hepatocyte uptake. The exchange of gallium-67 takes place between the lysosomes and the cytosol. After intravenous injection, blood pool activity remains high for up to 24 h [4]. Beyond 48 h, most gallium-67 is cell bound. About 10% of injected activity is excreted in the stool during the 1st week.

Increased capillary permeability facilitates gallium-67 entry into the site of acute inflammation, abscess, or tumor. In the case of an abscess, gallium-67 is found in association with the leukocytes, siderophores, and bacteria. *Staphylococcus aureus*, *Escherichia* coli, and other microorganisms are shown to ingest gallium-67, accounting for high uptake by the abscess [5, 6].

Because of normal uptake by bone, and slow excretion by mucosa into colon, bone and lower large bowel receive the largest radiation dose from gallium-67: 18 mGy/37 MBq to bone marrow and 8.4 mGy/37 MBq to lower large bowel (Table 3.3.1). Currently, ^{67}Ga-citrate imaging has reemerged in the evaluation of chemotherapy for lymphomas.

Table 3.3.1. Radiation absorbed dose from gallium-67 citrate

Organ	mGy/37 MBq	rads/mCi
Marrow	18	1.8
Lower colon	8.4	0.84
Spleen	7.0	0.70
Liver	6.3	0.63
Upper colon	5.5	0.55
Kidneys	5.4	0.54
Ovaries	3.0	0.30
Testes	2.5	0.25
Whole body	2.6	0.26

Modified from MIRD pamphlet no. 11, 1975

References

1. Edward CL, Hayes RL: Tumor scanning with 67 Ga citrate. J Nucl Med 1969;10:103–105
2. Lomas F, Dibos PE, Wagner HN Jr. Increased specificity of liver scanning with the use of 67-Gallium citrate. New Engl J Med 1972;286:1323–1329
3. Tsan MF. Mechanism of Gallium-67 accumulation in inflammatory lesions. J Nucl Med 1985;26:88–92
4. Aulbert E, Gebherdt A, Schutz E, Haubold U. Mechanism of Gallium-67 accumulation in normal rat liver lysosomes. Nuklearmedizin (Stuttg) 1976;15:185–194
5. Hammersley PA, Taylor DM, Cronshaw S. The mechanism of 67 Ga uptake in animal and human tumors. Eur J Nucl Med 1980;5:411–415
6. Scheffel U, Wagner HN Jr, Klein JL, Tsan MF. Gallium-67 uptake by hepatoma: studies in cell cultures, perfused livers and intact rats. J Nucl Med 1985;26:1438–1444

3.4 Somatostatin Receptor Imaging Agent

Somatostatin is a small peptide found in many normal tissues, and benign and malignant tumors. It was thought originally to regulate primarily the release of growth hormone [1]. Now it is evident that in addition to influencing growth hormone release, somatostatin regulates the release of cyclic neuropeptides and inhibits release of thyrotropin, insulin, glucagon, gastrin, secretin, and cholecystokinin [2]. The somatostatin receptors are present in the brain, thyroid, lung, gastrointestinal tract, liver, gallbladder, pancreas, adrenals, and activated leukocytes [3]. Two molecular forms of somatostatin are identified; one consists of 14 (Fig. 3.4.1) and the other 28 amino acids in the molecule. The longer one with 28 amino acids is a dimer formed by the union of two shorter molecules. The serum half-life of somatostatin is less than 3 min. Five subtypes of somatostatin receptors are recognized in the body. Both somatostatin 14 and 28 attach to all five subtypes with equal affinity. Octreotide is an analog of somatostatin with eight amino acids (octapeptide). It binds mainly to somatostatin receptor subtypes 2, 3 and 5 but not to subtypes 1 and 4 [3, 4].

Indium-111 Pentetreotide (OctreoScan)

Radiolabeled octreotide binds to somatostatin receptors on the surface of tumors enabling their detection [5]. Radiolabeling is achieved with either iodine-123 or indium-111. When iodine-123 is chosen, the amino acid tyrosine, a normal component of the analogue, is radiolabeled [6]. In the case of indium-111, a bifunctional chelate,

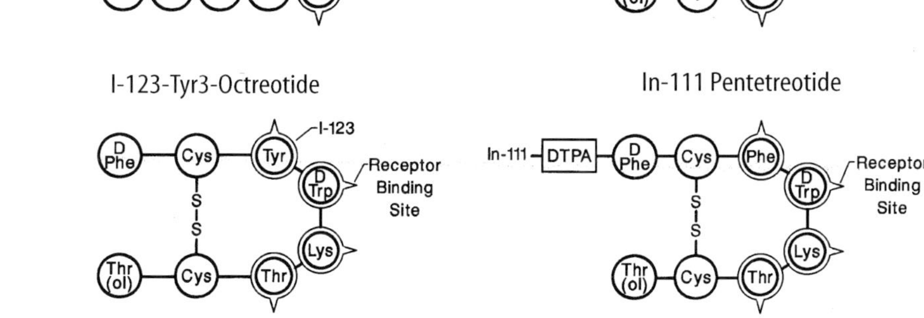

Fig. 3.4.1. Molecular structure of somatostatin and its radiolabeled analogues. Somatostatin consists of 14 amino acids. The receptor binding sites are located on four sequentially arranged amino acids. In labeled octreotide, radioiodine, iodine-123, attaches directly to tyrosine (*Tyr*), whereas indium-111 requires DTPA as chelate for its attachment

diethylenetriaminepentaacetic acid (DTPA) is required for radiolabeling (Fig. 3.4.1). As a bifunctional chelate, DTPA attaches to indium-111 (radiotracer) with one arm and to the amino acid, D-phenylalanine of somatostatin analogue (ligand), with the other arm. Four amino acids (phenylalanine, tryptophan, lysine, and threonine) arranged in a sequence provide the binding site for the radiolabeled analogue [7].

Following intravenous administration, ^{111}In-pentetreotide clears from blood rapidly. About 33% of the administered dose remains in circulation at the end of 10 min. Kidneys are the major route of excretion. About 50% of the injected dose is excreted in urine in 6 h, 85% in 24 h, and 90% in 48 h. Less than 2% of the dose is excreted in feces in 3 days. Stool radioactivity mostly represents biliary excretion. Kidneys are the target organs for radiation. About 7% of the dose accumulates in the kidneys by 4 h [8]. The recommended dose for scanning is 3 mCi for planar and 6 mCi for a SPECT study. Clinical studies usually require a SPECT study necessitating a 6 mCi (222 MBq) dose routinely [9]. Radiation to various organs from a diagnostic dose depends both upon the age and dose. Kidneys, spleen, and urinary bladder receive the largest radiation [10].

References

1. Krulich L, Dhariwal AP, McCann SM. Stimulatory and inhibitory effects of purified hypothalamic extract on growth hormone release from rat pituitary in-vitro. Endocrinology 1968;83:783–790
2. Reichlin S. Somatostatin. New Engl J Med 1983;309:1495–1501
3. Reubi JC, Kvols LK, Krenning E, Lamberts SWJ. Distribution of somatostatin receptors in normal and tumor tissue. Metabolism 1990;39:78–81 (suppl 2)
4. Lamberts SWJ, van der Lely AJ, deHerder WW, Hofland LJ. Octreotide. New Engl J Med 1996;334:246–254
5. Krenning EP, Bakker WH, Breeman WAP, Koper JW, Kooji PP, Ausema L, Lameris JS, Reubi JC, Lamberts SWJ. Localization of endocrine-related tumors with radioiodinated analog of somatostatin. Lancet 1989;1:242–244
6. O'Connor ML, Kvols LK, Brown ML, Hung JC, Hayostek RJ, Cho DS, Vetter RJ. Dosimetry and biodistribution of an I-123-labeled somatostatin analog in patients with neuroendocrine tumors. J Nucl Med 1992;33:1613–1619
7. Krenning EP, Bakker WH, Kooji PPM, Breeman WAP, Oei HY, deJong M, Reubi JC, Visser TJ, Bruns C, Kwekkeboom DJ, Reijs AEM, van Hagen PM, Koper JW, Lamberts SWJ. Somatostatin receptor scintigraphy with indium-111 DTPA-D-phe-1-octreotide in man: metabolism, dosimetry and comparison with iodine-123-Tyr-3 octreotide. J Nucl Med 1992;33:652–658
8. Somatostatin receptor imaging for neuroendocrine tumors. Product monograph. OctreoScan Mallinckrodt Medical Inc., St. Louis, MO, 1994
9. Jamar F, Fiasse R, Leners N, Pauwels S. Somastostatin receptor imaging with indium-111-pentetreotide in gastroenteropancreatic neuroendocrine tumors: safety, efficacy, and impact on patient management. J Nucl Med 1995;36:542–549
10. Stabin MG, Kooji PPM, Bakker WH, Inoue T, Endo K, Coveney J, deJong R, Minegishi A. Radiation dosimetry for Indium-111-pentetreotide. J Nucl Med 1997;38:1919–1922

Imaging of the Liver and Spleen Morphology

In most nuclear medicine departments throughout the world, gamma cameras have completely replaced rectilinear scanners. A large field of view gamma camera, single or dual head, fitted with a low energy, parallel hole, all purpose collimator is generally chosen for most planar studies using technetium-99m-labeled agents. The main advantage of the dual head gamma camera is patient convenience, where the data collection time is reduced by one-half as it allows simultaneous anterior and posterior image acquisition. The reduction in time often improves the spatial resolution due to less patient movement during the short acquisition interval. The triple head gamma camera, when available, is preferred for single photon emission computed tomography (SPECT) images. The gamma camera image acquisition parameters are identical for both the liver and spleen.

4.1 Imaging with Radiocolloid

Patient Preparation

In general, there is no special patient preparation required for morphology imaging with radiocolloid. This is a distinct advantage over functional imaging with ^{99m}Tc-HIDA, where the patient preparation requirements are quite stringent. The morphology imaging studies obtained immediately after a full meal may cause image artifacts and obscure the spleen in the anterior view due to photon attenuation by the gastric contents. The posterior and left lateral views usually clarify this situation.

Radiocolloid imaging introduced in the early 1950s with the use of rectilinear scanners marked the birth of nuclear hepatology. Morphology imaging with radiocolloid remained very popular until the early 1980s, when it was taken over by CT and ultrasound. Diagnosis of various diseases is made from assessing the changes in image pattern of the organ morphology. A thorough knowledge of normal morphology of liver and spleen and normal variant patterns is critical to be able to detect disease. This section deals mainly with liver and spleen morphology as seen on a radiocolloid image.

Normal Liver

Perfusion

Liver and spleen perfusion images are obtained either in the anterior or posterior view using ^{99m}Tc in any form. The aorta is the first abdominal organ to be seen, followed by the spleen, kidneys, and liver (Fig. 4.1.1). Aorta to spleen transit time is 2–4 s and aorta to kidney transit time is 3–6 s. Despite the fact that both the hepatic artery and the splenic artery arise from a common celiac artery, there is an apparent delay in appearance of liver perfusion due to dilution of hepatic artery radioactivity by the still non-radioactive portal venous blood. The portal vein receives its radioactivity much later than the hepatic and splenic arteries. The delay in arrival of the portal vein radioactivity is due to the delay in the intestinal capillary phase. The liver receives 25% of its blood supply through the hepatic artery and 75% through the portal vein. The liver portal perfusion is clearly seen 10–14 s after the appearance of the abdominal aorta [1].

Table 4.1.1. Data acquisition with ^{99m}Tc-sulfur colloid

Instrument	Single, dual, or a triple head, large field of view gamma camera
Collimator	Low energy, parallel hole, all purpose collimator
Agent	^{99m}Tc-Sulfur colloid, or ^{99m}Tc-albumin colloid
Dose	Adults, 2–4 mCi (74–148 MBq) for planar images, 4–10 mCi (148–370 MBq) for perfusion or SPECT images. Children, 30–50 µCi/kg (minimum 300 µCi)
Spectrometer setting	140 keV photopeak at 15–20% window
Perfusion images	At 1 or 2 s/frame for 60 s
Planar image data collection	500,000 to 1,000,000 counts for each of anterior, posterior, and two lateral views. Additional views are obtained as needed. A 5- or 10-cm-long lead marker is placed along the right costal margin to facilitate measurement of liver size and position. The same marker is used for measurement of spleen size using the posterior image.
SPECT data collection	Matrix 64×64 word or 128×128 word mode. Rotation, clockwise 360°, angle 3–6° for each stop (360/64=6°)
Filters	Depends upon the computer and gamma camera
Views	Transaxial, coronal, and sagittal

Perfusion images are obtained immediately after the injection of the radiotracer at 1 or 2 s/frame for 60 s using the setup for the planar mode described above and reformatted at 4–8 s/image for clinical interpretation. The planar and SPECT image data are collected 15–30 min after intravenous injection when all of the radiocolloid particles from blood are extracted by the RE cells

Shape, Surface, and Borders

There are wide variations in the shape of a normal liver and most of the variations occur along the superior and inferior margins [2, 3]. The most common shape of a normal liver is that of an approximate triangle consisting of a superior, inferior, and right lateral border (Fig. 4.1.2). Superior and right lateral borders form a smooth rounded contour at the right upper quadrant. The superior and inferior borders meet at an acute angle at the left tip of the left hepatic lobe. The inferior and right lateral borders meet at various angles. Often the inferior tip of the right hepatic lobe is elongated, forming a Riedel's lobe. The superior border of the liver is "S" shaped and the contour is influenced by the size of the heart, the exit of the hepatic vein, and the elevation of the dome of the right hemidiaphragm. The shape that appears like a Gendarme's hat is primarily due to the elevation of the right hemidiaphragm.

The contour of the inferior border is affected by the fossa for the gallbladder and the entrance of the structures at the porta hepatis. The gallbladder fossa is usually located

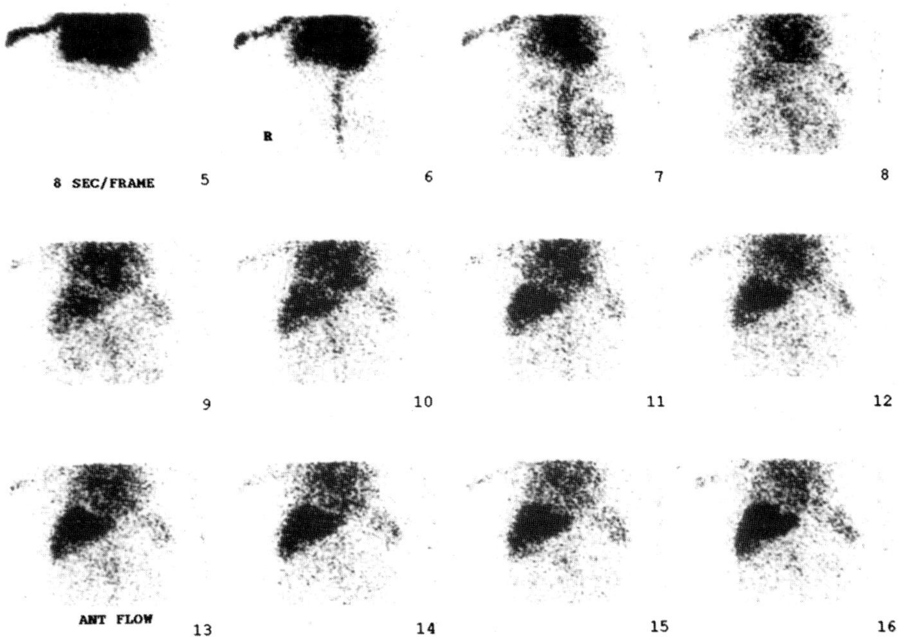

Fig. 4.1.1. Liver perfusion. Anterior perfusion image shows abdominal aorta *(#6 frame)*, followed by spleen and kidneys (*#7*). Liver appears faintly in the beginning (*#8*), representing hepatic artery perfusion, and becomes more clear in late images (#9) after the arrival of portal venous blood.

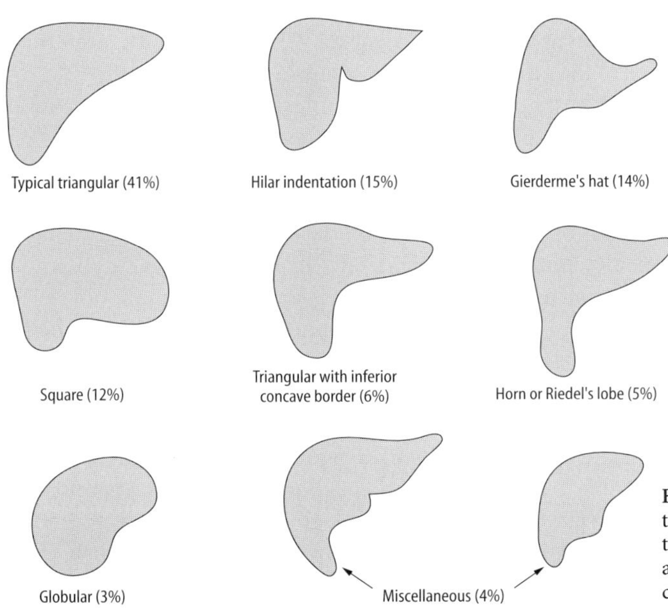

Fig. 4.1.2. Normal variations in liver shape and their frequency (%). Triangular shape is the most common type [2–4]

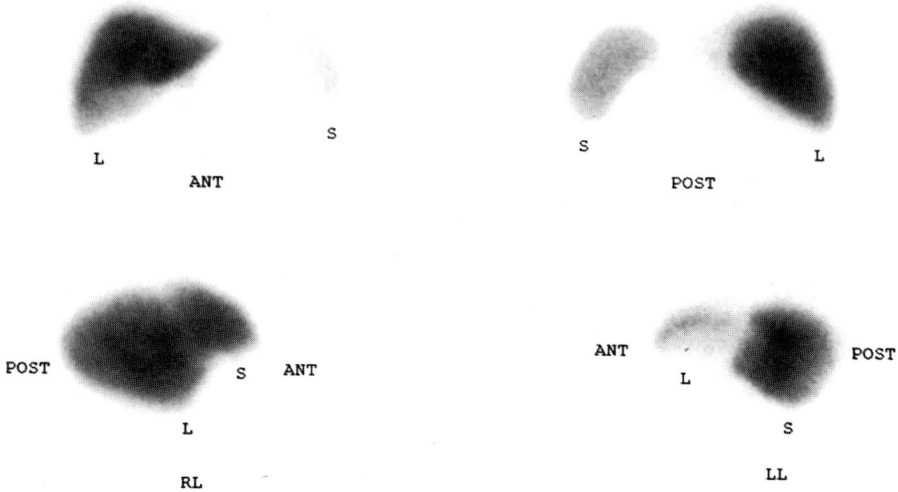

Fig. 4.1.3. Planar image. The liver (*L*) is seen clearly, and the spleen (*s*) faintly in an anterior (*ANT*) view. The spleen may project anterior to the liver in the right lateral (*RL*) view. In the left lateral (*LL*) view, the spleen appears clearly with the left lobe of the liver (*L*) projecting faintly anterior to it

at the junction of the lateral one-third with the medial two-thirds of the inferior border (Fig. 4.1.3). The position of the gallbladder can be marked during physical examination by drawing a straight line between the left anterior superior iliac spine and the umbilicus and extending it superiorly to meet the right costal margin. The position of the fundus of the gallbladder corresponds to the point where this line meets the right costal margin. The gallbladder can be situated anywhere along the inferior liver border and may be even intrahepatic. Intrahepatic gallbladders cause a "cold" filling defect in a radiocolloid scan and appear as a focal "hot" area in a ^{99m}Tc-HIDA study. Alteration in liver shape is usually due to the effect of extrinsic compression. The anterior and right lateral surfaces are smooth in outline whereas the inferior surface has grooves and fissures for the entrance and exit of vessels and ducts, respectively.

Lobes

The liver can be divided into right and left lobes on the basis of either morphology or physiology. The line of attachment of the falciform ligament marks the boundary between the morphologic right and left lobes. The division of the liver into physiologic right and left lobes is based on embryologic development of the bile ducts, hepatic artery, and portal vein. The line of physiologic division runs between the fossa for the gallbladder in the front to the deep fissure for the inferior vena cava in the back. The point of entrance of the porta hepatis also indicates the boundary between the physiologic right and left lobes. The line of physiologic division (porta hepatis) is situated on the right side of the anatomic line of division (falciform ligament). Therefore, the physiologic left lobe is much larger than the morphologic left lobe. In the anterior view, the line of attachment of the falciform ligament is shown by a slight decrease in counts due to photon attenuation.

The anterior view usually shows the entire liver and inferior part of the spleen. In the posterior view, the liver appears triangular in shape with a rounded superolateral corner. The posterior border in the right lateral view often shows an impression due to the right kidney. A wide vertical photopenic area between the right and left lobes is due to absorption of photons by the dense thoracic vertebrae (Fig. 4.1.3). Normally the uptake of the radiocolloid by the reticuloendothelial (RE) cells of the vertebral body is seen very faintly. The caudate lobe is situated posteriorly along the superior border but is not usually seen in the planar posterior image mainly due to absorption of photons by the vertebrae.

Dimensions of the Normal Liver and Spleen

The size of the liver is measured usually in the anterior view image and the size of the spleen in the posterior view (Fig. 4.1.4). A calibrated radioactive marker placed along the costal margin during data acquisition enables measurement of the organ size. The size is measured more accurately using the pixel number when images are recorded on the computer matrix. The position of the liver is assessed with reference to the right costal margin. A normal liver is situated above the right costal margin and the normal spleen above the left costal margin. The right lobe of the liver measures 10.0–15.5 cm in the right midclavicular line. The maximum vertical height from superior to inferior border of the right lobe is 10--20 cm. The horizontal length from the right lateral border to the tip of the left lobe is 14–24 cm [4, 5]. Because of wide variations in shape

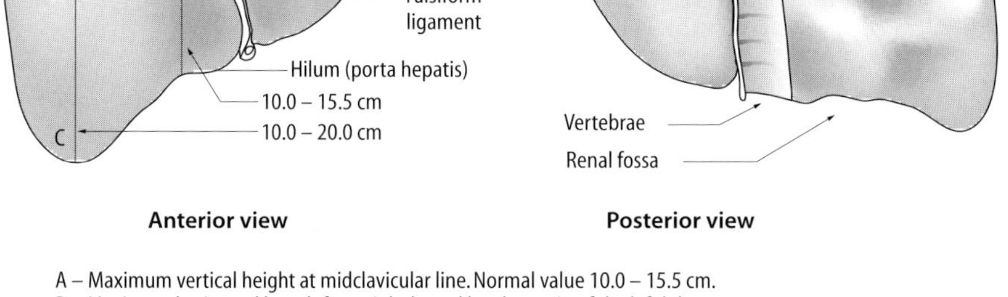

Fig. 4.1.4. Dimensions of the normal liver and spleen. In the anterior view, the right lobe measures 10.0–15.5 cm in the midclavicular line (*A*) and 10.0–20.0 cm from the dome to the inferior tip (*C*). The horizontal length from right lateral border to the tip of the left lobe ranges from 14.0 to 24.0 cm (*B*). In the posterior view, the upper limit of the normal spleen is 10.5 cm along the posterior oblique axis

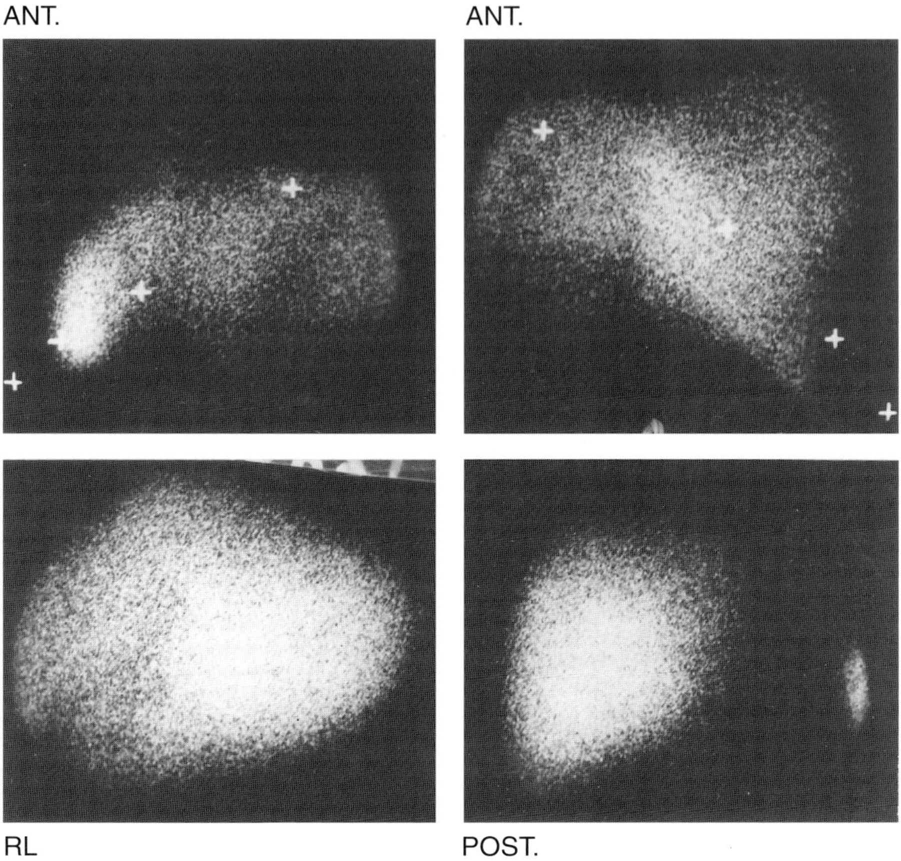

Fig. 4.1.5. Situs inversus. In the anterior (*ANT*) view, the spleen is located on the right and liver on the left side of the body. In the right lateral (*RL*) view, the spleen is superimposed at the posteroinferior part of the liver. Posterior (*POST*) view shows liver on the left and spleen (part of the spleen) on the right, separated by photon absorption by the vertebral bodies

at the tips, dimensions that include the tips tend to be less accurate as a measure of overall liver size. The measurement along the right midclavicular line serves a better reference point for estimating true liver size than measurements along other lines. For accurate measurement of the spleen size, an oblique line is drawn from superior to inferior tip using a posterior view image. The upper limit of the normal spleen is about 10.5 cm along this oblique axis [6]. The position of the liver and spleen are reversed in patients with situs inversus. (Fig. 4.1.5)

Pattern of Radiocolloid Uptake

A normal liver weighs 1500–1800 g and the spleen 150–200 g. The bone marrow is estimated to weigh about 1500 g [7]. The liver takes up about 90% of radiogold colloid (^{198}Au) and 85% of ^{99m}Tc-sulfur colloid. The spleen concentrates 3% of ^{198}Au-colloid and 7% of ^{99m}Tc-sulfur colloid. Bone marrow takes up about 7% of ^{198}Au-colloid and 5% of ^{99m}Tc-sulfur colloid (Chap. 3, Table 3.1.5). The differences in radiocolloid uptake among these three organs is a function of their overall size and the physicochemical nature of the radiocolloid particles [8]. The smallest particles are preferentially taken up by the bone marrow, medium size particles by the liver, and the largest particles by the spleen. As the liver disease progresses, there is shift in radiocolloid uptake from liver to the spleen and bone marrow. In moderate degree cirrhosis, radiocolloid uptake by the liver decreases (65–70%) and the uptake by the spleen and bone marrow increases. There is also more uptake by lung and other organs. In advanced cirrhosis, liver uptake may be as low as 30–35%. The spleen and bone marrow continue to show an increase in uptake of radiocolloid to as high as 25–30% of the dose by each organ. The remaining 10–12% of the injected radiocolloid dose is taken up by activated RE cells in lungs and other organs.

Spleen and Bone Marrow Uptake

In the posterior view, the intensity of radiocolloid uptake by a normal spleen is usually equal to that of the normal liver [9]. In cirrhosis, the intensity of splenic uptake increases in direct proportion to the degree of portal hypertension. In advanced cirrhosis, the intensity of spleen and bone marrow radiocolloid uptake often exceeds that of the liver. The intensity of thoracic and lumbar vertebral body radiocolloid uptake by the RE cells may match that of ^{99m}Tc-methylene diphosphate (MDP) uptake by the bone mineral matrix. Decreased radiocolloid uptake by the spleen is also abnormal and often is noticed in patients with Hodgkin's disease, reticulum cell sarcoma, poorly differentiated lymphocytic lymphoma, mycosis fungoides, or other types of lymphomas. In polycythemia rubra vera, the normal spleen/liver ratio is maintained despite an enormous increase in the size of the spleen.

The liver moves 1–3 cm up and down with each respiration. The size of the liver, therefore, may falsely appear large if the patient breathes deeply during scanning. When the liver enlarges and extends below the right costal margin, the radiocolloid uptake in the liver tissue extending below the right costal margin may appear greater than the tissue uptake behind the costal margin. This apparent effect is due to attenuation of photons by the ribs, and the right breast exaggerates the difference in women. The effect of extrinsic compression on the liver is ascertained by taking one image during deep inspiration and another during deep expiration. An intrinsic liver defect will not change its position, whereas a defect due to extrinsic compression moves with respiration [10]. Decreased radiocolloid uptake by the liver and increased uptake by the spleen, lungs, and other soft tissues are indicators of poor prognosis [11, 12]. Fatty infiltration of the liver causes irregular uptake of radiocolloid and accumulation of xenon-133 by the liver noticed serendipitously during a V/Q study obtained for the diagnosis of pulmonary embolism.

Appearance of the Normal Liver and Spleen on SPECT Images

Increased spatial resolution and high lesion to non-lesion contrast on SPECT show some of the normal structures much more prominently than in a planar image. Often such normal structures are misinterpreted as cold lesions in a radiocolloid scan or as hot lesions on a blood pool or ^{99m}Tc-HIDA study. The right and left branches of the portal vein, hepatic artery, and bile ducts pass through the middle of the liver in the opposite direction, 180° apart. The coronal, sagittal, and transaxial slices passing through these structures may depict these normal structures as cold or hot lesions depending upon the radiolabel used for the study. A cold lesion on a radiocolloid scan that fills in with ^{99m}Tc-red blood cells (RBCs) suggests a vessel or a hemangioma. A cold lesion that fills in with ^{99m}Tc-HIDA suggests a biliary origin (choledochal cyst). In the sagittal slice passing through the middle of the right lobe, the right portal vein may appear as a curvilinear defect in the radiocolloid scan. Sagittal slices over the lateral aspect of the right lobe show a linear defect which is usually due to the posterior branch of the right portal vein. The anterior branch of the right portal vein is slightly smaller and is not always evident on sagittal slices. These anatomical variants may not be evident in the planar images due to overlying or underlying liver tissue. The right and left portal veins and the right posterior segmental vein are 1.5–2 cm in diameter, large enough to be seen on the SPECT images as defects (Fig. 4.1.6). The medial and lateral segmental veins of the left lobe are too small to cause a defect [13]. Two or three of the most anterior coronal slices may show only the left lobe, confirming its more anterior location. Lower transaxial slices show the gallbladder fossa as a pear shaped defect along the anterior margin.

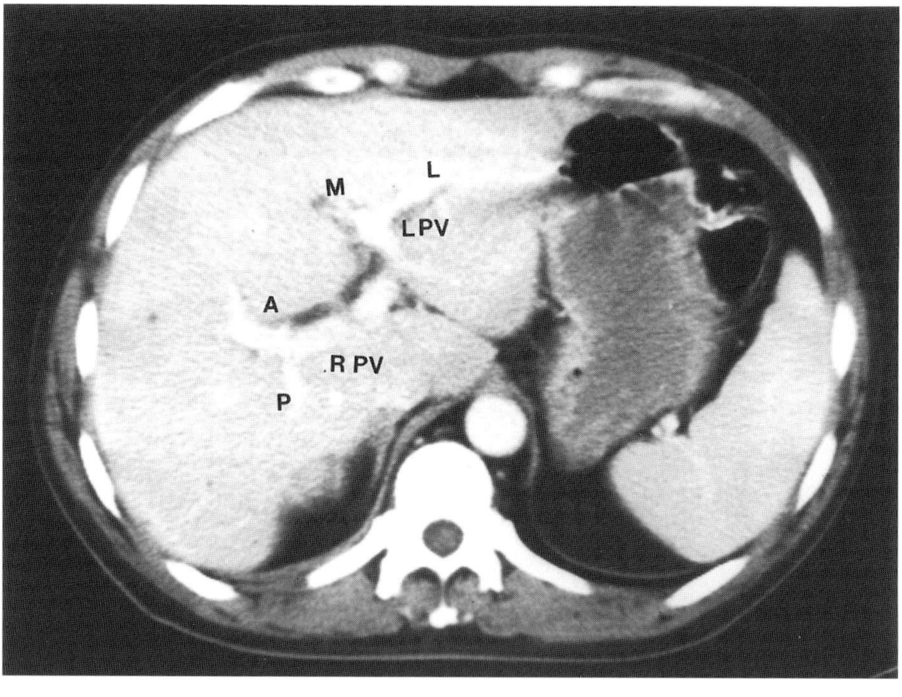

Fig. 4.1.6. Portal vein. Transaxial CT shows division of the portal vein in the middle of the liver into right portal vein (*RPV*) and left portal vein (*LPV*) branches. LPV divides into medial (*M*) and lateral (*L*), and RPV into anterior (*A*) and posterior (*P*), segmental branches

Abnormal Liver

Hepatomegaly

A general response of the liver to any type of injury is one of diffuse enlargement. Hepatomegaly usually disappears when the offending agent is removed. Metabolic diseases in children are generally associated with hepatomegaly (Table 4.1.2). The inferior border of most normal size livers does not extend below the right costal margin. In patients with chronic obstructive lung disease the liver may be pushed downwards to be palpable below the right costal margin. It is important to establish whether a clinically palpable liver is due to displacement or enlargement.

The space occupying lesions of the liver can be divided into four categories: (1) marginal lesions, (2) intrahepatic solitary focal lesions, (3) intrahepatic multiple focal lesions, and (4) intrahepatic diffuse lesions (Table 4.1.3).

Table 4.1.2. Causes of hepatomegaly

Common causes	Uncommon causes	Rare causes
1. Hepatitis	1. Hepatoma	1. Glycogen storage disease
2. Fatty infiltration	2. Hemochromatosis	2. Gaucher's disease
3. Cirrhosis	3. Granuloma	3. Cystic fibrosis
4. Metastatic tumors	4. Drug induced hepatitis	4. Galactosemia
5. Congestive heart failure	5. Wilson's disease	5. Kwashiorkor
6. Leukemia	6. Infections	6. Budd-Chiari syndrome
7. Lymphoma	7. Hemangioendothelioma	7. Amyloidosis
8. Abscess	8. Polycystic disease	8. Gangliosidosis
9. Biliary obstruction	9. Cholangiocarcinoma	

Table 4.1.3. Space occupying lesions of the liver

Marginal lesions	Intraparenchymal lesions		
(compression by adjacent organs)	Single focal	Multiple focal	Diffuse
Right kidney (hypernephroma)	Hepatoma	Metastasis	Hepatitis
Enlarged gallbladder	Abscess	Polycystic disease	Cirrhosis
Pancreatic carcinoma, pseudocyst	Adenoma	Fatty infiltration	Fatty infiltration
Intracapsular hematoma	Hemangioma	Hemangioma	Wilson's disease
Choledochal cyst	FNH	Multiple metastases	Lymphoma
Colon mass in hepatic flexure	Metastasis	Multicystic disease	Chemotoxins
Right costal margin	Simple cyst	Hydatid cyst	Hemochromatosis
Prominent porta hepatis	Hydatid cyst	Amebic abscess	Sclerosing cholangitis
Ascites	Infarction		Biliary cirrhosis
Right breast	Intrahepatic GB		
Enlarged heart	Pseudotumor		
Bile leak into GB fossa			

FNH, focal nodular hyperplasia

Marginal Lesions

Most marginal lesions are caused by compression of the liver margin by adjoining normal organs or lesions arising from them. A normal right kidney placed high in the posterior abdomen or a mass arising from it (hypernephroma) may cause a defect along the posterior border of the right lobe of the liver. Such lesions are seen as a focal defect in the posterior planar view or as a concave posterior border in the planar right lateral view. In a SPECT image it may appear as a round defect in the posterior slices of the coronal view and in the mid and lower slices of the transaxial views. A fully filled gallbladder may cause a cold defect in a radiocolloid scan along the inferior border in the anterior planar image. The gallbladder fossa appears as a pear shaped defect along the anterior border in the right lateral planar image. A large choledochal cyst arising from the common bile duct may compress the middle of the inferior liver margin, causing a cold defect near the porta hepatis in a radiocolloid scan.

A normal stomach after a full meal or a mass arising from the stomach or pancreas (pseudocyst, cancer) may cause a defect along the inferior border of the left lobe. Depressed right lateral ribs or a hematoma following an auto accident may cause a defect along the lateral surface of the right lobe. A lesion arising from the hepatic flexure of the colon may cause compression along the inferior liver margin of the right lobe. Post-traumatic subcapsular hematomas cause defects along any surface depending upon the point of impact, but most tend to occur along the right lateral or the anterior surface [14]. A large pendulous right breast or a breast prosthesis causes a concave defect along the superior border which may be misinterpreted as a filling defect or as hypoconcentration of radiocolloid. Breast artifact is corrected by taking a repeat image after lifting the pendulous breast or removing the prosthesis (Fig. 4.1.7). An enlarged heart due to congestive heart failure or cardiomyopathy causes an impression along the superior margin at the junction of the right and left lobes.

Marginal lesions of the spleen are seen mostly along the medial (hilum) or the lateral surface. Lateral surface lesions are mostly hematomas secondary to trauma due to auto accidents. Medial surface lesions are due to a large pancreatic pseudocyst, choledochal cyst, or postprandial fluid filled stomach. Most post-traumatic hematomas along the lateral surface resolve in 3–4 weeks [14].

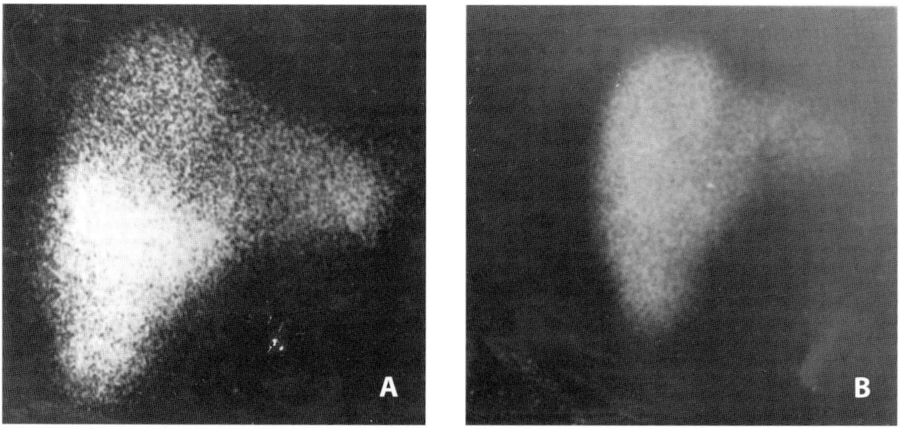

Fig. 4.1.7. Liver artifact. A large defect over the superior part of the right lobe caused by a breast prosthesis (**A**) disappears in the repeat image after its removal (**B**)

Intrahepatic Solitary Focal Lesions

These are the most common type of liver lesions seen when scintigraphy is obtained early in the course of liver disease. They tend to be associated with normal or mildly abnormal liver function tests. Most focal liver lesions appear as round. Infarction appears as wedge shaped and radiation necrosis causes a characteristic appearance (quadrangular) depending upon radiation port. A thorough knowledge of the mode of clinical presentation, clinical findings, and changes in liver function tests is necessary to arrive at an etiological diagnosis. This is true for all types of liver imaging procedures including radiocolloid scan, computerized tomography, ultrasound, or magnetic resonance imaging. No single imaging test or even a combination of imaging tests is capable of making an etiological diagnosis all of the time [15–18].

Intrahepatic Multiple Focal Lesions

Multiple metastases, polycystic or multicystic liver disease, and fatty infiltration are examples of multiple intrahepatic focal lesions. Multiple metastatic lesions are the most common (Fig. 4.1.8). In a patient with a known primary cancer elsewhere, multiple liver lesions are considered secondary until proven otherwise. Polycystic liver disease is associated with cysts in the kidney, spleen, and other organs and has an autosomal dominance pattern of inheritance. Fatty infiltration may cause focal or diffuse defects. On ultrasound, fatty infiltration appears as a hypoechoic mass with angulation and interdigitating margins [19]. Liver with fatty infiltration shows xenon-133 retention after a lung ventilation study obtained to rule out pulmonary embolism. Xenon-133 retention by the liver is specific for fatty infiltration [20].

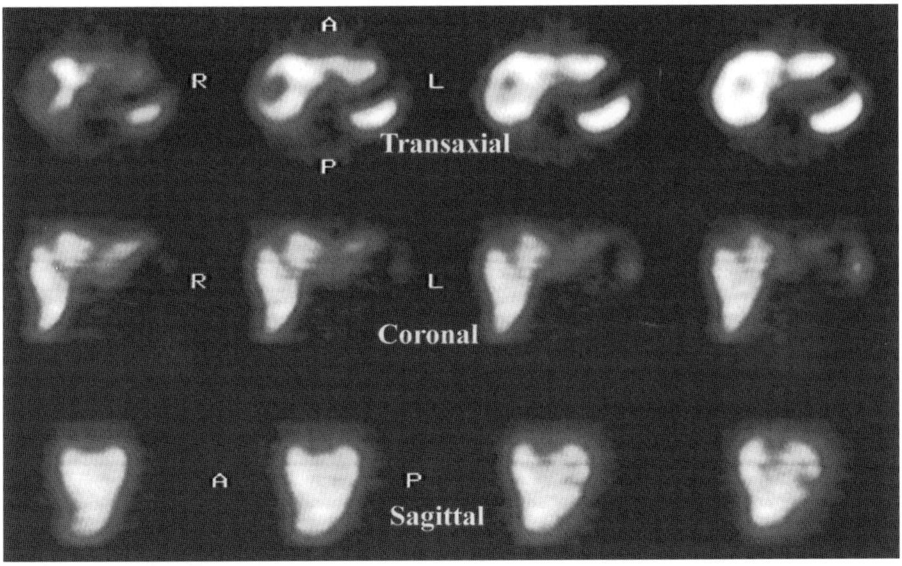

Fig. 4.1.8. Multiple metastatic liver disease. Transaxial, coronal, and sagittal SPECT images with radiocolloid show multiple intrahepatic metastasis from colon cancer. (Courtesy of Dr. Kumaresan, Hyderabad, India)

Intrahepatic Multiple Diffuse Lesions

Alcoholic hepatitis, viral hepatitis, and cirrhosis are the most common causes followed by other rare diseases, such as hemochromatosis, Wilson's disease, primary biliary cirrhosis, primary sclerosing cholangitis, and drugs (chemotherapy) or toxin induced hepatitis. Many of these diseases are associated with a changing image pattern, depending upon the phase of parenchymal liver disease. Viral and alcoholic hepatitis often heal completely when the offending agent is removed completely. Defects due to chemotherapy usually disappear after the completion of the course. The role of radiocolloid imaging in the detection of liver lesions has diminished recently and has been replaced by CT and ultrasound, which have better spatial resolution and provide additional information about structural changes in organs around the liver [21, 22]. Radiocolloid imaging is now requested mostly to clarify an abnormality already seen with the CT or ultrasound study to confirm whether the lesion is hepatic in origin. The posterior view image shows all three organs that take up radiocolloid, the liver, spleen, and bone marrow in the thoracic and lumbar vertebral bodies, and provides information related to their relative function. Bone marrow replacement by a tumor causes a "cold" defect in the vertebra in a radiocolloid image and a "hot' lesion in a ^{99m}Tc-MDP image at the corresponding site (Fig. 4.1.9).

Relative Merits of the Diagnostic Tests

The positive predictive and negative predictive values are similar for CT, ultrasound, and radiocolloid scan. The sensitivities of CT and radiocolloid scan are similar, but is slightly lower for ultrasound (Table 4.1.4). Any one of the three imaging modalities is capable of detecting a solitary liver lesion, but the choice of one over another depends upon local expertise, availability, reproducibility, and cost [22]. Because CT and ultrasound studies provide additional information about nearby organs, they have become clinically popular and have almost completely replaced radiocolloid scans for liver

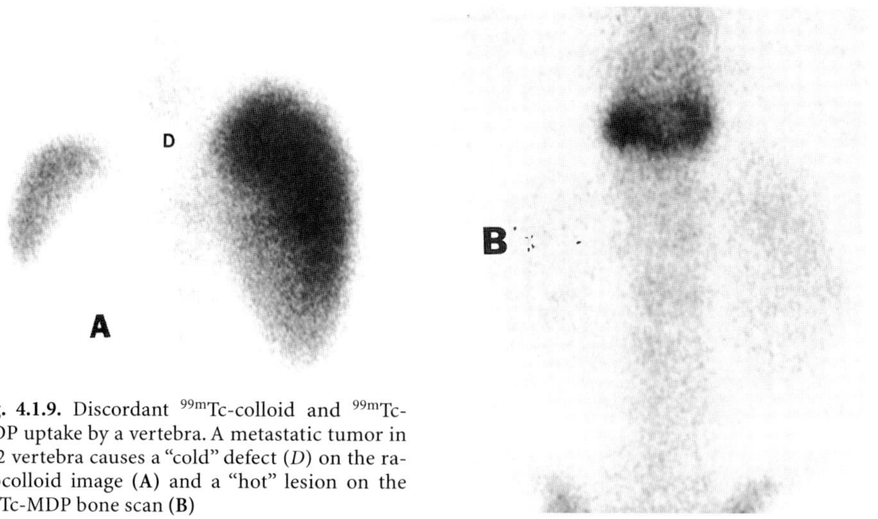

Fig. 4.1.9. Discordant ^{99m}Tc-colloid and ^{99m}Tc-MDP uptake by a vertebra. A metastatic tumor in T12 vertebra causes a "cold" defect (*D*) on the radiocolloid image (**A**) and a "hot" lesion on the ^{99m}Tc-MDP bone scan (**B**)

imaging today. Once a lesion is detected by one imaging modality, incremental information from the second or third imaging test is not substantial enough to justify obtaining more than one morphologic imaging procedure. This factor is observed more critically by insurance companies and other third party payers than by physicians and patients. The information obtained from a combination of one morphology and one physiologic imaging may be better for patient management than the information gathered from a combination of two or more morphological imaging procedures.

Table 4.1.4. Sensitivity, specificity, positive predictive and negative predictive value of radiocolloid scan (RN), CT, and ultrasound (US) studies in the detection of space occupying lesions of the liver

No. of patients	Sensitivity RN	CT	US	Specificity RN	CT	US	+ predictive value RN	CT	US	– predictive value RN	CT	US	Refs.
1438	86	75	75	79	91	82	82	90	81	83	77	76	[15]
122	86	93	82	83	88	85	83	83	76	86	86	78	[16]
80	79	76	61	81	89	94	74	83	87	84	84	77	[17]
Total 1640	84	81	73	81	89	87	80	85	81	84	82	77	

Biochemical tests specific for a disease may offer clues in arriving at an etiological diagnosis from an imaging procedure. Most hepatomas are associated with a rise in serum alpha-fetoprotein and the tumor size correlates with serum levels [23]. However, a slight rise in serum alpha-fetoproteins levels is often seen in viral hepatitis, postnecrotic cirrhosis, chronic active hepatitis, drugs, and a variety of other liver diseases. Hepatomas may cause diffuse irregular radiocolloid uptake or present as a solitary or multiple focal liver lesion [24].

References

1. DeNardo GL, Stadalnik RC, DeNardo SJ, Raventos A. Hepatic scintiangiographic patterns. Radiology 1974;111:135–141
2. Quinn JL III. Nuclear medicine in gastroenterology. Hospital practice 1972. pp 115–122
3. McAfee JG, Ause RG, Wagner HN Jr. Diagnostic value of scintillation scanning of the liver. Follow-up of 1,000 studies. Arch Intern Med 1965;116:95–110
4. Mould RF. An investigation of the variations in normal liver shape. Br J Radiol 1972;45:586–590
5. Rosenfield AT, Schneider PB. Rapid evaluation of hepatic size on radioisotope scan. J Nucl Med 1974;15:237–240
6. Siegel RM, Becker DV, Hurley JR. Evaluation of spleen size during routine liver imaging with Tc-99m and the scintillation camera. J Nucl Med 1970;11:689–692
7. MIRD. Summary of current radiation dose estimates to humans with various liver conditions from Tc-99m-sulfur colloid. J Nucl Med 1975;16:108A–108B
8. MIRD. Dose estimate report number 4. Summary of current radiation dose estimate to humans with various liver conditions from Au-198 colloid. J Nucl Med 1975;16:173–174
9. Bekerman C, Gottschalk A. Diagnostic significance of the relative uptake of liver compared with spleen in ^{99m}-Tc-sulfur colloid scintiphotography. J Nucl Med 1971;12:237–240
10. Oppenheim BE, Hoffer PB, Gottschalk A. The use of inspiration-expiration scintiphotos to determine the intrinsic or extrinsic nature of liver defects. J Nucl Med 1972;13:554–556
11. Keyes JW Jr, Wilson GA, Quinones JD. An evaluation of lung uptake of colloid during liver imaging. J Nucl Med 1973;14:687–691
12. Ahmad M, Witztum KF, Fletcher JW, Hendershott LR, Klos D, George EA, Donati RM. Xenon-133 accumulation in hepatic steatosis. J Nucl Med 1977;18:881–885

13. Pettigrew RI, Witztum KF, Perkins GC, Johnson ML, Burks RN, Verba JW, Halpern SE. Single photon emission computed tomography of the liver: normal vascular intrahepatic structures. Radiology 1984;150:219–223
14. Froelich JW, Simone JF, McKussick KA, Winzelberg GC, Strauss HW. Radionuclide imaging and ultrasound in liver/spleen trauma: a prospective comparison. Radiology 1982;145:457–461
15. McClees EC, Gedgaudas-McClees RK. Screening for diffuse and focal liver disease: the case for hepatic scintigraphy. J Clin Ultrasound 1984;12:75–81
16. Anderson PO, Adams DF, McNeil BJ, Sanders R, Siegelman SS, Finberg HJ, Hessel SJ, Abrams HL. Computed tomography, ultrasound, and scintigraphy of the liver in patients with colon or breast carcinoma: a prospective comparison. Radiology 1983;149:225–230
17. Kemeny MM, Sugarbaker PH, Smith TJ, Edwards BK, Shawker T, Vermess M, Jones AE. A prospective analysis of laboratory tests and imaging studies to detect hepatic lesions. Ann Surg 1982;195:163–167
18. Brendel AJ, Leccia F, Drouillard J, San Galli F, Eresue J, Wynchank S, Barat JL, Ducassou D. Single photon emission computed tomography (SPECT), planar scintigraphy, and transmission computed tomography: a comparison of accuracy in diagnosing focal hepatic disease. Radiology 1984;153:527–532
19. Quinn SF, Gosink BB. Characteristic sonographic signs of hepatic fatty infiltration. Am J Roentgenol 1985;145:753–755
20. Patel S, Sandler CM, Rauschkolb EN, McConnell BJ. Xe-133 uptake in focal hepatic fat accumulation: CT correlation. Am J Roentgenol 1982;138:541–544
21. Krishnamurthy S, Krishnamurthy GT. Evolution of nuclear hepatology as a clinical subspeciality. J Nucl Med Tech 1995;23:35S–45S
22. McGarrity TJ, Samuels T, Wilson FA. An analysis of imaging studies and liver function tests to detect hepatic neoplasia. Dig Dis Sci 1987;32:1113–1117
23. Tonami N, Aburano T, Hisada K. Comparison of alpha 1 fetoprotein radioimmunoassay method and liver scanning for detecting primary hepatic cell carcinoma. Cancer 1975;36:466–470
24. Bloomer JR, Walman TA, McIntire KR, Klastskin G. Alpha-fetoprotein in non-neoplastic hepatic disorders. JAMA 1975;233:38–41

4.2 Adenoma and Focal Nodular Hyperplasia

Adenoma and focal nodular hyperplasia (FNH) are relatively rare solitary liver tumors in women found mostly during their reproductive years and both have a close association with the use of oral contraceptives [1]. The tumors remain usually asymptomatic, and are discovered incidentally during an abdominal CT or ultrasound examinations obtained to assess some other organ in the abdomen. When these tumors become symptomatic they often present with acute onset of abdominal pain, hemorrhage, and hypotension [2]. Bleeding is more frequent in adenoma than focal nodular hyperplasia. One study reported bleeding at presentation in 4 of 27 patients with adenoma and none of 23 patients with focal nodular hyperplasia [3]. Liver function tests are usually normal with both tumors.

Both tumors appear as a non-specific space occupying lesion in a radiocolloid scan, ultrasound, MRI, or CT examination. Arteriography, contrast CT, or blood pool imaging may show hypervascularity in FNH. Adenoma, on the other hand, usually shows no hypervascularity. However, these morphologic and arteriographic characteristics are not distinct enough to separate FNH reliably from adenoma (Table 4.2.1) or from other space occupying lesions of the liver listed in Table 4.1.2.

Adenoma

Adenoma is a well encapsulated, round, solitary lesion, varying in size from 8 to 15 cm. It consists of sheets of hepatocytes without any bile ducts or fibrous septa (Fig. 4.2.1).

Kupffer cells are either absent or markedly decreased in number. Few of these Kupffer cells that are present lack phagocytic function and hence the nodule appears as "cold" in a radiocolloid scan [4]. The hepatocytes are able to concentrate ^{99m}Tc-HIDA but cannot secrete into bile due lack of bile ducts [5]. About 80% of adenomas show mixed echogenicity on the ultrasound examination and about 86% appear as a hypodense mass on non-contrast CT examination [4]. The consistent pattern of hepatic adenoma is one of a well circumscribed solitary mass lesion on CT or US with no uptake on radiocolloid scintigraphy. Atypical forms with functioning Kupffer cells are rare [6]. Some adenomas may show a nodule-in-nodule pattern on CT and MRI and are indistinguishable from hepatocellular carcinoma. Adenomas may be separated from carcinomas by depicting its functional characteristics. Lack of gallium-67 citrate uptake (in contrast to hepatocellular carcinoma) and no radiocolloid uptake, and late uptake with no excretion of ^{99m}Tc-HIDA, may distinguish adenoma from hepatoma, FNH or other types of focal liver lesions [7].

Table 4.2.1. Characteristic features of hepatic adenoma and focal nodular hyperplasia

Parameter	Adenoma	Focal nodular hyperplasia
Age	30–40 years	30–40 years
Female: male ratio	30:0	10:1
Oral contraceptive association	+++	++
Well defined capsule	Present	Absent
Bile ducts	Absent	Decreased and narrowed
Fibrosis	Absent	Present
Hypervascularity	++	++++
Hepatocyte number (in lesion)	Normal or increase	Normal or decrease
Kupffer cells	Absent or decrease	Normal or decrease
Radiocolloid uptake	Absent	Normal or decrease
^{99m}Tc-HIDA uptake	Increase or normal	Normal
^{99m}Tc-HIDA excretion	Absent	Slow
^{99m}Tc-GSA receptors	Not known	Increase or normal

HIDA, hepatic iminodiacetic acid; GSA, galactosyl human serum albumin

Focal Nodular Hyperplasia

In contrast to hepatic adenoma which consists mostly sheets of hepatocytes, focal nodular hyperplasia (FNH) usually consists of all types of cells of a normal liver, including the hepatocytes, Kupffer cells, bile ducts and other supporting cells. There is a central fibrosis with radiating fibrous connective tissue which divides the nodule into several smaller sections of varying size, mimicking the pattern seen with pseudonodules of cirrhosis [8]. A capsule is absent, a clear distinction from adenoma (Fig. 4.2.1). Bile ducts show proliferation with narrow lumen impeding bile flow through them. The hepatocytes show clear to dark cytoplasm with sparse bile canaliculi [2]. Most FNH are found just beneath the liver surface and some are pedunculated. The size of the lesions vary from 1 to 15 cm. Malignant transformation is uncommon. About 90% of FNH are hypervascular, and the rest are hypovascular on the angiogram. On the ultrasound examination, 50% are hyperechoic, 40% hypoechoic, and 10% show a mixed pattern [9, 10].

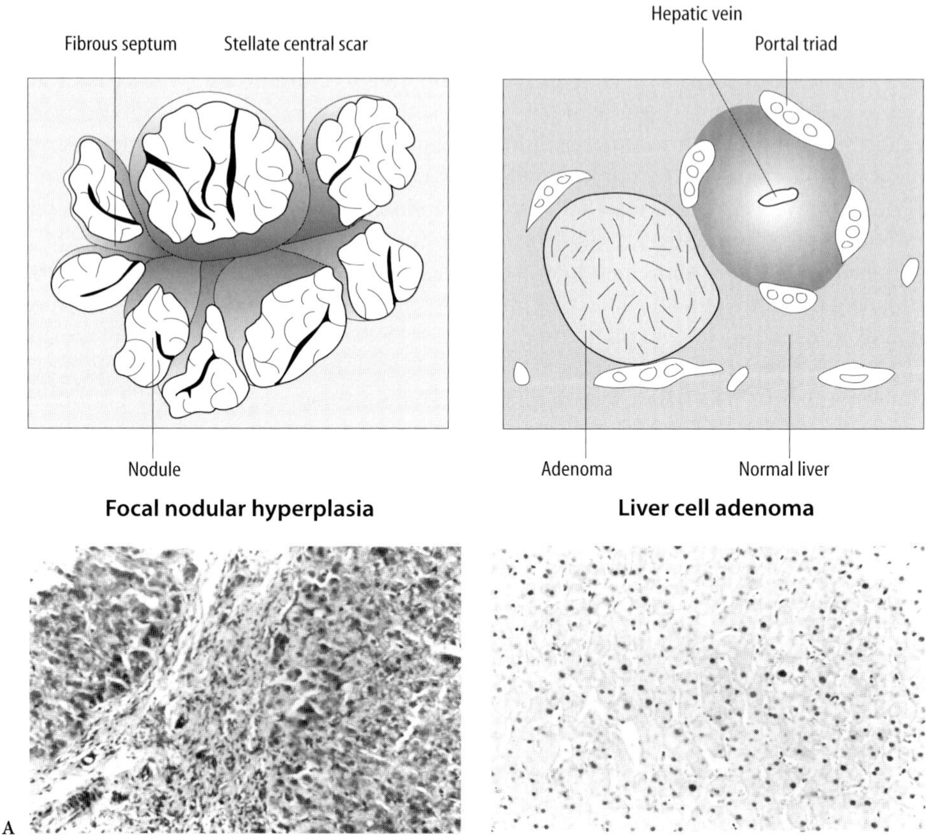

Fig. 4.2.1. A schematic diagram (*top*) of focal nodular hyperplasia and liver cell adenoma. Focal nodular hyperplasia (**A**) consists of radiating dense fibrous tissue with all types of liver cells but without any capsule. Histology (*bottom*) shows the hepatocytes, Kupffer cells, and fibrous tissue with formation of small nodules. Adenoma (**B**), on the other hand, consists of a capsule with monotonous sheets of hepatocytes without any Kupffer cells or fibrous tissue (Courtesy of Dr. Ted Pinkert)

Scintigraphic Features

Both focal nodular hyperplasia and a regenerating nodule of cirrhosis contain Kupffer cells. Most of the other focal liver lesions (adenoma, hemangioma, primary and metastatic liver lesions) do not contain any Kupffer cells, or those few Kupffer cells that are present lack phagocytic function. A normal radiocolloid uptake pattern is seen in 64% of FNH and the remaining 34% show decreased uptake [11]. A characteristic feature of FNH includes a hypervascularity seen on contrast CT (Fig. 4.2.2a). About 76% of them show hypervascularity in a perfusion study with ^{99m}Tc-HIDA (Fig. 4.2.2b). Early phase functional images (within 10 min) show ^{99m}Tc-HIDA uptake by the nodule equal to that of the adjoining normal liver (Fig. 4.2.2c). Late phase images (after 45 min) show slow clearance by the nodule and a normal clearance from adjoining normal liver. By 60 min, the radioactivity retained by FNH is about twice as much as the adjoining normal liver and hence it appears as "a hot nodule" on the late image (Fig. 4.2.2d,e). A normal mean excretion half-time of 18 min increases to 40 min for FNH, explaining its appearance as a "hot lesion" [11]. The slow excretion is due to narrowing of the cholangioles draining the FNH. The time of appearance of the "hot nodule" is a function of both how rapidly the radiotracer is cleared from the normal liver and how slowly it is cleared from the nodule. Routine inclusion of the perfusion phase as an integral part of hepatobiliary imaging enhances the nodule detectability by showing its hypervascularity. The radiocolloid image depicts the lesion as "cold" (Fig. 4.2.2f).

The overall detectability of FNH is 92% with ^{99m}Tc-mebrofenin cholescintigraphy, 84% with CT, and 84% with MRI [10]. Despite hypervascularity around the periphery, some large FNH lesions remain hypo- or avascular centrally. Demonstration of this feature helps to differentiate it from a hemangioma (Fig. 4.2.3).

Surface Receptors

The hepatocytes of FNH show an increase in the number of asialoglycoprotein surface receptors which bind to ^{99m}Tc-galactosyl-human serum albumin much more intensely than the adjoining normal liver parenchyma. In a study of 12 patients with focal nodular hyperplasia, 9 with hepatocellular carcinoma, and 3 patients with metastatic liver cancer, the authors were able to distinguish FNH from primary and metastatic liver lesions by calculating a nodule/normal liver ratio obtained with ^{99m}Tc-neoglycoalbumin. Eight of 12 patients with FNH showed an increase in ratio and the remaining 4 showed an uptake equal to that of the adjoining normal liver tissue. The nodule/normal liver mean ratio was 1.7±0.3 in patients with FNH and 0.4±0.2 in patients with primary and metastatic cancer, enabling clear separation of benign from malignant liver lesions [12]. Imaging with other tumor seeking agents like ^{67}Ga-citrate and ^{201}Tl-chloride, combined with ^{99m}Tc-phytate (radiocolloid) or ^{99m}Tc-pyridoxyl-5-methyltryptophan (a hepatobiliary agent) also aids in separating benign from malignant hepatic lesions [13, 14].

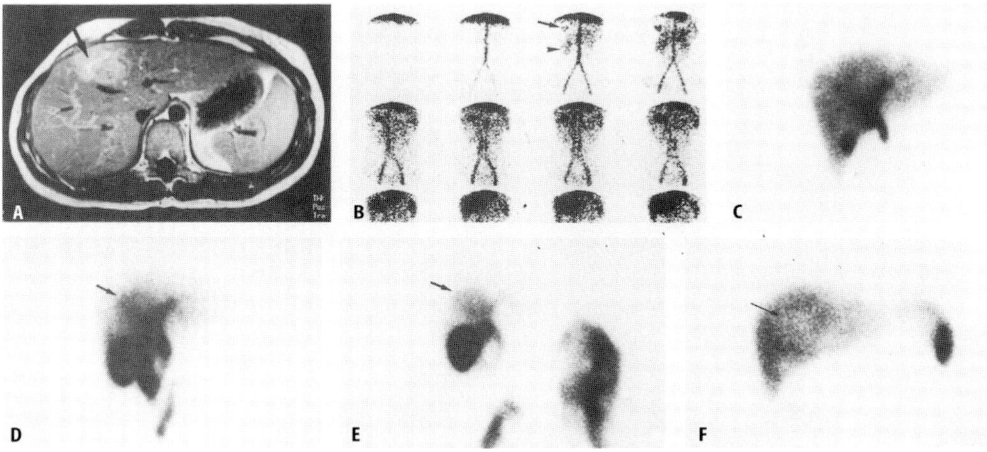

Fig. 4.2.2. Functional characteristics of focal nodular hyperplasia. It shows its hypervascularity on a contrast CT (**A**) and a perfusion study with ^{99m}Tc-HIDA (**B**). Early images show normal uptake (**C**) and late images at 45 min (**D**) and 60 min (**E**) show retention *(arrows)* of the radiotracer. It appears as "cold" *(arrow)* on a radiocolloid image (**F**) due to paucity of Kupffer cells [11]

A
B
C

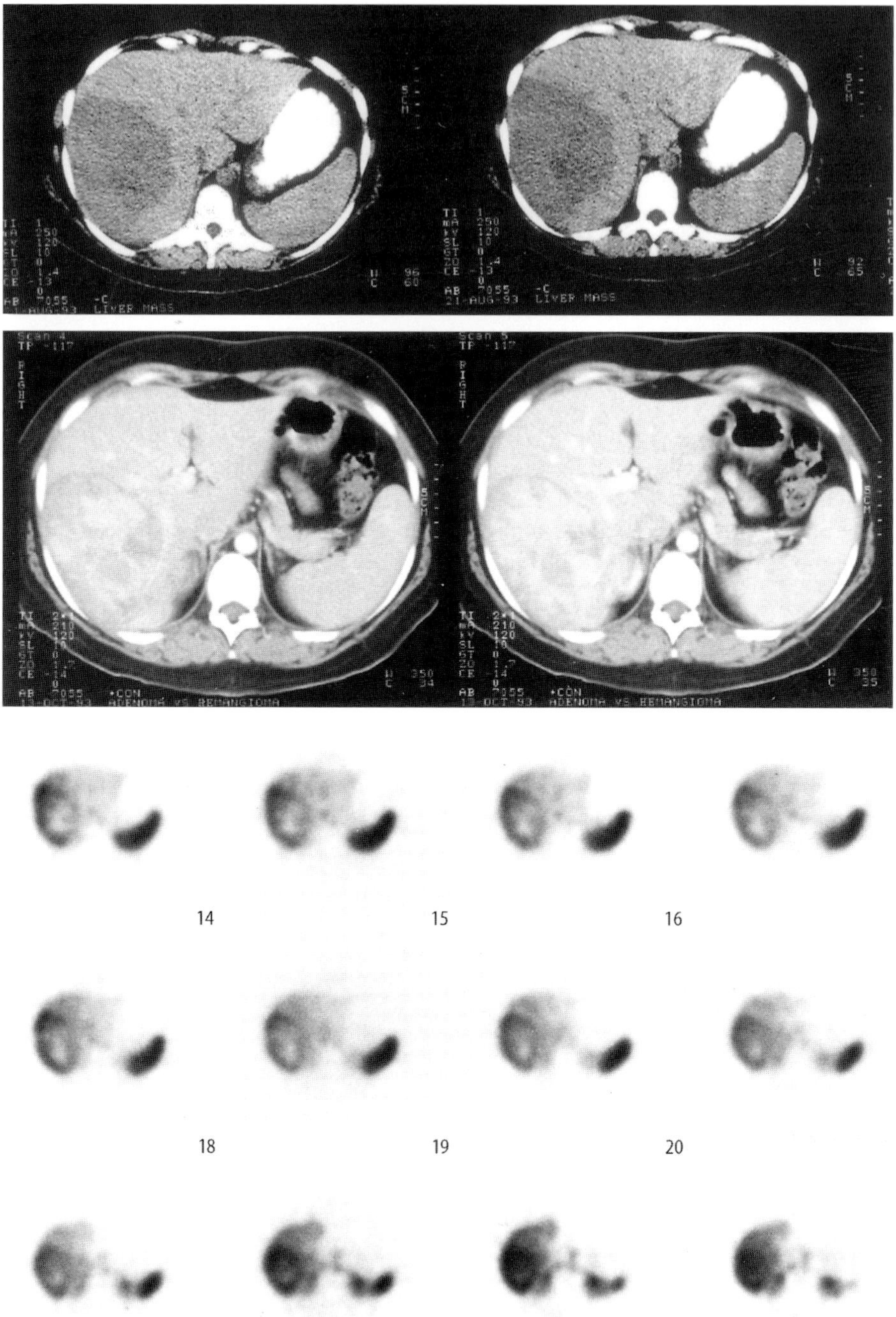

Fig. 4.2.3A–C. Blood pool features of focal nodular hyperplasia. A large focal nodular hyperplasia in the posterior right lobe appears as hypodense on a CT scan without the contrast (**A**), and as non-uniform hyperdense with the contrast agent (**B**). Blood pool imaging with autologous ^{99m}Tc-RBCs shows a non-filling center (**C**)

Treatment

The treatment approach needs flexibility. Asymptomatic patients are managed conservatively [15]. Some nodules regress spontaneously on discontinuation of oral contraceptives [16]. Surgical resection is recommended when the nodule grows rapidly in size or becomes acutely symptomatic. Because both hepatic adenoma and FNH occur more frequently in women during their reproductive years and are often detected serendipitously on US or CT, done for unrelated reasons, proper management strategy requires clear differentiation of adenoma from FNH, and both need differentiation from other types of space occupying liver lesions before deciding on a specific form of therapy [17, 18]. Biopsy is not mandatory.

Adenomatosis (multiple small adenomas) is a distinct entity and behaves much differently from adenoma and focal nodular hyperplasia in terms of its clinical presentation. Adenomatosis occurs equally in both sexes, shows no association with oral contraceptives, and is associated with elevation of serum alkaline phosphatase and gamma glutamyl transpeptidase. Hemorrhage is uncommon, and it requires no specific form of therapy [19].

References

1. Baum JK, Holtz F, Brookstein JJ, et al. Possible association between benign hepatoma and oral contraceptives. Lancet 1973, 2:926–929
2. Stauffer JQ, Lapinski MW, Donold DJ, Myers TK. Focal nodular hyperplasia of the liver and intrahepatic hemorrhage in young women on oral contraceptives. Ann Intern Med 1975;83:301–306
3. Mathieu D, Bruneton JN, Drouillard J, Pointreau CC, Vasile N. Hepatic adenoma and focal nodular hyperplasia: Dynamic CT study. Radiology 1986;160:53–58
4. Welsh TJ, Sheedy PF, Johnson CM, Stephen D, Charboneau JW, Brown ML, May GR, Adson MA, McGill DB. Focal nodular hyperplasia and hepatic adenoma: comparison of angiography, CT, US, and scintigraphy. Radiology 1985;156:593–595
5. Drane WE, Krasicky GA, Johnson DA, Radionuclide imaging of primary tumors and tumor like conditions of the liver. Clin Nucl Med 1987;12:569–582
6. Lubbers RP, Ros PR, Goodman ZD, Ishak KG. Accumulation of technetium-99m sulfur colloid by hepatocellular adenoma: scintigraphic pathologic correlation. Am J Roentgenol 1987;148:1105–1108
7. Kume N, Suga K, Nishigauchi K, Shimizu K, Matsunaga N. Characterization of hepatic adenoma with atypical appearance on CT and MRI by radionuclide imaging. Clin Nucl Med 1997:22;825–831
8. Knowles DM, Wolff M. Focal nodular hyperplasia of the liver, a clinicopathologic study and review of the literature. Human Pathol 1976;7:533–545
9. Biersack HJ, Thelen M, Torres JF, Lackner K, Winkler CG. Focal nodular hyperplasia of the liver as established by Tc-99m-sulfur colloid and HIDA scintigraphy. Radiology 1980;137:187–190
10. Rogers JV, Mack LA, Freeny PC, Johnson ML, Sones PJ. Hepatic focal nodular hyperplasia: angiography, CT, sonography, and scintigraphy. Am J Roentgenol 1981;137:983–990
11. Boulahdour H, Cherque D, Charlotte F, Rahmouni A, Dhumeaux D, Zafrani E, Meignan M. The hot spot hepatobiliary scan in focal nodular hyperplasia. J Nucl Med 1993;34:2105–2110
12. Kurtaran A, Muller C, Novacek G, Kaserer K, Mentes M, Raderer M, Pidlich J, Eibenberger K, Angelberger P, Virgolini I. Distinction between hepatic focal nodular hyperplasia and malignant liver lesions using technetium-99m-galactosyl-neoglycoalbumin. J Nucl Med 1997;38:1912–1915
13. Bernard EJ, Nicholls W, Howman-Giles R, Kan A, Stevens M. Tl-201 positive, Ga-67 negative hepatoblastoma: a case report of a 12-year-old boy. Clin Nucl Med 1997:22;835–837
14. Shuke N, Yoshikawa D, Saito Y, Sato J, Ishikawa Y, Yoshida H, Kino S, Miyokawa N, Aburano. Focal nodular hyperplasia of the liver. Scintigraphic demonstration using three imaging agents. Clin Nucl Med 1999;24:451–453
15. Pain JA, Gimson AE, Williams R, Howard ER. Focal nodular hyperplasia of the liver: results of treatment and options in management. Gut 1991;32:524–527
16. Ross D, Pina J, Mirza M, Galvan A, Ponce L. Regression of focal nodular hyperplasia after discontinuation of oral contraceptives. Ann Intern Med 1976;85:203–204

17. Sandler MA, Petrocelli RD, Marks DS, Lopez R. Ultrasonic features and radionuclide correlation in liver cell adenoma and focal nodular hyperplasia. Radiology 1980;135:393–397
18. Sherlock S, Dooley J. Diseases of the liver and biliary system. Blackwell Science, Malden, MA 1997. 10th edition, pp 337–369
19. Flejou J Barge J, Menu Y, Degott C, Bismuth H, Potet F, Benhamou J. Liver adenomatosis. An entity distinct from liver adenoma? Gastroenterology 1985;89:1132–1138

4.3 Hemangioma

Hemangiomas are the most common liver lesions, accounting for nearly 5–7% of all benign tumors [1]. They are congenital vascular malformations at birth which increase in size with the growth of the liver. Hemangiomas affect both sexes, occur at all ages, but manifest clinical symptoms, if at all, usually in the 3rd and 5th decades of life. They are relatively more common in women than men, with a ratio of 4:1 to 6:1 [2]. They are found more frequently in multiparous women and increase in size during pregnancy, and after administration of estrogens [3].

Histopathology

Cavernous hemangioma is usually a solitary lesion consisting of multiple vascular channels, lined by a single layer of flat endothelial cells, and supported by an intervening fibrous tissue. Lesions vary in size from a few millimeters to several centimeters, some as large as 20–30 cm. Hemangiomas larger than 4 cm are referred to as giant cavernous hemangiomas. Most are sessile without a capsule and are located superficially inside the superior part of the right lobe of the liver. Occasionally a pedunculated lesion may be seen well separated from the main liver mass. Hemangiomas consist of a large blood pool but show a reduction in rate of blood flow (ml/g/min) when compared to the adjoining normal liver tissue [4].

Clinical Presentation

Most hemangiomas remain asymptomatic. In the past they were discovered usually at autopsy [2]. Today hemangiomas are discovered serendipitously while performing an ultrasound or CT scan of the abdomen [5]. Large hemangiomas may cause abdominal pain due to compression of the adjoining organs or thrombosis within the lesion. Acute onset of severe abdominal pain may indicate hemorrhage.

Diagnosis

Most hemangiomas are discovered today during their asymptomatic phase with ultrasound or CT, as space occupying lesions of the liver. The real challenge, therefore, is not one of discovery but that of differentiation from other types of liver lesions, such as adenoma, focal nodular hyperplasia, and primary or metastatic tumors. Blood pool imaging with ^{99m}Tc-RBC, contrast CT, MRI, and contrast angiography have been used for diagnosis [6–9]. Imaging with ^{99m}Tc-labeled autologous red blood cells carries the highest specificity and is considered the diagnostic modality of choice for confirmation of hemangiomas [10].

Blood Pool Scintigraphy

Patient red blood cells are labeled with ^{99m}Tc using an in vitro method as described in detail in Chap. 3.2. A rapid sequence perfusion study is obtained after injecting 15–30 mCi (555–740 MBq) autologous ^{99m}Tc RBC (or ^{99m}Tc-pertechnetate for the in vivo method) by collecting data at one frame/2 s for 60 s. Planar blood pool images in the anterior, posterior, and two lateral views are obtained 10 min after the perfusion study. Delayed images are obtained at 30 or 60 min by collecting at least one million counts per image. When not seen clearly in planar images by 60 min, SPECT imaging study is obtained between 1 and 2 h. The SPECT data are collected over a 360° rotation by obtaining 64 frames at 30 s/frame using a 64×64×8 matrix. After appropriate correction for camera non-uniformity and center of rotation deviation, the projections are reconstructed with the vendor specific filtered backprojection algorithm. Transaxial, coronal, and sagittal slices are obtained with known pixel size to be able to measure size accurately.

Scintigraphic Features

A normal study (Fig. 4.3.1) clearly shows the blood pool in the abdominal aorta, inferior vena cava, two kidneys, liver, and spleen. The inferior vena cava in general is seen more prominently than the aorta. The heart is the hottest organ in the chest in the anterior view, and the spleen is the brightest organ in the abdomen in the posterior view.

Hemangiomas typically show a decreased perfusion followed by a delayed filling, reflecting their basic pathophysiology. Despite an enormous increase in blood pool, blood flow (ml/g/min) is generally reduced relative to the surrounding normal liver tissue. Due to a reduction in blood flow, mixing of radiolabeled RBCs with the unlabeled RBCs within the hemangioma occurs slowly over several minutes or hours, depending upon the size of the hemangioma. Very large hemangiomas are often missed when sufficient time is not allowed for complete mixing or equilibration, prior to acquisition of SPECT data. Giant hemangiomas are delineated better in delayed SPECT images obtained 2–4 h after injection of the labeled red blood cells.

Small hemangiomas in the peripheral liver equilibrate early and are seen faintly on planar blood pool images and become very clear on the SPECT images (Fig. 4.3.2). They manifest varied characteristics on the ultrasound and CT images. Many appear as hypodense on CT without contrast, and become isodense (Fig. 4.3.3) or hyperdense after the contrast. Some fill in only partially and others not at all. These varied features make it difficult to distinguish hemangioma from other benign and malignant liver lesions from a CT scan.

Giant hemangiomas often involve one complete segment or lobe of the liver (Fig. 4.3.4). Rapid sequence perfusion study shows markedly decreased blood flow, followed by delayed equilibration. Some may equilibrate only partially even after 3–4 h of equilibration, and may require images at 18–24 h.

The sensitivity and accuracy of an imaging test depends very much on the size of the hemangioma. For lesions larger than 2 cm, the sensitivity and accuracy of ^{99m}Tc-RBC perfusion and SPECT blood pool imaging varies from 89% to 92% and from 89% to 94%, respectively. For similar size lesions, MRI sensitivity varies from 85% to 100% and accuracy from 81% to 100% [10]. For lesions less than 2 cm in size, scintigraphic

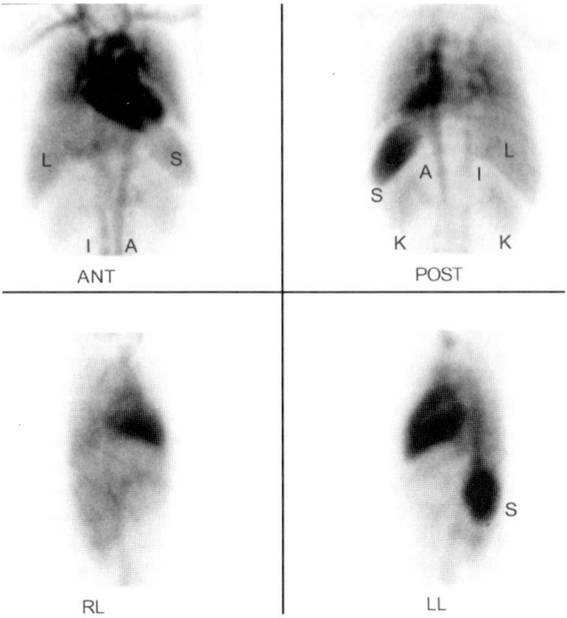

Fig. 4.3.1. Normal abdominal blood pool. Anterior (*ANT*) and posterior (*POST*) planar images show inferior vena cava (*I*), aorta (*A*), liver (*L*), spleen (*S*), and two kidneys (*K*). Liver appears faint in the right lateral (*RL*) view and spleen appears bright in the left lateral (*LL*) view

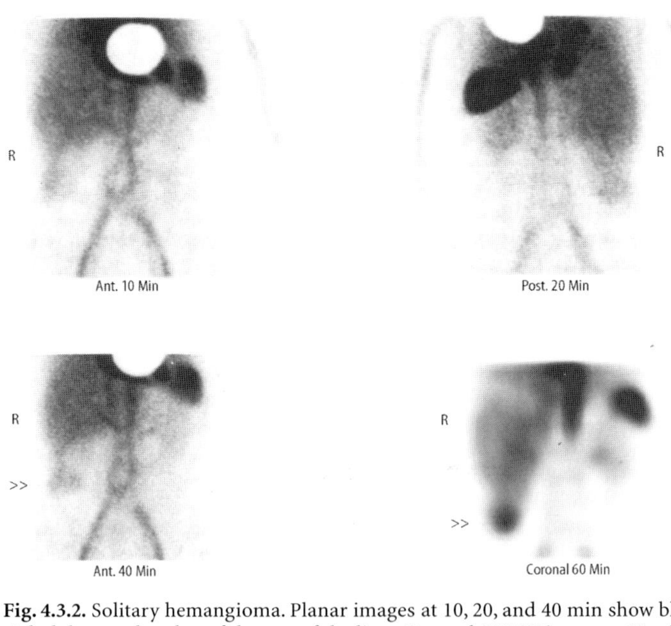

Fig. 4.3.2. Solitary hemangioma. Planar images at 10, 20, and 40 min show blood pool at the tip of the right lobe equal to that of the rest of the liver. Coronal SPECT image at 60 min clearly shows increased blood pool at the tip *(arrowheads)* and confirms hemangioma

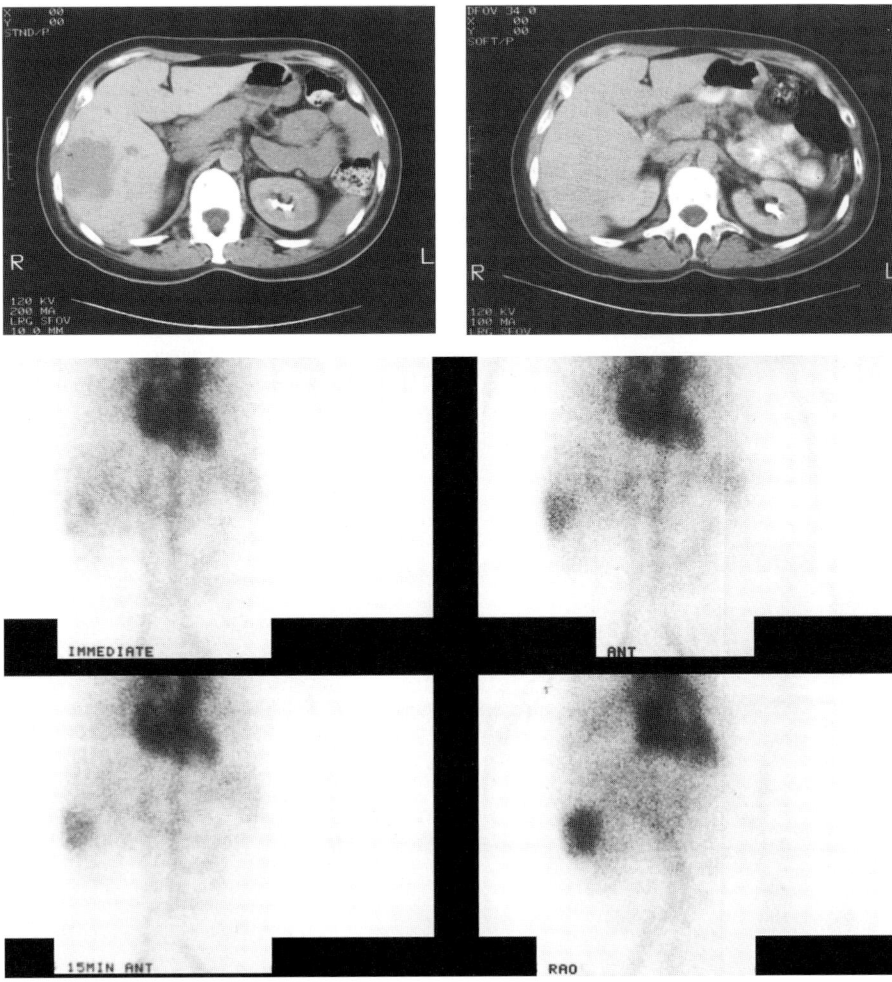

A B C

Fig. 4.3.3. Variable pattern hemangioma. A CT without contrast (**A**) shows a hypodense lesion in the right lobe which becomes isodense (**B**) after injection of the contrast agent. Immediate planar ^{99m}Tc-RBC blood pool scintigraphy shows hemangioma faintly, which becomes much clearer at 5 and 15 min (**C**)

sensitivity is 58% and accuracy 60% and MRI carries a sensitivity of 83% and an accuracy of 84% (Table 4.3.1). As MRI often fails to differentiate hemangioma from hypervascular neoplasm or focal nodular hyperplasia, blood pool imaging with SPECT is considered the method of choice for confirmation of hemangioma [6, 10]. Angiography is necessary only in those patients who do not show a blood pool pattern typical for hemangioma. Needle biopsy is avoided in most patients unless the lesion is small and the diagnosis is not confirmed from blood pool imaging. MRI with contrast may be preferred over angiography and needle biopsy for small lesions not seen on the blood pool study [10].

A

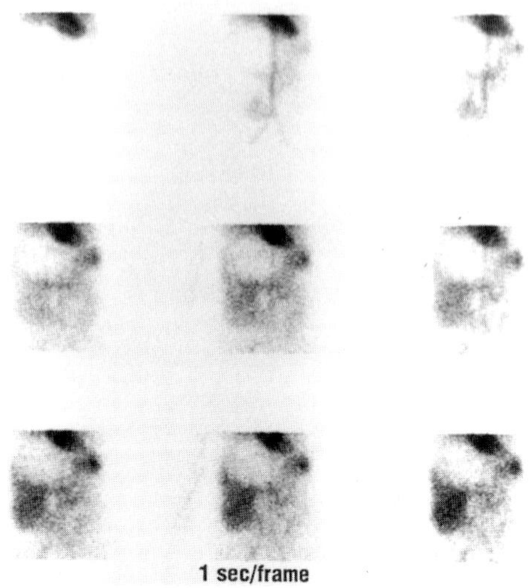

B

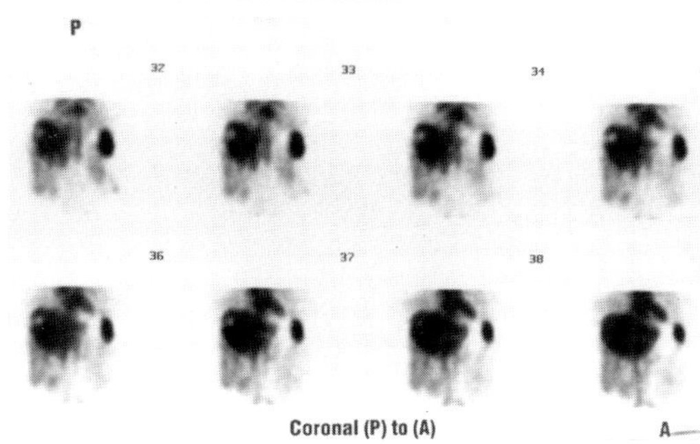

C

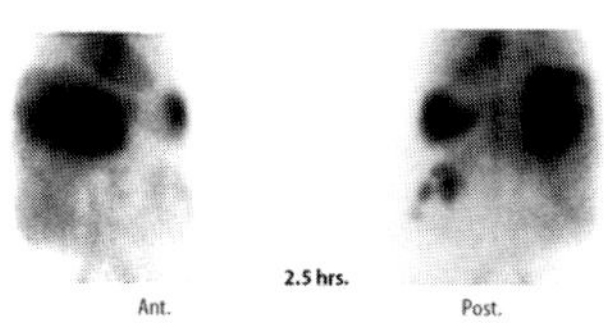

D

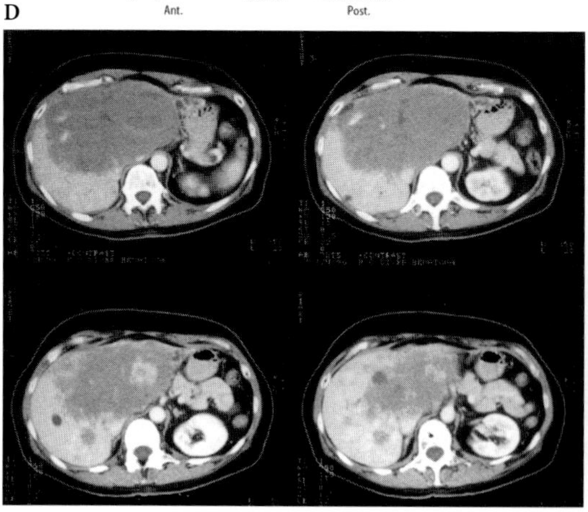

E

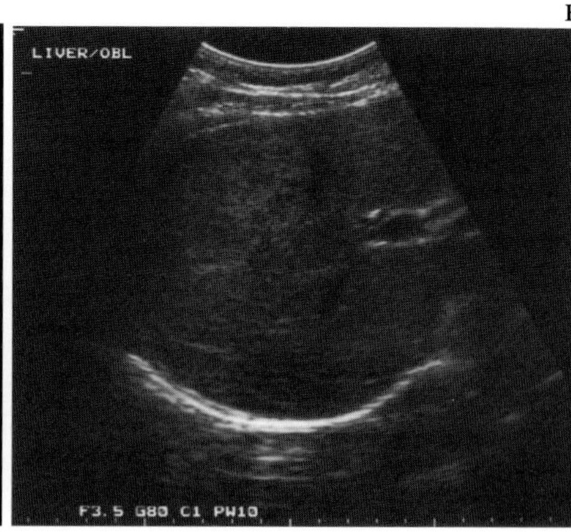

Fig. 4.3.4. Giant cavernous hemangioma. A perfusion scintigraphy **(A)** shows no blood flow through a giant hemangioma involving the superior right lobe and the medial left lobe in a patient with breast cancer. Coronal view SPECT at 60 min shows hemangioma with a small superolateral region not yet in equilibrium **(B)**. Anterior (*ANT*) and posterior (*POST*) planar images at 2.5 h show complete filling of the hemangioma **(C)**. A CT with contrast **(D)** shows a variable blood pool within the hemangioma and an ultrasound study **(E)** shows mixed hyper- and hypoechoic regions. (Courtesy of Dr. Ronald Hagelman, Tucson, AZ)

Table 4.3.1. Comparison of ^{99m}Tc red blood cell SPECT and MR imaging in the diagnosis of hepatic hemangioma [10]

	Hemangioma size (cm) (n=64)		
	1.0–1.9 (n=24)	2.0–2.9 (n=13)	3.0–13.0 (n=27)
SPECT			
No. positive (n=50)	14	12	24
No. negative (n=14)	10	1	3
Sensitivity (%)	58	92	89
Accuracy (%)	60	94	89
MR imaging			
No. positive (n=58)	20	11	27
No. negative (n=6)	4	2	0
Sensitivity (%)	83	85	100
Accuracy (%)	84	81	100

About 90% of hemangiomas are single. They are found in both hepatic lobes, the right lobe 9 times more frequently than the left (Table 4.3.2). Most are situated in the superior areas of both lobes [11]. Multiple hemangiomas may involve both lobes at different locations (Fig. 4.3.5). A typical pattern of a "cold" lesion on blood flow and a delayed filling (hot) on the blood pool image is found in 66% of hemangiomas. Others show an atypical pattern of early incomplete and delayed complete filling [12]. For lesions between 1 and 2 cm, SPECT increases sensitivity by 11% over the planar image. On ultrasound examination, 59% appear as hyperechoic, 11% as hypoechoic, and 30% show a mixed pattern

Table 4.3.2. Features of 130 hemangiomas [11]

Feature	Number (%)
Distribution	
Single	116 (89)
Multiple	14 (11)
Right lobe	118 (91)
Subdiaphragmatic	103 (87)
Left lobe	12 (9)
Superficial	109 (84%)
Deep	21 (16)
Posterior	83 (64)
Anterior	47 (36)
Scintigraphic features	
Typical filling pattern	86 (66)
Atypical filling pattern	44 (34)
Ultrasound features	
Hyperechoic	76 (59)
Hypoechoic	14 (11)
Mixed pattern	39 (30)

Treatment

No treatment is required for most patients without symptoms. Lobectomy or segmentectomy is recommended for patients with recent onset of pain or for a rapidly expanding lesion [13, 14].

A

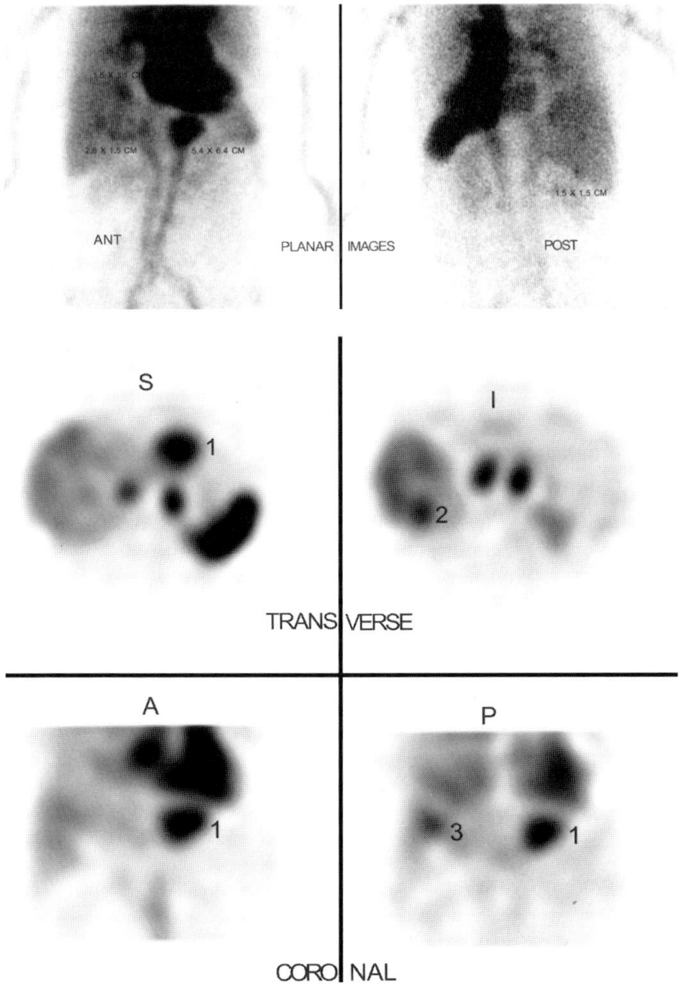

B

C

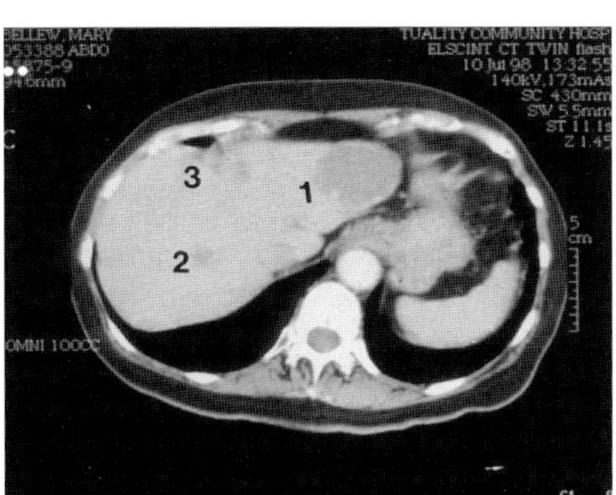

Fig. 4.3.5. Multiple hemangiomas. Anterior (*ANT*) and posterior (*POST*) view planar images (**A**) show three hemangiomas of variable sizes. Superior (*S*) and inferior (*I*) section transverse SPECT images (**B**) show one hemangioma in the left lobe (#1) and another in the posterior part of the right lobe (#2). Anterior (*A*) and posterior (*P*) coronal slices confirm #1 lesion but the posterior slice shows an additional (#3) hemangioma. A CT with contrast (**C**) shows three hypodense lesions, only #1 showing slight enhancement at the periphery

References

1. Ishak KG, Rabin L. Benign tumors of the liver. Med Clin North Am 1975;59:995–1013
2. Edmondson HA. Tumors of the liver and intrahepatic bile ducts. In: Atlas of tumor pathology. Section VII, Fascicle 25. Washington DC, Armed Forces Institute of Pathology, 1958;113
3. Kew MC. Tumors of the liver. In: Zakim D, Boyer TD (eds) Hepatology. A textbook of liver disease. W.B. Saunders Co, Philadelphia, 1996
4. Taylor RD, Anderson PM, Winston MA, Blahd WH. Diagnosis of hepatic hemangioma using multiple radionuclide and ultrasound technique. J Nucl Med 1976;17:362–364
5. Sherlock S, Dooley J. Hepatic tumors. In: Diseases of the liver and biliary system. 10th edn. Blackwell Science, Malden, MA 1997
6. Rabinowitz SA, McKusick KA, Strauss HW. Tc-99m red blood cell scintigraphy in evaluating focal liver lesions. Am J Roentgenol 1984;143:63–68
7. Brodsky RI, Friedman AC, Maurer AH, Radecki PD, Caroline DF. Hepatic cavernous hemangioma: diagnosis with Tc-99m labeled red cells and single photon emission CT. Am J Roentgenol 1987;148:125–129
8. Bree RL, Schwab RE, Glazer GM, Fink-Bennett D. The varied appearance of hepatic hemangioma with sonography, computed tomography, magnetic resonance imaging and scintigraphy. Radiographics 1987;7:1153–1175
9. Whitney WS, Herfkens RJ, Jeffrey RB, McDonnell CH, Li KCP, Van Dalsem WJ, Low RN, Francis IR, Dabatin JF, Glazer GM. Dynamic breath-hold multiplanar spoiled gradient-recalled MR imaging with gadolinium enhancement for differentiating hepatic hemangiomas from malignancies at 1.5 T. Radiology 1993;189:863–870
10. Birnbaum BA, Weinreb JC, Megibow AJ, Sanger JJ, Lubat E, Kanamuller H, Noz ME, Bosniak MA. Definitive diagnosis of hepatic hemangiomas: MR imaging versus Tc-99m labeled red blood cell SPECT. Radiology 1990;176:95–101
11. El-Desouki M, Mohamadiyeh M, Al-Rashed R, Othman S, Al-Mofleh. Features of hepatic hemangioma on planar and SPECT Tc-99m-labeled red blood cell scintigraphy. Clin Nucl Med 1999,24:583–589
12. Randor M, Petrozzo P. Hepatic Hemangioma. N Engl J Med 2000; 312:791
13. Belli L, DeCarlis L, Beati C, et al. Surgical treatment of symptomatic giant hemangiomas of the liver. Surg Gyn Obstet 1992;174:474
14. Sinanan MN, Marchioro T. Management of cavernous hemangioma of the liver. Am J Surg 1989;157:519

4.4 Somatostatin Receptor Scintigraphy

Somatostatin Source

Somatostatin belongs to a multigene family peptide, synthesized, stored, and released by many cells in the body [1]. Upon release from cells, somatostatin acts as an autocrine, paracrine, and endocrine hormone. Two forms of somatostatin are identified: one with 14 (Chap. 3, Fig. 3.4.1) and the other with 28 amino acids. The larger molecule is a dimer formed by the union of two shorter ones attached at the N-terminal end [2, 3]. The cells secreting somatostatin are distributed throughout the body, the heaviest concentration found in the anterior pituitary, thyroid, lungs, liver, spleen, gastrointestinal tract, pancreas, kidneys, adrenal medulla, and paraganglions of the nervous system. Somatostatin secreting cells were once called APUD (amine precursor uptake decarboxylation) cells and have now been renamed as neuroendocrine cells [4].

Action of Somatostatin

In contrast to most hormones, which generally have a stimulatory effect on their target cells in the body, somatostatin has predominantly an inhibitory effect on its target cells. Its serum half-life is less than 3 min. Somatostatin inhibits secretion of: (1)

growth hormone and thyrotropin from the anterior pituitary gland; (2) insulin, glucagon, and exocrine secretion from the pancreas; (3) gastrin, vasoactive intestinal polypeptide (VIP), secretin, and cholecystokinin from the gastrointestinal tract; and (4) excessive production of the basic hormone secreted by tumors arising from various organs (Table 4.4.1). By its ability to inhibit production and release the basic hormone by the endocrine gland, somatostatin either reduces or totally abolishes the hormonal effect on the target cells and often reduces the size of the primary and metastatic tumors. Other physiological actions of somatostatin include reduction of hepatic blood flow, inhibition of gallbladder contraction and bile emptying, and inhibition of gastrointestinal motility. It increases absorption of water and electrolytes from the intestine [5].

Table 4.4.1. Somatostatin receptor positive tumors

Gastrinoma	Carcinoid
Insulinoma	Medullary thyroid cancer
Glucagonoma	Pituitary adenoma
Small cell lung cancer	Neuroblastoma
VIPoma	Paraganglioma
Cholangiocarcinoma	Meningioma
Pheochromocytoma	Motilinoma

Somatostatin Receptors

Five subtypes of somatostatin receptors have been recognized [5]. Each subtype has its own chromosome location and manifests a different level of affinity for somatostatin uptake (Table 4.4.2). The organs that are seen faintly on a normal ^{111}In-pentetreotide (OctreoScan) scan include the lungs, anterior pituitary, and GI tract, and the organs that are seen intensely include the thyroid, liver, and spleen. Neuroendocrine tumors with the heaviest concentration of somatostatin receptors and are visible on a ^{111}In-pentetreotide (OctreoScan) scan are shown in Table 4.4.3.

Octreotide

Somatostatin with a serum half-life of less than 3 min is unsuitable for diagnostic or therapeutic application. This problem is solved by making chemical substitutions at its basic molecule and creating somatostatin analogues of longer serum half-life. The first successful synthetic compound created was octreotide with eight amino acids. It behaves much like the parent hormone with 14 or 28 amino acids in inhibiting somatostatin secretion by the tumor. The serum half-life of octreotide is about 2 h after subcutaneous administration. In order to accomplish both the task of binding to the receptors and at the same time carry its physiological action, all somatostatin analogues must retain the basic loop structure and four receptor binding amino acids, phenylalanine (Phe), tryptophan (Trp), lysine (Lys), and threonine (Thr). Octreotide differs from somatostatin in not only having only eight amino acids but also by carrying D-Phe in place of -Phe. Vapreotide (RC-160) and lanreotide (BIM-23014) are newer synthetic analogues of somatostatin used in the treatment of somatostatin receptor positive tumors [5].

Table 4.4.2. Characteristics of human somatostatin receptor subtypes [5]

Character	Subtype 1	Subtype 2	Subtype 3	Subtype 4	Subtype 5
Chromosome #	14	17	22	20	16
G protein binding	+	+	+	+	+
Receptor affinity to:					
Somatostatin-14	+++	+++	++	++++	+++
Octreotide	±	+++	++	±	++
Vapreotide	±	++	+	+	+++
Lanreotide	±	++	+	+	++++
Distribution in normal organs	Brain, lungs, stomach, jejunum, kidneys, liver, pancreas	Brain, kidneys, bile ducts	Brain, pancreas	Brain, lungs	Brain, heart, adrenals, pituitary, small intestine, skeletal muscl

Table 4.4.3. Somatostatin receptor positivity by in vivo scintigraphy and in vitro autoradiography [12]

Tumor type	In vivo scintigraphy (%)	In vitro autoradiography (%)
Meningioma	100	98
Paraganglioma	100	92
Small cell lung cancer	100	57
Hodgkin's disease	98	100
Carcinoid	95	88
Gastrinoma	93	100
Unclassified APUDoma	89	100
Neuroblastoma	89	65
Pheochromocytoma	87	73
Non-Hodgkin's lymphoma	83	87
Non-functioning pituitary adenoma	75	55
Pituitary GH producing tumor	70	98
Medullary thyroid cancer	69	38
Breast cancer	68	46
Insulinoma	46	67
Sarcoidosis	100	100
Tuberculosis	100	100
Rheumatoid arthritis	100	86

Radiolabeling of Octreotide

Octreotide was radiolabeled first with radioiodine, ^{123}I. The loop structure and three of the four receptor binding amino acids were retained, the fourth receptor binding amino acid, phenylalanine, was replaced by tyrosine to enable easy radioiodination [6, 7]. The radiolabeling technique is cumbersome, and the cost of production and delivery very high due to the short physical half-life of ^{123}I (13 h). Because of these drawbacks, imaging did not become clinically very popular. Replacement of radioiodine ^{123}I with ^{111}In appeared logical and was readily accomplished (see Chap. 3, Fig. 3.4.1).

Indium-111 Pentetreotide (OctreoScan)

A bifunctional chelate, diethylenetriaminepentaacetic acid (DTPA), attaches to the ligand (Octreotide) at one end, and to the radiotracer indium-111 at the other end [8]. The loop structure and the four receptor binding amino acids, Phe, D-Trp (in place of Trp), Lys, and Thr, are retained. To facilitate firm chelation with DTPA, Phe is replaced by D-Phe [9]. Following intravenous injection, ^{111}In-pentetreotide (OctreoScan) distributes rapidly in the extravascular space with only 33% of the dose remaining in the intravascular pool at the end of 10 min and less than 1% at the end of 20 h. About 50% of the dose is excreted in urine in 6 h, 85% in 24 h, and more than 90% in 72 h. A very small amount is secreted into bile which is excreted in the stool, about 2% of the dose in 72-h stool. The biokinetics of ^{111}In-pentetreotide differ slightly from those of ^{14}C-octreotide. In rats, most of ^{14}C-octreotide enters the liver to be excreted in bile [9], whereas most of ^{111}In-pentetreotide enters the kidney to be excreted in urine [9, 10]. The usual scan dose of ^{111}In-pentetreotide is 3–6 mCi (111–222 MBq) bound to 10 μg of the peptide. The biological half-time of ^{111}In-pentetreotide is about 6 h [9]. In the beginning, most of ^{111}In is attached to the receptors on the surface of the cell. After about 6 h, 50% of the cell radioactivity becomes internalized. Autoradiographic studies show that ^{111}In inside the cell remains with the cytoplasm and the nucleus of cultured cells from carcinoid and glucagonoma [11]. This feature indicates a therapeutic potential for ^{111}In-pentetreotide.

OctreoScan Imaging Protocol

Patient Preparation. Therapy with somatostatin analogues is discontinued for 24–48 h prior to the injection and through the duration of imaging. The patient is hydrated with 16–24 oz. liquids just before and after the dose.

Table 4.4.4. OctreoScan image acquisitotion protocol

Agent	^{111}In-pentetreotide
Dose	3 mCi (111 MBq) for planar and 6 mCi (222 MBq) for SPECT images
Route	Intravenous
Imaging time	4, and 24 h. Repeat at 48 and 72 h if necessary
Bowel preparation	Laxatives (Bisacodyl, fleet enema) before scan
Image acquisition parameters	
Gamma camera	Large field of view camera
Collimator	Medium energy parallel hole collimator
Spectrometer settings	One set over 172 keV and the other over 245 keV energy, 20% window
Matrix	64×64 or 128×128 word matrix
Counts per image	300,000 for head and neck or 10-min image Chest and abdomen, each 500,000 counts or 10 min per view
SPECT protocol	
Matrix	64×64 or 128×128 matrix, 360°, with 4° or 6°, 60–90 stops
Filter	Hamming or Wiener

Somatostatin Receptor Positive Tumors

Successful detection of hepatic and extrahepatic somatostatin receptor positive tumors with ^{111}In-OctreoScan depends upon several factors including tumor size, histology, location, and receptor subtype within the tumor. A clear distinction must be drawn between tumor somatostatin receptor content vs tumor positivity with ^{111}In-OctreoScan. Tumors may have a differing concentration of receptor subtypes with a varying affinity level for somatostatin-14 or somatostatin-28 vs ^{111}In-pentetreotide (Table 4.4.2). Octreotide has a relatively higher affinity for receptor subtypes 2, 3, and 5 than for subtypes 1 and 4. Since ^{111}In-pentetreotide differs in structure slightly from that of octreotide, it could have a slightly different affinity for tumor uptake than octreotide and may explain a lower or higher rate of scintigraphic tumor detection rate in clinical studies.

Overall detection and localization of somatostatin receptor positive tumors with ^{111}In-pentetreotide scintigraphy alone varies from 98% to 100% for Hodgkin's disease, meningioma, lung cancer, and paraganglioma, from 90% to 95% for gastrinoma and carcinoid, and from 80% to 89% for pheochromocytoma and neuroblastoma [12]. The detection and localization of metastatic gastrinoma in the liver (Fig. 4.4.1) is 92% by ^{111}In-pentetreotide scintigraphy alone compared to a sensitivity of 83% by multimo-

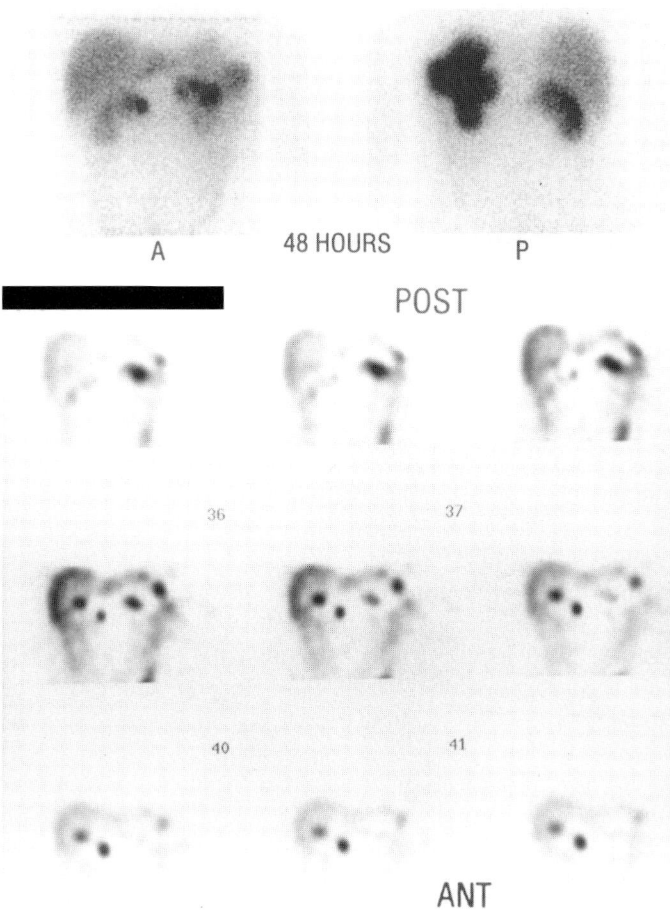

Fig. 4.4.1. Metastatic gastrinoma. Planar images (*top*) in the anterior and posterior view show lesions in parapancreatic and paragastric lymph nodes. Normal activity is seen in the kidneys and spleen. Coronal view SPECT images show (*bottom*) multiple intrahepatic lesions in the liver, not shown by planar images. *Post*, posterior; *Ant*, anterior slices

dality imaging consisting of ultrasound, CT, MRI, and contrast angiogram [13]. Overall, in vivo scintigraphy shows an excellent correlation with in vitro autoradiography, but wide variations are seen in a few specific types of tumors (Table 4.4.3). In vivo scintigraphy with ^{111}In-pentetreotide may often show results much better than those predicted from in vitro autoradiographic studies, suggesting a role for factors other than somatostatin receptor binding alone. Such findings are commonly seen in the case of carcinoid, small cell lung cancer, paraganglioma, neuroblastoma, pheochromocytoma, and medullary thyroid cancer. In the case of insulinoma, growth hormone producing pituitary adenoma, and unclassified APUDomas, scintigraphy may detect lesions less often than predicted from autoradiographic results.

Several factors, both technical and physiological, contribute towards false-positive results which occur in one in ten patients with Zollinger-Ellison syndrome [14]. A high specificity of ^{111}In-somatostatin receptor scintigraphy can be achieved by reducing false-positive results through a clear understanding of the disease and circumstances that cause false-positive scans. An intrahepatic gallbladder may mimic hepatic metastasis by accumulating the radiotracer secreted into bile. An improvement in specificity aids the proper management of patients.

Radiation Dosimetry

Following intravenous injection, ^{111}In-OctreoScan is distributed diffusely throughout the body. Good hydration and frequent urination reduce the radiation dose to the organs [15]. A dose of 3 mCi ^{111}In-pentetreotide is sufficient for planar imaging and a dose of 6 mCi is required for a SPECT study. SPECT imaging has now become a routine standard for achieving the best sensitivity and specificity of the test. SPECT of chest, abdomen, and pelvis is obtained routinely. Kidneys are the critical organs receiving the largest dose, followed by the spleen, urinary bladder, and liver [16]. The radiation to the kidneys from a 6-mCi (222 MBq) dose is 11.4 rad (115 mGy). The effective dose equivalent is 2.28 rem/6 mCi (22.8 mSv/222 MBq). Internalization of ^{111}In into cytoplasm and nucleus of the cells from carcinoid and glucagonoma from ^{111}In-pentetreotide raises the therapeutic potential for ^{111}In [11].

The somatostatin receptor status of the tumor may have a great impact on clinical diagnosis and management, especially in the selection of type of therapy. Documentation of somatostatin receptor positivity can reduce the number and necessity of other diagnostic imaging tests. It is suggested that somatostatin receptor scintigraphy be used as the imaging modality of first choice in the case of gastrinoma because of its cost-effectiveness and also for its impact on patient management [17, 18]. Somatostatin receptor positive tumors have been successfully treated medically with a combination of octreotide and prednisone [19]. Attempts are being made to label somatostatin analogues with technetium-99m, which should further impact favorably on cost containment [20].

References

1. Krulich L, Dhariwal APS, McCann SM. Stimulatory and inhibitory effects of purified hypothalamic extracts on growth hormone release from rat pituitary in-vitro. Endocrinology 1968;83:783–790
2. Reichlin S. Somatostatin. (First of two parts). N Engl J Med 1983;309:1495–1501
3. Reichlin S. Somatostatin. (Second of two parts). N Engl J Med 1983;309:1556–1563
4. Reubi JC, Kvols L, Krenning E, Lamberts SWJ. Distribution of somatostatin receptors in normal and tumor mice. Metabolism 1990;39:78–81
5. Lamberts SWJ, Vanderlely A, De Herder WW, Hofland LJ. Octreotide. N Engl J Med 1996;334:246–254
6. Krenning EP, Bakker WH, Breeman WAP et al. Localization of endocrine-related tumors with radioiodinated analogue of somatostatin. Lancet 1989;1:242–244
7. Kvols LK, Brown ML, O'Connor MK et al. Evaluation of a radiolabeled somatostatin analogue (I-123 octreotide) in the detection and localization of carcinoid and islet cell tumors. Radiology 1993;187:129–133
8. Krenning EP, Bakker WH, Kooiji PPM et al. Somatostatin receptor scintigraphy with Indium-111 DTPA-D-Phe-1-Octreotide in man. Metabolism, dosimetry, and comparisons with Iodine-123-Tyr-3-Octreotide. J Nucl Med 1992;33:652–658
9. Somatostatin receptor imaging for neuroendocrine tumors. Product monograph. OctreoScan. Mallincrodt Medical Inc. Mallincrodt Nuclear Medicine Division, St. Louis, MO. 1994
10. Krenning EP, Kwekkeboom DJ, Bakker WH, et al. Somatostatin receptor scintigraphy with (In-111-DTPA-D-Phe-1) and (I-123-Tyr-3)-Octreotide: the Rotterdam experience with more than 1,000 patients. Eur J Nucl Med 1993;20:716–731
11. Andersson P, Forssel-Aronsson E, Johanson V, Wangberg B, Nilsson O, Fjalling M, Ahlman H. Internalization of Indium-111 into human neuroendocrine tumor cells after incubation with Indium-111-D-Phe-1-Octreotide. J Nucl Med 1996;37:2002–2006
12. Krenning EP, Kwekkeboom DJ, Pauwels S, Kvols K, Reubi JC. Somatostatin receptor scintigraphy. In: Freeman LM (ed) Nuclear Medicine Annual 1995. Raven Press Ltd., New York 1995, pp 1–50
13. Gibril F, Reynolds JC, Doppman JL, Chen CC, Venzon DJ, Tremanini B, Weber HC, Stewart CA, Jensen RT. Somatostatin receptor scintigraphy: its sensitivity compared with that of other imaging methods in detecting primary and metastatic gastrinoma; A prospective study. Ann Intern Med 1996;125:26–34
14. Gibril F, Reynolds JC, Chen CC, Yu F, Goebel SU, Serrano J, Doppman JL, Jensen RT. Specificity of somatostatin receptor scintigraphy: a prospective study and effects of false-positive localization on management in patients with gastrinomas. J Nucl Med 1999;40539:553
15. Yamada T, Niinuma K, Lemaire M, Terasaki T, Sugiyama Y. Mechanism of the tissue distribution and biliary excretion of the cyclic peptide octreotide. J Pharmacol Exp Ther 1996;279:1357–1364
16. Stabin MG, Kooji PPM, Bakker WH, Inoue T, Endo K, Coveney J, deJong R, Minegishi A. Radiation dosimetry for Indium-111-pentetreotide. J Nucl Med 1997;38:1919–1922
17. Termanini B, Gibril F, Reynolds JC, Doppman JL, Chen CC, Stewart CA, Sutliff VE, Jensen RT. Value of somatostatin receptor scintigraphy: A prospective study in gastrinoma of its effects on clinical management. Gastroenterology 1997;112:335–347
18. Jamar F, Fiasse R, Laners N, Pauwels S. Somatostatin receptor imaging with Indium-111-pentetreotide in gastroenteropancreatic neuroendocrine tumors: Safety, efficacy and impact on patient management. J Nucl Med 1995;36:542–549
19. Palmieri G, Lastoria S, Colao A, Vergara E, Varrella P, Biondi E, Selleri C, Catalano L, Lombardi G, Bianco AR, Salvatore M. Successful treatment of a patient with a thymoma and pure red-cell aplasia with octreotide and prednisone. N Engl J Med 1997;336:263–265
20. Vallabhajosula S, Moyer BR, Lister-James J, McBride BJ, Lipszyc H, Lee H, Bastidas D, Dean RT. Preclinical evaluation of Technetium-99m-labeled somatostatin receptor-binding peptides. J Nucl Med 1996;37:1016–1022

Imaging and Quantification of Hepatobiliary Function

5.1 Hepatobiliary Imaging

The liver is one of the most frequently imaged organs in the body using ultrasound, CT, MRI, or scintigraphy. The first three of these imaging techniques depend upon morphological changes to detect disease, whereas scintigraphy uses both morphological and physiological changes to discover liver pathology. Since physiological changes usually precede morphological alterations by several weeks or months, there is great potential for early diagnosis by scintigraphy, well before irreversible functional changes take place. Once very popular, imaging with radiocolloids has now been almost completely replaced by quantitative hepatobiliary functional imaging with ^{99m}Tc-HIDA [1].

Functional studies are obtained with the protocol outlined in Table 5.1.1, by using any one of several ^{99m}Tc-HIDA agents, which delineates the entire hepatobiliary tree as it travels from the hepatocyte to enter the duodenum (Fig. 3.1.2, Chap. 3]. Time of appearance of various normal biliary structures depends upon many factors of which the tonus of the sphincter of Oddi plays the major role [2]. Following intravenous injection of ^{99m}Tc-disofenin or ^{99m}Tc-mebrofenin, the liver peak uptake is reached within 10 min, and the common bile duct is seen by 20 min. Both the gallbladder and small intestine are seen within 30 min in the great majority of patients (Table 5.1.2). Some patients show a reciprocal relationship between the time of appearance of the gallbladder and small intestine, the intestine appearing late when the gallbladder appears early and vice versa. Normally about 50% of gallbladders are seen within 15 min, 90% within 30 min, and 95% within 50 min. In the remaining 5%, gallbladders appear between 50 and 60 min after injection of the radiotracer [3].

Identification of Lobes, Segments, and Areas from ^{99m}Tc-HIDA Images

Physiologically, the liver is divided into three lobes (including the caudate lobe), four segments, and eight areas (Fig. 5.1.1). The right lobe is divided into anterior and posterior segments; and the left lobe into medial and lateral segments. The right and left branches of the portal vein travel through the middle of the liver in opposite directions and divide the liver into a superior and inferior area. The right and left lobe each consists of four areas. The caudate lobe is situated along the superior margin of the posterior surface and is considered an independent lobe because of its unique blood supply. Its veins drain blood directly into the inferior vena cava.

Liver division into physiologic right and left lobes is currently preferred over anatomic division because it serves as a useful boundary line during surgical resection of the liver. The lobes, segments, and areas are identified on an anterior, right lateral, and a posterior view image, much like identifying the lobes and segments of a lung from a perfusion scan. Obstruction of a segment or an area bile duct is seen as bile stasis over the corresponding region, similar to identifying a lack of perfusion of a lobe or segment in a lung scan due to pulmonary embolism. The numbers shown in Fig. 5.1.1 are adopted from Table 1.1.1 of Chap. 1, as developed by different authors over the years. Healy and Schroy suggested a directional nomenclature after careful dissection of nearly 100 cadaver livers [4].

Table 5.1.1. Hepatobiliary imaging protocol

Patient preparation	Patient should fast overnight (6–10 h optimal), minimum 4 h, and maximum 24 h. Give 0.01 μg/kg (10 ng/kg) CCK-8 intravenously when patient is fasting for longer than 24 h or on parenteral nutrition. Wait for 60 min after CCK-8 to begin hepatic phase imaging with ^{99m}Tc-HIDA
Agent	^{99m}Tc-Mebrofenin or ^{99m}Tc-disofenin
Dose	Adults: 2–4 mCi (74-148 MBq) for serum bilirubin less than 2 mg% 5–8 mCi (185-296 MBq) for serum bilirubin 3–10 mg% 10 mCi (370 MBq) for serum bilirubin greater than 11 mg% Children: 200 μCi/kg (7.4 MBq/kg) (minimum 1 mCi (37 MBq))
Position	Supine
Camera	Large field of view gamma camera
Collimator	Low energy, all purpose, parallel hole
Window	20% at 140 keV photopeak
Matrix	64+64+16
Computer data acquisition	Data acquisition is separated into two parts: (1) hepatic phase and (2) gallbladder phase.
Hepatic phase	1 frame/min for 60 min (0–60 min). Obtain a right lateral view when gallbladder appearance is not certain at 60 min
Gallbladder phase	1 frame/min for 30 min (61–90 min). Delayed images are obtained at 2–4 h or at 24 h when needed
Cholecystokinin dose preparation and administration	The dose is prepared as per instructions in the package insert (Kinevac, Bracco Diagnostics, Princeton, NJ). The recommended dose in the package insert is for oral cholecystogram and for stimulating pancreatic enzyme secretion. This dose is too large for cholescintigraphy and should be avoided. The recommended dose for cholescintigraphy is 10 ng/kg infused slowly over 3 min (3.3 ng/kg/min for 3 min) through an infusion pump

Table 5.1.2. Time of appearance of normal common bile duct, gallbladder, and small intestine [3]

Appearance of common bile duct	
Within 20 min	100%
Appearance of gallbladder	
Within 15 min	50%
Within 30 min	90%
Within 50 min	95%
Within 60 min	100%
Appearance of small intestine	
Within 60 min	80%

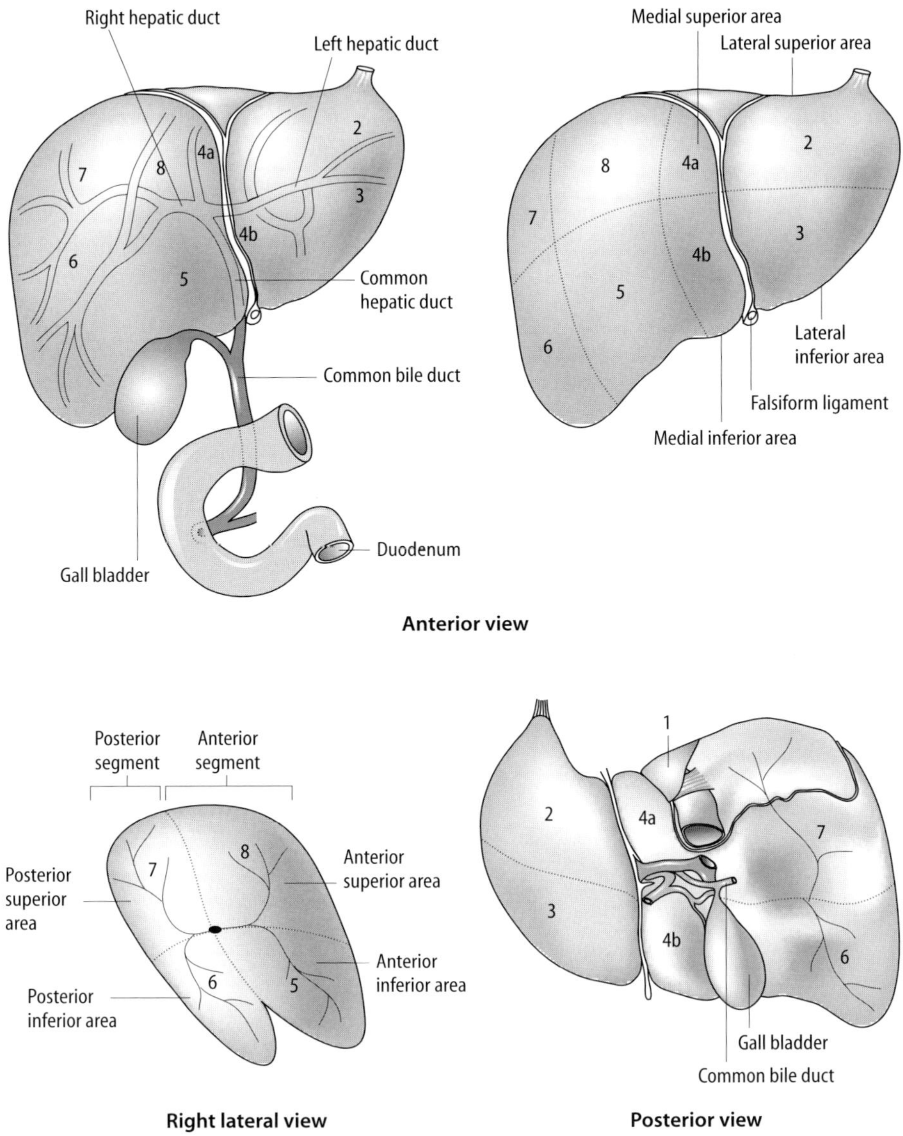

Fig. 5.1.1. Biliary anatomy. The bile ducts from the medial (#4a, 4b) and lateral (#2, 3) segments of the left lobe unite to form the left hepatic duct (LHD), and are seen separately in an anterior image. The ducts from the anterior (#5, 8) and posterior (#6, 7) segments of the right lobe join to form the right hepatic duct (RHD), and a right lateral view is required to separate them and their branches. RHD and LHD unite to form the common hepatic duct which in turn forms the common bile duct after joining with the cystic duct from the gallbladder. The caudate lobe in the posterior view is usually obscured by photon attenuation by vertebral bodies

The medial segment of the physiologic left lobe (4a, 4b) becomes a part of the right lobe when the liver is divided morphologically into right and left lobes on the basis of the attachment of the falciform ligament. The caudate lobe (#1) is posterior in location, but usually not seen on a posterior view image due to attenuation of photons by the vertebrae. The inferior area of the medial segment of the physiologic left lobe (4b) is often referred to as the quadrate lobe.

There are many variations in the manner in which the segmental ducts unite to form lobar ducts. The right hepatic duct is formed by the union of its anterior and posterior segmental ducts and the left hepatic duct by the union of its medial and lateral segmental ducts in 72% of patients. The posterior segmental duct from the right lobe joins the left hepatic duct directly in 22% of patients. In the remaining 6%, the anterior segmental duct from the right lobe joins with the left hepatic duct directly [4]. It is very rare for the bile from either the medial or lateral segmental duct of the left lobe to drain directly into one of the segmental ducts of the right lobe (Fig. 1.1.6, Chap. 1).

The distal 0.5–1.5 cm of the right and left hepatic ducts, and the entire common hepatic and common bile ducts, are outside the liver parenchyma (extrahepatic), although they may appear as intrahepatic in an anterior view ^{99m}Tc-HIDA study. This apparent depiction is due to extension of the inferior liver border in front of these ducts. The common hepatic duct usually measures about 2–7 cm and the common bile duct about 7–17 cm in length. The total length of the common duct (common hepatic plus common bile ducts) from its origin at the union of the right and left hepatic ducts to its termination in the duodenum varies from 10 to 20 cm. On a ^{99m}Tc-HIDA image, however, total length of the common duct is about 6.6±1.3 cm [3]. This foreshortening is caused by the position of the gamma camera (placed anteriorly) and its relationship with the direction of the common hepatic and common bile duct.

Duct Asymmetry

Asymmetry in appearance of the right and left hepatic duct is common on cholescintigraphy. Normally the left hepatic duct appears more prominent than the right in 55% of subjects, the right hepatic duct more prominent than the left in 13%, and both ducts appear equal in 10% of subjects (Table 5.1.3). In the remaining 22% of subjects neither duct is seen because of rapid bile flow through a lax sphincter of Oddi [3]. Several reasons are offered for duct asymmetry and these include: (1) a more anterior location of the left liver lobe than the right, (2) a more anterior location of the left hepatic duct in comparison to the right hepatic duct, (3) a variant bile flow pattern where either the posterior or the anterior segmental duct from the right lobe drains bile directly into the left hepatic duct, (4) an undivided portion of left hepatic duct is twice as long as that of the right duct and hence prone to tortuosity, impeding bile flow through it, and (5) a short right hepatic duct which lies in direct line with the common hepatic duct offers less impedance to bile flow through it. A slower bile flow allows relatively more counts to accumulate in the image to manifest an apparent prominence.

Hepatobiliary studies are usually carried out 6–10 h after the fast which establishes the basal state. Fasting less than 4 h or more than 24 h is avoided. Cholecystokinin reaches its lowest serum level during fasting, promoting a maximum increase in the tonus of the sphincter of Oddi and maximum relaxation of the smooth muscle of the gallbladder wall. Both of these factors acting together promote rapid filling of the gallbladder to its full volume of 50 ml. The liver normally secretes about 600 ml bile per day (0.4 ml/min) continuously, of which about 70% (0.3 ml/min) enters the gallbladder, and the remaining 30% (0.1 ml/min) enters the duodenum directly during fasting [5, 6]. A fully filled gallbladder is still able to accommodate this constant inflow of hepatic bile (0.3 ml/min) by absorbing an equal volume of water through the wall. The lateral intercellular spaces between the columnar epithelial calls are kept widely open during fasting allowing free passage of water from the gallbladder lumen into the interstitium. Fasting for less than 4 h results in either non-visualization or low ^{99m}Tc-HIDA counts within the gallbladder due to preferential flow of bile directly into the duodenum through a lax sphincter of Oddi.

Table 5.1.3. Variations in the appearance of the normal right and left hepatic ducts [3]

Left hepatic duct more prominent than right hepatic duct	55%
Right hepatic duct more prominent than left hepatic duct	13%
Right hepatic duct = left hepatic duct	10%
Neither duct seen clearly	22%

Effect of Food Intake on Uptake and Excretion of ^{99m}Tc-HIDA

Physiological changes that take place soon after a meal affect some of the functional parameters obtained with ^{99m}Tc-HIDA and should be taken into account during data interpretation. In the immediate postprandial state, time to peak hepatic uptake of ^{99m}Tc-HIDA decreases, compared to studies performed after 6–10 h of fasting (Fig. 5.1.2). These changes are attributed to an increase in postprandial liver blood flow and faster extraction of ^{99m}Tc-HIDA by the liver [7]. The radiotracer also clears from the liver parenchyma much more rapidly in the immediate postprandial state, which is attributed to an increase in ductal bile flow induced by endogenous release of secretin, cholecystokinin, and other gastrointestinal hormones. Faster uptake combined with rapid clearance shifts the peak of the hepatic curve to an earlier time. The gallbladder does not fill in due to its contraction induced by postprandial release of endogenous cholecystokinin. When the gallbladder is the organ for study, it is essential to maximize hepatic bile entry into it by fasting for at least 8–10 h, when both the absorption of water through the wall and the tonus of the sphincter of Oddi are at their peak [8]. Longer duration of fasting provides a better counting statistics due to preferential entry of ^{99m}Tc-HIDA mixed hepatic bile into the gallbladder [9]. Fasting longer than 24 h has an adverse effect on gallbladder filling due to formation of bile sludge.

Quantification of Liver Function

Besides providing an excellent morphology of the entire hepatobiliary system, imaging with ^{99m}Tc-HIDA enables simultaneous quantification of liver function as an integral part of imaging. Traditionally the liver function is monitored by obtaining the serum level of various substances handled by the liver including albumin, bilirubin, alkaline phosphatase, and transaminase. Serum levels are indirect indicators of liver function and are influenced by the status of the cardiac and renal function, and hence may not reflect

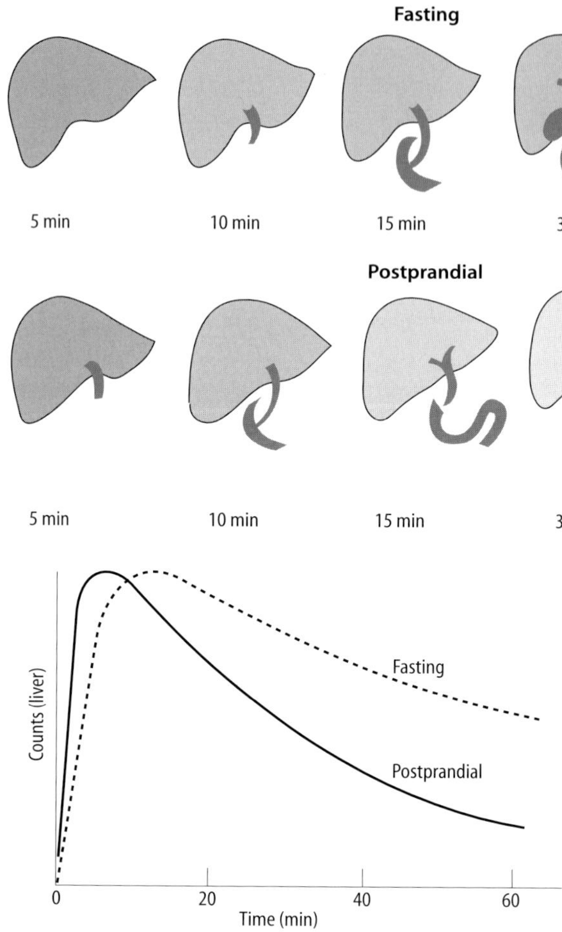

Fig. 5.1.2. Effect of feeding on the kinetics of ^{99m}Tc-HIDA: In the fasting state (*top*), increased tonus of the sphincter of Oddi diverts much of the hepatic bile into the gallbladder. There is some residual radioactivity in the liver at 60 min. In the postprandial state (*bottom*), there is more rapid hepatic uptake and excretion, shifting the peak of the curve to an earlier time, and very little residual radioactivity remains in the liver beyond 15 min. The gallbladder does not fill in due to a lax sphincter of oddi

accurately the hepatocyte function in the presence of heart or kidney failure. Measurement of radioactivity emitted from the liver serves as a direct indicator of the physiological status of the hepatocyte, unaffected by renal function. The biokinetic pathways of ^{99m}Tc-HIDA which involve several steps before its elimination from the liver into small intestine (Chap. 3.1) enable not only quantification but also differentiation of hepatocyte from biliary disease. Hepatic extraction fraction and excretion half-time are two of the functional parameters measured routinely as an integral part of hepatobiliary imaging [1].

Hepatic Extraction Fraction (HEF). The patient is positioned supine underneath a large field of view gamma camera and the data are collected as described in Table 5.1.1.

Regions of interest (ROI) are drawn over the heart, liver, and spleen (Fig. 5.1.3). Each ROI consists of at least 75–100 pixels. The heart ROI includes both ventricles. The liver ROI includes mostly the right upper lobe, right lower lobe, and left lobe. Care is taken to avoid inclusion of heart and bile ducts within the liver ROI. Superior and right lateral liver margins, which move in and out of ROI during deep inspiration or upon coughing, and the gallbladder, are also excluded from the liver ROI. The spleen is seen only in a few of the early images (0- to 4-min frames) and its ROI may be superimposed by jejunal bile radioactivity in late images. After selecting ROI, the entire 60-min study is reviewed in cine display to insure separation of the regions. Regions are altered if there is superimposition by other structures.

The liver curve is smoothed first and then subjected to deconvolution. The liver true response curve is deconvoluted from the input (heart) and output (liver) curve using the Fourier transformation technique. The deconvolution corrects for systemic recirculation of the injected radiotracer [10]. A smooth decreasing long tail in the shape of one-half of a cosine wave is appended to the end of the input and output curve. This long tail avoids errors due to abrupt data termination at 30 min. The append begins at the 30th frame and falls to zero at the 128th added frame, giving approximately 6 times the duration of acquisition [11]. A duration of such a length is a minimum to avoid artifacts in the deconvolution process. The formula for the appended tail in frame *i* of the heart or liver curve is given by:

$$\text{Tail} = 0.5 \times \text{AMP} \times (\cos\,[\pi \times (i-30)/(128-30)]+1).$$

where $i = 30$–128 and AMP is the heart or liver curve value (counts per pixel) at frame 30.

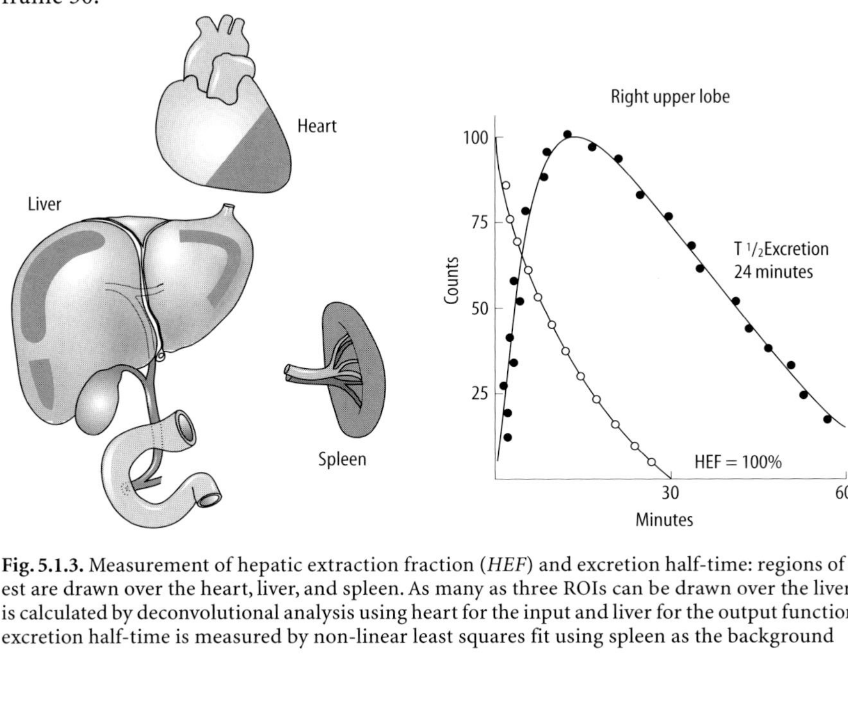

Fig. 5.1.3. Measurement of hepatic extraction fraction (*HEF*) and excretion half-time: regions of interest are drawn over the heart, liver, and spleen. As many as three ROIs can be drawn over the liver. HEF is calculated by deconvolutional analysis using heart for the input and liver for the output function. The excretion half-time is measured by non-linear least squares fit using spleen as the background

The hepatic extraction (HEF) is the ratio of the *Y* intercept of the exponential fit to the maximum data point in the liver response curve. The exponential fit is by linear least square, working in reverse from 30 min to the first frame which visually departs significantly from the exponential fit. HEF is calculated by the following equation:

$$\text{Hepatic Extraction Fraction (HEF)} = \frac{\text{Y intercept exponential fit liver response curve}}{\text{Y-MAX data value liver response curve}}$$

When the gamma camera collects counts over the liver, the counts come from both the hepatocytes and the hepatic blood pool. Deconvolutional technique separates hepatocyte counts from the hepatic blood pool counts. A deconvoluted liver curve, therefore, represents a hypothetical true response as though ^{99m}Tc-HIDA was injected directly into the hepatic artery or portal vein. Normal hepatic extraction fraction with ^{99m}Tc-mebrofenin and ^{99m}Tc-disofenin varies from 92% to 100%. Extraction fraction decreases as the hepatocyte function decreases. Functional changes show good correlation with Child's classification (Table 5.1.4) of the severity of liver disease [11].

Table 5.1.4. Child's classification of liver disease

Clinical and laboratory findings	Child's class		
	A	B	C
Ascites	None	Controlled	Uncontrolled
Neurological findings	None	Minimal	Advanced
Nutrition	Excellent	Good	Poor
Bilirubin (mg%)	<2.0	2.0–3.0	>3.0
Albumin (g%)	>3.5	3.0–3.5	<3.0

Hepatic Excretion Half-time. After the uptake, ^{99m}Tc-HIDA is secreted by the hepatocytes in its native state into bile canaliculi, where it mixes thoroughly with the bile. Secretion of radioactive bile into canaliculi serves as the direct in vivo, non-invasive method of radiolabeling hepatic bile, without altering basal liver physiology. After mixing with the canalicular bile, ^{99m}Tc-HIDA follows the path taken by the hepatic bile. Excretion half-time is a measure of how fast the radiotracer is secreted by the hepatocyte into bile canaliculi, and how rapidly it moves through the intrahepatic bile ducts to enter the common hepatic duct and common bile duct, and finally into the gallbladder and duodenum. Measurement of excretion half-time uses the liver and spleen ROI (Fig. 5.1.3). Since both the liver and spleen receive their arterial blood supply from a common source, the celiac artery, the spleen serves as the most appropriate organ for subtraction of the blood background. Background subtracted liver curve is modeled by an uptake and excretion compartment and is given by the following equation [11]:

$$L(t) = k\,(e^{-0.693\, t/\mathrm{TE}} - e^{0.693\, t/T\,U}),$$

where $L(t)$ = background corrected liver counts/pixel at time t, k = a constant of the model, TE = excretion effective $T_{1/2}$, and TU = uptake effective $T_{1/2}$.

The hepatic phase data are collected for 60 min. Calculation of HEF uses only the first 30 min data, whereas excretion $T_{1/2}$ uses all 60-min data points. Only right upper lobe values are shown here for clarity and simplicity. In patients with normal liver function or with mild liver disease with serum bilirubin levels less than 5 mg%, both HEF and $T_{1/2}$ excretion can be obtained by collecting data for only 30 or 45 min. In patients with moderate to severe liver disease (serum bilirubin levels above 5 mg%), it is necessary to collect data for a minimum of 60 min to obtain a reliable excretion half-time [12]. The normal $T_{1/2}$ excretion value for ^{99m}Tc-mebrofenin and ^{99m}Tc-disofenin ranges from 11 to 32 min. Both HEF and $T_{1/2}$ excretion can be calculated using semiautomatic software which is shown to be highly reproducible, both within and between institutions, and among different technologists [13]. HEF values remain within a normal range in early biliary disease, but decrease in hepatocellular disease. When the biliary disease is severe and progressive, the HEF value begins to decrease. Excretion half-time, on the other hand, increases in both hepatocyte and biliary disease, starting from the very beginning. Both parameters provide a measure of the severity of hepatobiliary disease, irrespective of the etiology (Fig. 5.1.4A–C).

Effect of Bile Duct Obstruction on Liver Function. In the case of hyperacute or acute total obstruction of the common bile duct, HEF values remain within a normal range for 4–5 days, as long as the serum bilirubin level remains below 8 mg% (Fig. 5.1.4A). HEF begins to decrease when obstruction persists and serum bilirubin level rises above 8 mg% [14]. Excretion half-time continues to increase from the very beginning (Fig. 5.1.4B). Prolongation of excretion half-time in biliary obstruction is due to bile stasis within the canaliculi and intrahepatic bile ducts. In congenital biliary atresia, a condition due to extrahepatic bile duct obstruction, HEF remains high for about 2 months after birth and then begins to decrease if the obstruction is not relieved [15, 16]. Excretion half-time and HEF show an inverse relationship; as the HEF decreases, excretion half-time increases and vice versa (Fig. 5.1.4C). A high serum bilirubin level decreases HEF by two mechanisms; first it displaces ^{99m}Tc-HIDA from its carrier protein, albumin, and, second, bilirubin competes with ^{99m}Tc-HIDA for the hepatocyte uptake by receptor mediated endocytosis.

Differential Hepatic Bile Flow and Gallbladder Filling. A normal gallbladder which measures about 50 ml in volume requires at least 3–4 h to fill to its full capacity, after a complete emptying. Since the gallbladder is already filled to its full capacity after an overnight fasting, two mechanisms are responsible for accommodating a constant inflow of 0.3 ml/min of the hepatic bile: (1) absorption of water through the gallbladder wall and (2) an increase in tonus of the sphincter of Oddi. During fasting, the gallbladder wall absorbs water from the lumen through widely opened lateral intercellular spaces between the columnar cells of the mucosa. Bile salts, bile pigments, cholesterol, and other bile constituents are not absorbed. This process of selective absorption of water resulting in higher concentration of solutes is called concentration function of the gallbladder [8]. The second mechanism responsible for hepatic bile entry into the gallbladder is the tonus of the sphincter of Oddi. After an overnight fast, the mean pressure within the sphincter of Oddi is 15 mmHg, 12 mmHg in the common bile duct

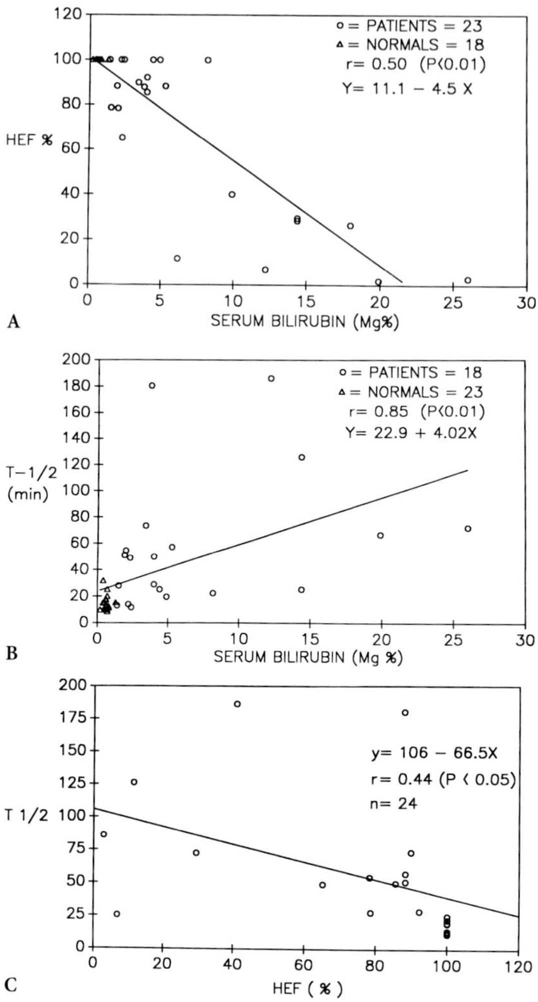

Fig. 5.1.4. Hepatic extraction fraction (*HEF*) and excretion half-time in health and disease (11). HEF remains near normal level in early obstruction and begins to decrease as bilirubin increases (**A**). Excretion half-time increases from the very beginning, and rises further as serum bilirubin value increases (**B**). HEF and excretion half-time show an inverse relationship (**C**)

and 10 mmHg inside the gallbladder. Because of the pressure difference at various levels, hepatic bile follows the path of least resistance and enters the gallbladder. The volume of hepatic bile that partitions between the gallbladder and small intestine is primarily controlled by the tonus of the sphincter of Oddi.

Bile secreted by the liver during a 60-min period of ^{99m}Tc-HIDA hepatobiliary imaging enters the gallbladder and small intestine. The quantity of bile that partitions between these two structures is measured using the hepatic phase data. One ROI is drawn over the gallbladder and another over the rest of the abdomen, excluding the liver and the gallbladder (Fig. 5.1.5A). Time/activity curves are generated over both regions and the counts are decay corrected (Fig. 5.1.5B). Bile produced during each minute is obtained by summing the gallbladder and intestinal counts for that minute [6, 17]. Total bile produced during 60 min of imaging is obtained by adding gallbladder and intestinal counts at 60 min. The percentage of the hepatic bile entering the gallbladder is obtained by the following formula:

$$\text{Hepatic Bile Flow into gallbladder (\%)} = \frac{\text{Gallbladder total counts at 60 min} \times 100}{\text{Gallbladder total counts at 60 min} + \text{Intestinal total counts at 60 mins}}$$

$$= \frac{49{,}700 \times 100}{49{,}700 + 50{,}300}$$

$$\text{Hepatic bile flow into gallbladder} = 49.7\ \%$$

$$\text{Hepatic bile flow into small intensine} = 50.3\ \%$$

Bile from the common hepatic duct enters the gallbladder in a stepwise fashion and corresponds to the phasic waves passing through the sphincter of Oddi [17]. After passing through the cystic duct, the radioactive hepatic bile first collects at the gallbladder neck and then mixes thoroughly with the rest of the bile in the body and fundus. Often a septum divides the gallbladder into two separate compartments when mixing of the radiolabeled hepatic bile occurs first with the proximal compartment bile, followed by mixing with bile in the distal compartment. By drawing one ROI over the proximal compartment and the other over the distal compartment, a differential bile entry into each compartment can be measured. Compartments are easy to recognize in the early images, but become more difficult in late images as radioactivity equilibrates with bile in both compartments. It is essential to recognize such compart-

A

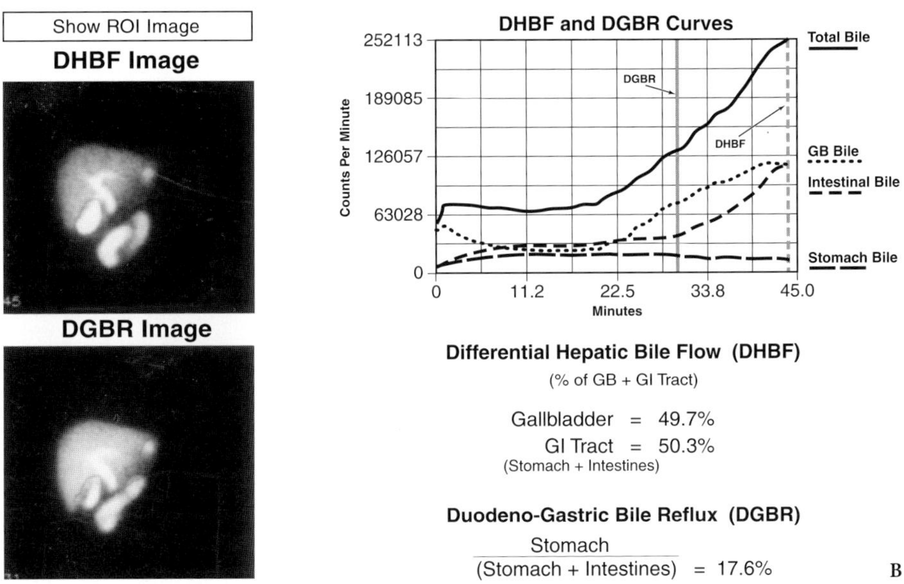

B

Fig. 5.1.5. Differential hepatic bile flow and duodenogastric bile reflux. One ROI is drawn over each of the gallbladder, stomach, and intestine (**A**). Total bile counts are obtained by adding gallbladder, stomach, and intestinal counts. Differential bile flow into the gallbladder vs intestine is calculated. Duodenogastric bile reflux is obtained by dividing the stomach counts by stomach plus intestinal counts (**B**).

ments while measuring the gallbladder ejection fraction, as the two compartments may show different degrees of emptying. By marking a separate ROI over the stomach region, duodenogastric bile reflux can be calculated (see 5.4).

Quantification of Gallbladder Function

Gallbladder Emptying (Ejection Fraction). Measurement of gallbladder emptying has become popular recently primarily due to availability of a simple and reliable diagnostic test. Gallbladder volume was estimated in the past using an oral cholecystogram by applying a technique called the sum of the cylinder method, introduced first in 1949 by De Silva [18]. On the oral cholecystogram, the gallbladder is divided into several small cylinders and the volume of each cylinder is computed by applying a mathematical formula for the volume of a cylinder. By summing the volume of all cylinders, gallbladder total volume is estimated. A slightly modified version of the sum of the cylinder method has been adopted for measuring the gallbladder volume with ultrasound [19]. Both the oral cholecystogram and ultrasound are geometric techniques and are based on an assumption that the gallbladder is a cylinder before, during, and after contraction. It is frequently seen that the gallbladder is not a cylinder before contraction and it often changes its shape during and after contraction. A count based, non-geometric technique overcomes these shortcomings [20]. Cholescintigraphy with ^{99m}Tc-HIDA is a non-geometric method and enables precise measurement of both ejection fraction and ejection rate. The scintigraphic method uses ^{99m}Tc-HIDA counts, which show a linear relationship with bile within the gallbladder (Fig. 5.1.6).

Data Collection. The gallbladder phase data are acquired on the computer using the protocol outlined in Table 5.1.1, at 1 frame/min for 30 min when CCK-8 is used. The data should be collected for a minimum of 60 min, preferably 60–120 min, when a fatty meal is used as the stimulus to induce gallbladder contraction. A magnification factor of 1.2–2.4 may be used during data acquisition. The gamma camera angle is changed to a degree that maximally separates the CBD from the gallbladder and the duodenum [9]. Infusion of CCK-8 is begun at 5 min and continued for 3 min. The first 5-min counts represent the gallbladder basal volume.

Dose and Duration of Cholecystokinin Infusion

In the United States, a fragment of the hormone cholecystokinin is available for clinical use as CCK-8. In Europe and other continents, the entire molecule with 33–39 amino acids is made available. The hormone is prepared as per the manufacturer's instructions in the package insert (sincalide, Bracco Lab., Princeton, NJ). Volume is adjusted with saline to achieve the desired dose rate and duration of infusion. Most clinical protocols adopt a 3-min infusion. Some prefer a longer duration of infusion of 45–60 min. Selection of a proper dose and dose rate within the physiologic range is critical; duration of infusion then becomes a matter of personal preference. A CCK-8 dose of 10 ng/kg (0.01 μg/kg) is infused slowly over 3 min (a dose rate of 3.3 ng/kg/min for 3 min). Before the test begins, the patient is instructed to raise the hand as soon as the symptoms begin, and raise the hand again when symptoms abate. The technologist notes the time of onset and total duration of symptoms on a work sheet. Usual symptoms in-

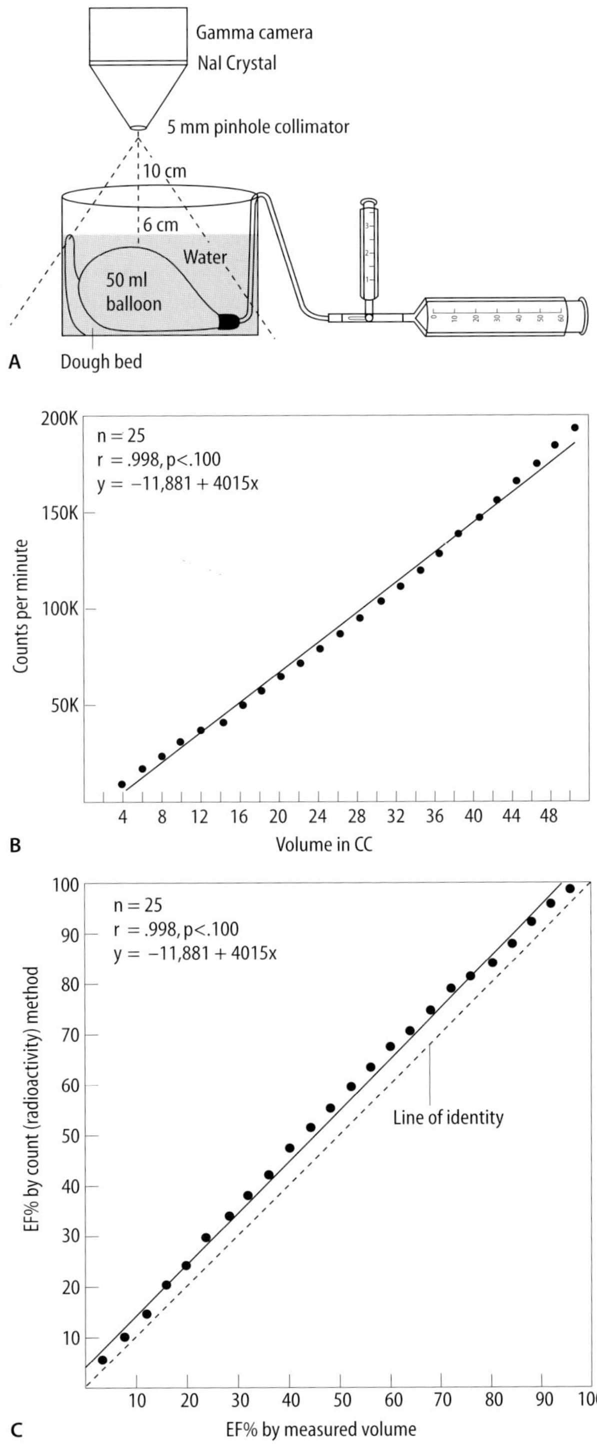

Fig. 5.1.6. Gallbladder bile volume and ^{99m}Tc-HIDA count relationship. A rubber balloon filled with 50 ml water and ^{99m}Tc representing the gallbladder is placed inside a container placed underneath a gamma camera. One milliliter of water is removed at a time through the syringe and counts are taken with the gamma camera after each withdrawal (**A**). Counts show a linear relationship with the bile volume (**B**). Ejection fraction measured by volume and ^{99m}Tc-HIDA counts methods show a perfect linear (**C**) relationship [20]

clude abdominal pain, nausea, and/or abdominal discomfort. Symptoms may also be indicated on the gallbladder time/activity curve [21].

Effect of Non-Physiologic Dose of Cholecystokinin

The package insert in the kit (sincalide, Kinevac by Bracco Diagnostics, Princeton, NJ) suggests a CCK-8 dose of 0.02 μg/kg (20 ng/kg) infused over 30 or 60 s. This dose rate was originally developed for the oral cholecystogram and for induction of pancreatic enzyme secretion for duodenal aspiration. Recent studies have demonstrated that this dose rate is too large for cholescintigraphy and often produces a low ejection fraction in 20–26% of normal subjects [22–25]. A normal gallbladder ejection fraction value of 35% or higher is based on a CCK-8 dose of 10 ng/kg, infused over 3 min (3.3 ng/kg/min for 3 min). A change in dose, dose rate, and/or duration of infusion may produce different values for the gallbladder ejection fraction (Table 5.1.5). It is preferable to establish local values when the technique chosen is different from that in the published literature [26].

Table 5.1.5. Effect of dose and duration of CCK-8 infusion on gallbladder ejection fraction (means ± SE)

CCK-8 dose rate [ref.]	Duration of CCK-8 infusion 3 min	30 min	60 min
0.5 ng/kg/min [27]	–	79.3%±6.9%	91.3%±5.3%
3.3 ng/kg/min (10 ng/kg/3 min) [23]	59.4%±4.0%	–	–
5.0 ng/kg/min [27]	–	82.4%±6.7%	94.0%±5.1%

Calculation of Gallbladder Ejection Fraction

Any one of the first five frames, or a summed image of the first five frames of the gallbladder phase data, is chosen for selection of five ROI: (1) gallbladder, (2) common bile duct, (3) a Y-shaped region encompassing the common hepatic duct and right and left hepatic ducts, (4) duodenum, and (5) background region over the liver. The background ROI is superior and lateral to the gallbladder (Fig. 5.1.7). Net gallbladder counts are obtained after subtraction of the background counts and decay corrected [9]. The ejection fraction is calculated by noting counts before and after emptying of the gallbladder (Fig. 5.1.8):

$$\text{Gallbladder ejection fraction (GBEF) (\%)} = \frac{\text{Net GB Peak counts (A)} - \text{First minimum net GB counts (B)} \times 100}{\text{Net GB Peak counts (A)}}$$

$$\text{GBEF} = \frac{A - B \times 100}{A}$$

Ejection period = Time from GB Peak counts to first minimum counts (B–A)
Ejection rate = % Ejection fraction/Ejection period
= %/ minute

Normal values for 3-min infusion of 10 ng/kg of CCK-8:
- Ejection fraction ≥35%
- Ejection period = 6–12 min
- Ejection rate ≥3.5%/min

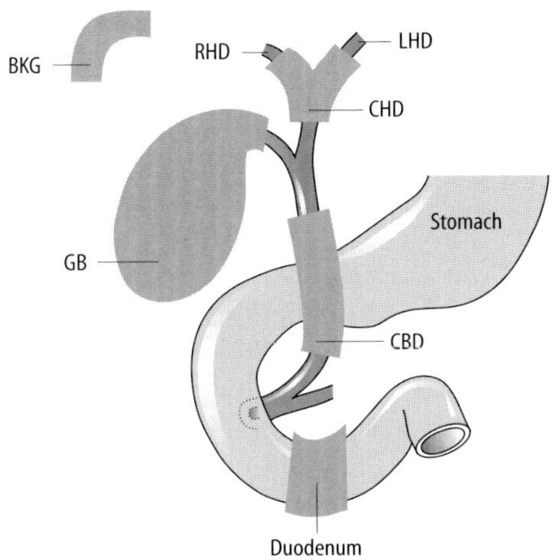

Fig. 5.1.7. Quantitative biliary dynamics. Time/activity curves are generated by drawing ROIs over the gallbladder (*GB*), common bile duct (*CBD*), common hepatic duct (*CHD*) including the right hepatic duct (*RHD*) and left hepatic duct (*LHD*), duodenum, and a background (*BKG*) over the liver. Net counts are obtained after subtracting the background

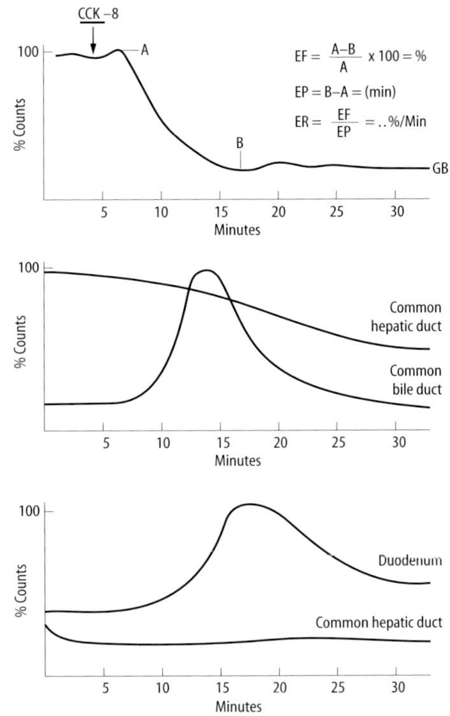

Fig. 5.1.8. Calculation of gallbladder ejection fraction. Occasionally counts may increase just before the gallbladder begins to empty (*A*). First minimum counts represents end of emptying (*B*). Ejection fraction (*EF*) is calculated by dividing *A–B* counts by counts at *A*. Time from *A* to *B* is the ejection period (*EP*). Ejection rate (*ER*) is calculated by dividing %*EF* by *EP*

Ejection Fraction with a Fatty Meal Stimulation

A fatty meal stimulates release of endogenous cholecystokinin from the endocrine cells lining the mucosa of the duodenum, jejunum, and upper ileum. It may take as long as 6–26 min after a meal for the endogenous CCK level to rise above the serum threshold required to initiate gallbladder contraction and emptying. Once the gallbladder emptying begins it continues for 1–3 h postmeal. The duration of data collection with the fatty meal, therefore, should be for a minimum of 60 min, preferably for 120 min. The data are collected at 1 frame/min for 60 or 120 min (Fig. 5.1.9). A standardized meal of known nutritional and caloric value is ingested at 5–10 min, such that a baseline count representing volume is established prior to the meal [27, 28]. Half and half (H&H) milk (carbohydrate 11 g, fat 28 g, and protein 8 g with total calories of 325), at a dose of 8 oz/70 kg body weight, has been used as a meal to stimulate release of endogenous CCK.

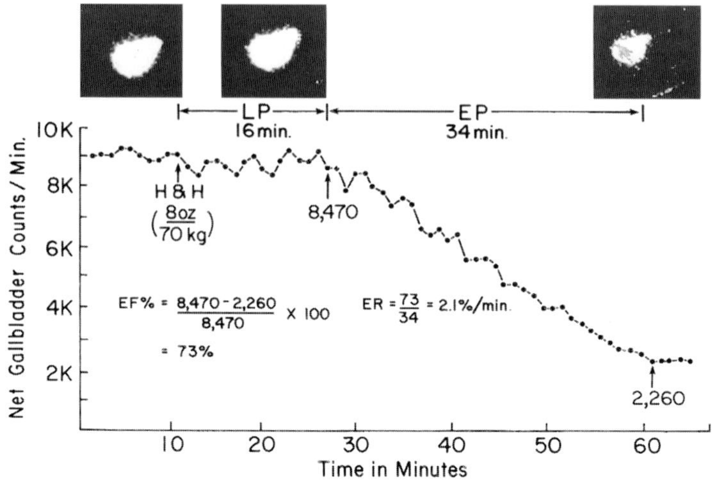

Fig. 5.1.9. Gallbladder emptying with fatty meal stimulation: Meal is ingested at 10 min. There is a latent period of 16 min before the gallbladder begins to empty. Ejection fraction is 73% with an ejection period of 34 min, and an ejection rate of 2.1%/min [28]

Data Analysis. Two regions of interest, one over the gallbladder and the other over the liver as background, are drawn. Due to the slow rate of bile emptying, CBD and CHD are not well delineated with the fatty meal stimulation. The value of the gallbladder ejection fraction with a fatty meal is reported with reference to its time of measurement, i.e., at 60 min or 120 min, postmeal. A 30-min continuous infusion of CCK-8 or 60-min post fatty meal appear to produce an ejection fraction of about 80% (Table 5.1.6). The latent period (the time from meal ingestion to beginning of gallbladder emptying) is variable depending upon the time for release of endogenous CCK [28]. A delay in onset of gallbladder emptying may also be caused by a delay in gastric emptying. Since there are no CCK-secreting cells in the esophagus and stomach [29], hormone induced gallbladder emptying does not begin until the food reaches the duodenum. Gallbladder ejection fraction is low in patients with gallstones and diabetes [30]. Obese diabetics have a much more pronounced reduction in EF compared to non-obese diabetic patients [31]. A cephalic phase emptying due to cholinergic nerve stimulation, independent of hormonal action, should be taken into account when found [32].

Table 5.1.6. Effect of type of meal and duration of emptying on gallbladder ejection fraction (%) (means ± SE)

Meal type	Meal volume	Duration from meal ingestion 30 min	60 min	120 min
Fatty meal [28] (half and half)	8 oz/70 kg	–	64.4±6.7	–
Fatty meal [27] (lipomul)	15 ml	49.8±5.2	71.7±3.6	77.8±2.0

References

1. Krishnamurthy S, Krishnamurthy GT. Technetium-99m iminodiacetic acid organic anions: review of biokinetics and clinical application in hepatology. Hepatology 1989;9:139–153
2. Bobba VR, Krishnamurthy GT, Kingston E, Brown PH, Eklem M, Turner FE. Comparison of biokinetics and biliary imaging parameters of four Tc-99m iminodiacetic acid derivatives in normal subjects. Clin Nucl Med 1983;8:70–75
3. Williams W, Krishnamurthy GT, Brar HS, Bobba VR. Scintigraphic variations of normal biliary physiology. J Nucl Med 1984;25:160–165
4. Healey JE, Schroy PC. Anatomy of the biliary ducts within the human liver. Analysis of the prevailing pattern of branchings and the major variations of the biliary ducts. Arch Surg 1953;66:599–616
5. Sherlock S, Dooley. Diseases of the liver and biliary system. 10th edition. Blackwell Science, Malden, MA. 1997, pp 217–237
6. Krishnamurthy GT, Bobba VR, McConnell D, Turner FE, Mesgarzadeh M, Kingston E. Quantitative biliary dynamics: introduction of a new non-invasive scintigraphic technique. J Nucl Med 1983;24:217–223
7. Klingensmith WC III, Spitzer CM, Fritzberg AR, Kuni CC. The normal fasting and post-prandial diisopropyl-IDA Tc-99m hepatobiliary study. Radiology 1981;141:771–776
8. Wheeler HO. Concentrating function of the gallbladder. Am J Med 1971;51:588–595
9. Krishnamurthy S, Krishnamurthy GT. Evolution of nuclear hepatology as a clinical subspeciality. J Nucl Med Technol 1995;23:35S–44S
10. Tagge EP, Campbell DA Jr, Reichle R, Averill DR, Jr. Merion RM, Dafoe DC, Turcotte JG, Juni JE. Quantitative scintigraphy with deconvolutional analysis for the dynamic measurement of hepatic function. J Surg Res 1987;42:605–612
11. Brown PH, Juni JE, Lieberman DA, Krishnamurthy GT. Hepatocyte versus biliary disease: a distinction by deconvolutional analysis of technetium-99m IDA time-activity curves. J Nucl Med 1988;29:623–630
12. Doo E. Krishnamurthy GT, Eklem MJ, Gilbert S, Brown PH. Quantification of hepatobiliary function as an integral part of imaging with technetium-99m-mebrofenin in health and disease. J Nucl Med 1991;32:48–57
13. Spackman J, Bartlett ME, Ryals L, et al. Reproducibility of technetium-99m-mebrofenin hepatic functional parameters obtained with a semiautomatic software. J Nucl Med Technol 1991;19:228–231
14. Juni JE, Reichle R. Measurement of hepatocellular function with deconvolutional analysis: application in the differential diagnosis of acute jaundice. Radiology 1990;177:171–175
15. Howan-Giles R, Moase A, Gaskin K, Uren R. Hepatobiliary scintigraphy in a pediatric population: Determination of hepatic extraction fraction by deconvolution analysis. J Nucl Med 1993;34:214–221
16. Howman-Giles R, Uren R, Bernard E, Dorney S. Hepatobiliary scintigraphy in infancy. J Nucl Med 1998;39:311–319
17. van der Linden W, Kempi V. Filling of the gallbladder as studied by computer-assisted Tc-99m-HIDA scintigraphy: Concise communication. J Nucl Med 1984;25:292–298
18. deSilva GS. A simple method for computing the volume of the human gallbladder. Radiology 1949;52:94–102
19. Everson GT, Braverman DZ, Johnson ML, Kern F Jr. A critical evaluation of real-time ultrasonography for the study of gallbladder volume and contraction. Gastroenterology 1980;79:40–46
20. Krishnamurthy GT, Bobba VR, Kingston E. Radionuclide ejection fraction: a technique for quantitative analysis of motor function of the human gallbladder. Gastroenterology 1981;80:482–490
21. Krishnamurthy S, Krishnamurthy GT. Biliary dyskinesia: role of the sphincter of Oddi, gallbladder and cholecystokinin. J Nucl Med 1997;38:1824–1830
22. Krishnamurthy S, Krishnamurthy GT. Cholecystokinin and morphine pharmacological intervention during Tc-99m-HIDA cholescintigraphy: a rational approach. Semin Nucl Med 1996;26:16–24
23. Krishnamurthy GT, Bobba VR, Kingston E. Optimization of octapeptide of cholecystokinin (OP-CCK) dose for gallbladder emptying. In: Raynaud C (ed) Proceedings of the third world congress of nuclear medicine and biology, Paris, France. Pergamon Press, New York, 1982, pp 2244–2247
24. Ziessman HA, Fahey FH, Hixson DJ. Calculation of a gallbladder fraction: advantage of continuous sincalide infusion over the three-minute infusion method. J Nucl Med 1992;33:537–541
25. Toftdahl DB, Hojgaard L, Winkler K. Dynamic cholescintigraphy: induction and description of gallbladder emptying. J Nucl Med 1996;37:261–266
26. Krishnamurthy S, Krishnamurthy GT. Gallbladder ejection fraction: a decade of progress and future promise (editorial). J Nucl Med 1992,32:542–544

27. Fisher RS, Rock E, Levine G, Malmud L. Effects of somatostatin on gallbladder emptying. Gastroenterology 1987;92:885–890
28. Bobba VR, Krishnamurthy GT, Kingston E, Turner FE, Brown PH, Langrell K. Gallbladder dynamics induced by a fatty meal in normal subjects and patients with gallstones: concise communication. J Nucl Med 1984;25:21–24
29. Sjolund K, Sanden G, Hakanson R, Sundler F. Endocrine cells in human intestine. an immunocytochemical study. Gastroenterology 1983;85:1120–1130
30. Fisher RS, Stelzer F, Rock F, Malmud LS. Abnormal gallbladder emptying in patients with gallstones. Dig Dis Sci 1982;27:1019–1024
31. Shreiner DP, Sarva RP, Van Thiel D, Yingvorapant N. Gallbladder function in diabetic patients. J Nucl Med 1986;27:357–360
32. Hopman WPM, Jansen JBM, Rosenbusch G, Lamers CB. Cephalic stimulation of gallbladder contraction in humans: role of cholecystokinin and the cholinergic system. Digestion 1987;38:197–203

5.2 Measurement of Hepatic Arterial vs Portal Venous Blood Flow

The liver has a dual blood supply, through the hepatic artery and portal vein. The hepatic artery supplies about 400 ml arterial blood/min at 100–120 mmHg systolic blood pressure. The portal vein supplies about 1200 ml/min venous blood at 7–10 mmHg pressure. Thus, approximately 25% of the total liver blood supply comes via the hepatic artery and the remaining 75% through the portal vein. After injection into a peripheral vein, the radiotracer arriving via the portal vein takes 7–10 s more to reach the liver than the radiotracer arriving via the hepatic artery. This delay via the portal vein is primarily due to time taken for the radiotracer to traverse through the intestinal veins and portal vein.

The hepatic arterial vs portal venous blood supply to the liver is measured using a first pass curve obtained with any radiotracer that passes through the liver [1]. Technetium-99m-pertechnetate, ^{99m}Tc-DTPA, and ^{99m}Tc-MDP have been used. These tracers that merely pass through, but not retained by the liver, to do not allow any additional liver imaging. The agents that both pass through and are retained by the liver (^{99m}Tc-S-colloid or ^{99m}Tc-HIDA) allow follow-up imaging of the liver. Immediately upon an antecubital vein injection, the radiotracer mixes thoroughly with blood in the ventricles before its arrival at the liver. The quantity of the radiotracer reaching the liver is directly proportional to the volume of blood supplied to the liver. The differential blood flow to the liver, via the hepatic artery vs portal vein, is calculated by two methods. One method is based on analysis of the slope of the uptake and washout [2] and the other method employs the area under the curve by deconvolutional analysis [3].

Data Collection

A fasting patient is positioned supine underneath a large field of view gamma camera fitted with a low energy, all purpose, parallel hole collimator. The position of the gamma camera in either the anterior or posterior view is adjusted to make sure that it covers the lower part of the lungs, entire liver, spleen, and kidneys. A simultaneous anterior and posterior perfusion can be obtained with a dual head gamma camera (Fig. 5.2.1A,B). About 10–15 mCi (370–555 MBq) ^{99m}Tc-labeled agent is injected intravenously as a rapid bolus followed by a 30 ml saline flush. Data is collected on 64+64 word

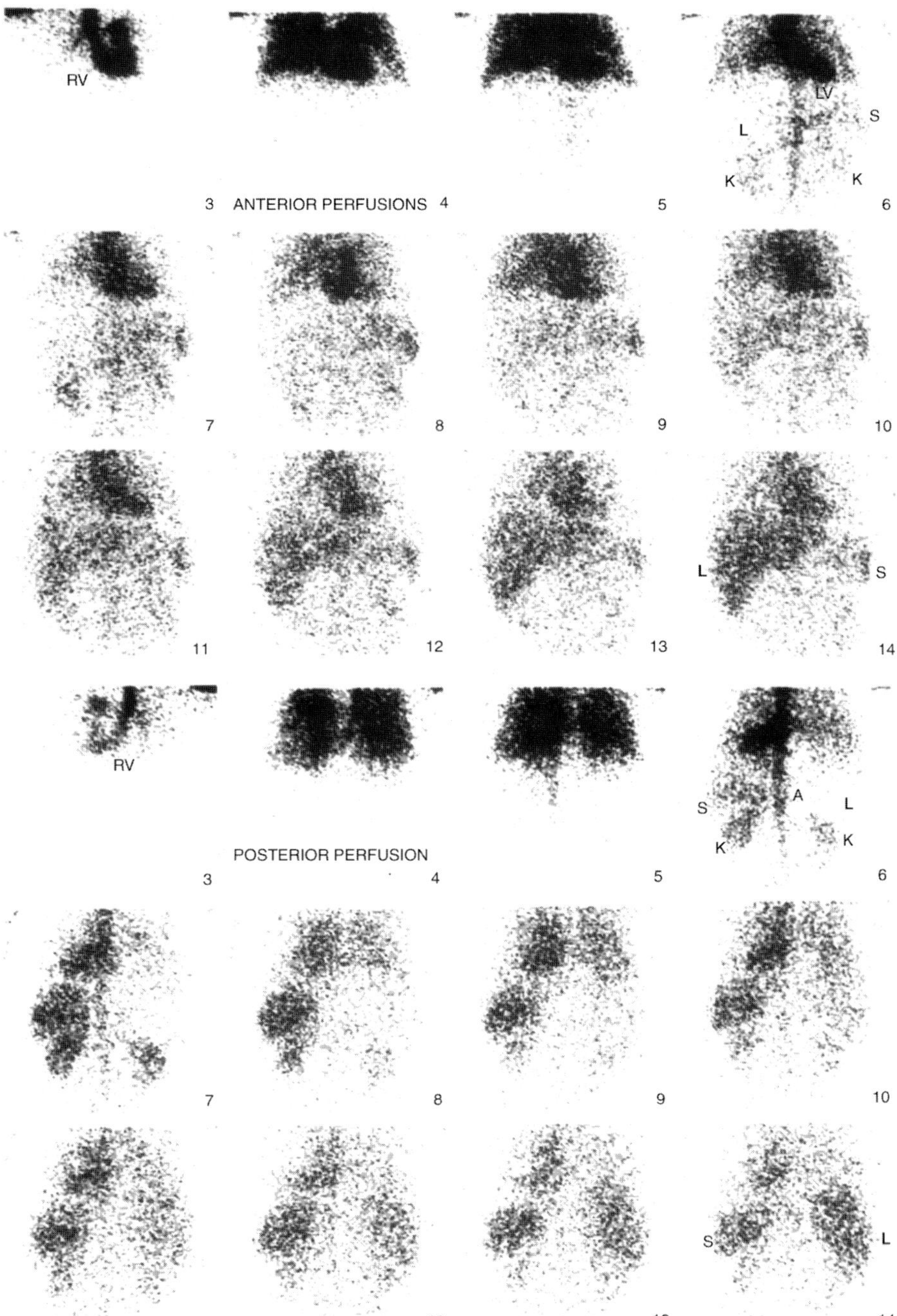

Fig. 5.2.1. Liver perfusion study. Anterior *(top)* and posterior *(bottom)* view liver perfusion study shows the passage of radiotracer serially through the right ventricle (*RV*), left ventricle (*LV*), abdominal aorta (*A*), spleen (*S*), kidneys (*K*), and liver. Left lobe perfusion is seen better in the anterior view and the perfusion of the spleen and kidneys is seen better in the posterior view

mode matrix at 1 frame per 0.5 s for 100 s [2]. Data acquisition is begun just before the injection of the radiotracer. The first 30 frames are summed to form a composite image on which 4 regions of interest are drawn: (1) liver (mid part of the right lobe excluding the right kidney and aorta), (2) lower right lung, (3) spleen, and (4) cross-talk region between the right lung and the liver (Fig. 5.2.2). The left kidney is substituted for the spleen in patients with splenectomy.

Slope Method

Time/activity curves are generated over all four regions as outlined above (Fig. 5.2.3A). The cross-talk curve from the region between the right lung and liver (Fig. 5.2.3B) is scaled to the same height as the early part of the liver curve (before the arrival of the liver arterial phase, usually between 0 and 20 s) and subtracted from the liver and spleen curve to generate the corrected liver and spleen curves (Fig. 5.2.3C). Corrected liver and spleen curves are displayed separately (Fig. 5.2.3D,E). Three time points are identified on the corrected time/activity curve. The initial arrival of radioactivity at the liver is denoted by Ta, which corresponds to the beginning of the hepatic arterial phase. Because the hepatic and splenic artery have a common origin from the celiac artery, the time of peak activity on the spleen curve (Sp) is considered the end of the arterial phase and beginning of the portal venous phase, and corresponds to time, Tp, on the liver curve (Fig. 5.2.3D). Normally, there is 7±2-s delay between the arrival of the

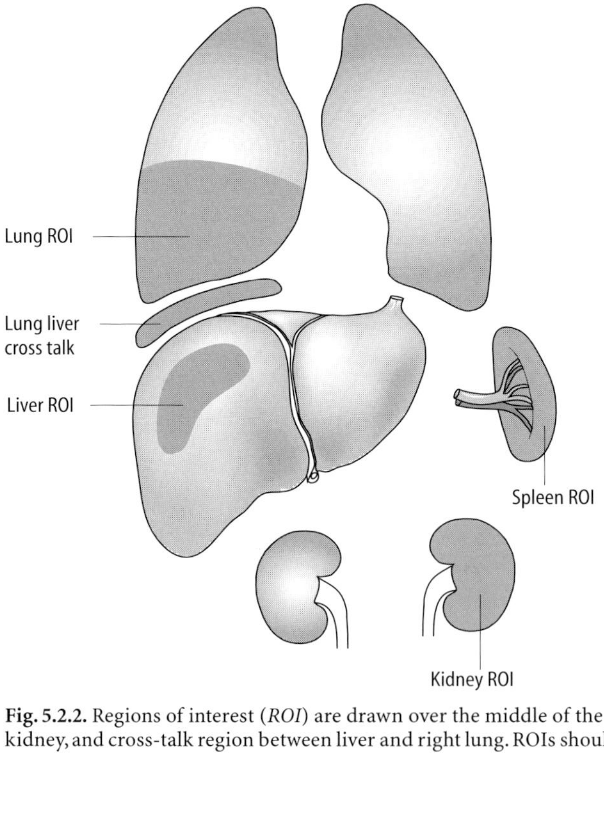

Fig. 5.2.2. Regions of interest (*ROI*) are drawn over the middle of the liver, right lower lung, spleen, left kidney, and cross-talk region between liver and right lung. ROIs should exclude liver margins and aorta

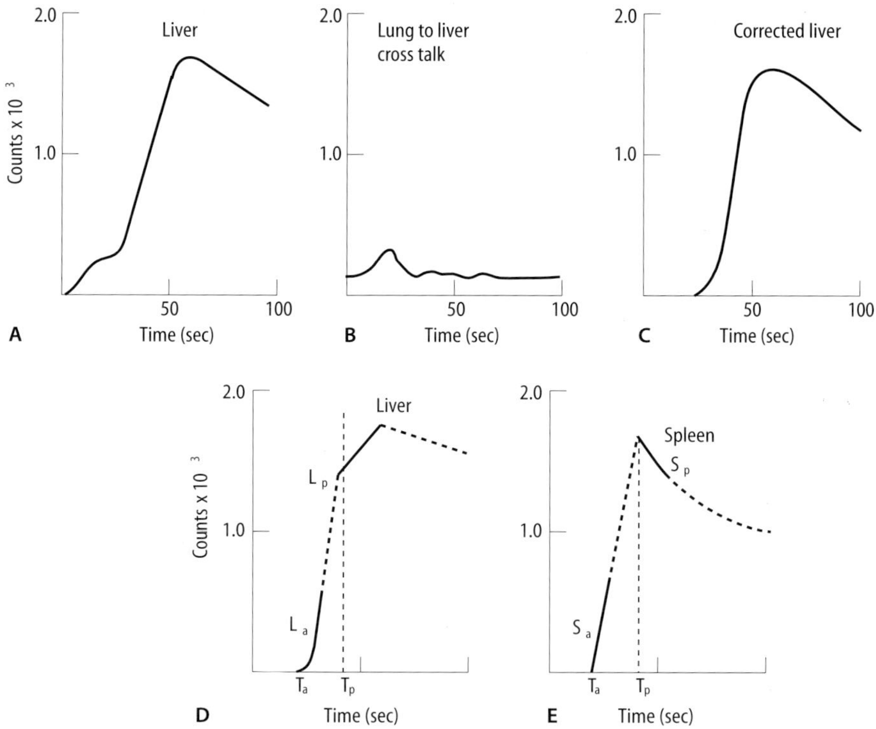

Fig. 5.2.3. Hepatic arterial vs portal venous blood flow by the slope method. Time-activity curves are generated over the liver (**A**) and cross-talk region between the lung and liver (**B**). Both curves are scaled to the same height, and the corrected liver curve (**C**) is obtained after subtracting the cross-talk counts. The onset of the arterial (*Ta*) and portal venous (*Tp*) are noted on the corrected liver curve (**D**). *La* and *Lp* represent the slope of the arterial and portal venous phases measured over 7 s from *Ta* and *Tp*, respectively. Spleen curve (**E**) shows the onset of arterial (*Ta*) and peak arterial flow (*Tp*); *Sa* and *Sp* represent the slopes of the curve in a manner similar to *La* and *Lp* [2, 4]

hepatic arterial and portal venous blood supply to the liver. The slope of the arterial phase, La, is measured from Ta to Ta+7 s and the slope of the portal venous phase, Lp, is measured from Tp to Tp+7 s. Total counts are integrated and percent arterial blood flow to the liver is measured using the following formula from a linear fit to the curve [2]:

$$\text{Percent arterial liver blood flow} = La/(La+Lp)\times 100$$

where La = slope of the hepatic arterial phase and Lp = slope of the portal venous phase.

To correct for the fraction of hepatic arterial component still present during the portal venous phase in the liver curve, the slope of the splenic curve is used with the following modification. The ratio of Sa/Sp of the splenic curve is assumed to represent the fraction of the arterial flow present during the portal venous phase of the liver curve [2].

Corrected portal slope (Lp correct) = Lp–La (Sp/Sa)

Percent arterial liver blood flow = La/[La+Lp correct]×100

Area Method

This method uses deconvolutional analysis [2, 4]. Like the slope method, it is dependent upon the temporal separation between the arrival of the hepatic arterial and portal venous blood to the liver. It takes into account the role of recirculation of the injected radiotracer. Data acquisition is identical to the slope method described above (Fig. 5.2.1). Using a large of field of view gamma camera, computer data are collected on a 64+64 word matrix at one frame per 0.5 s for 100 s. The data collection is started just before injection of 10–15 mCi (370–555 MBq) of the radiotracer. On the first 30-frame composite image, regions of interest are drawn and time/activity curves are generated over: (1) liver, mid right lobe excluding the right kidney and aorta, (2) lower right lung, (3) spleen, and (4) cross-talk region between right lung and liver (Fig. 5.2.2). The cross-talk curve is scaled to the same height as the initial part of the liver curve (before the arrival of the radiotracer to the liver) and subtracted from the liver and spleen curve to generate a corrected liver and spleen curve (Fig. 5.2.4A). Liver and spleen curves are deconvoluted with the lung curve using the modified Fourier transformation technique (Fig. 5.2.4B). The curve is expanded from 200 to 1024 data points by addition of an exponentially decreasing tail which eliminates artifacts due to a sharp cutoff at the end of data termination. An assumption is made that the spleen blood flow pattern is similar to that of the hepatic artery. The spleen curve is used to approximate hepatic arterial blood flow. The spleen curve is multiplied by a constant so that the upslope superimposes over the early part of the liver curve (Fig. 5.2.4C). The liver and modified spleen curves are integrated to give the areas under the curve, AL and As, respectively.

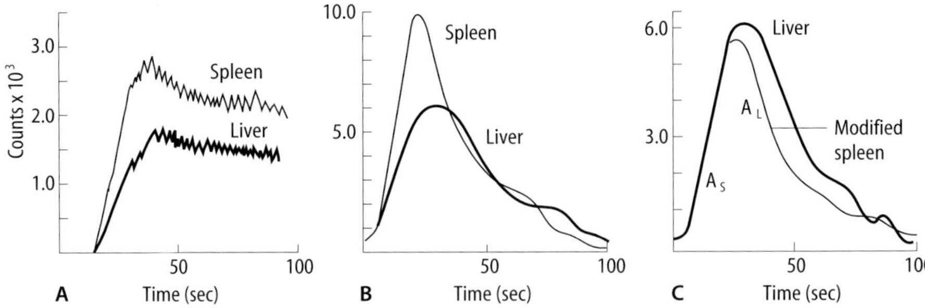

Fig. 5.2.4. Hepatic arterial vs portal venous blood flow by the area method. Corrected spleen and liver curves are obtained first (**A**) after subtracting the background counts from the lung to liver cross-talk region and then subjected to deconvolutional analysis (**B**). Magnitude of the spleen curve is modified so that its upslope matches with that of the liver (**C**). *As* and A_L represent the area under the modified spleen and liver curves, respectively

$$\text{Arterial liver blood flow (\%Ha)} = \frac{\text{As}}{\text{AL}} \times 100$$

$$\text{Portal venous blood (\%)} = 100\text{–\%Ha}$$

Both the slope and area methods are found clinically useful and have been validated in experimental animals [5]. The slope method technically is much simpler but has a wider variability between studies. The area method using the deconvolutional analysis provides the best separation between normal subjects and patients with increasing severity of liver disease. Arterial to venous ratio increases as the severity of liver disease increases from Child's class A to C (Table 5.1.3). In cirrhosis, low pressure (7–10 mmHg) portal venous blood flow is affected much earlier than the high pressure (100–120 mmHg) hepatic arterial blood flow. Portal venous blood flow decreases as the portal venous pressure raises (Fig. 5.2.5). Measurement of the hepatic arterial vs portal venous blood flow is found useful in the diagnosis of hepatic vein thrombosis and also in following patients treated for portal hypertension [4].

The final shape of the liver and spleen curve depends upon whether or not the chosen agent is retained by these organs. Technetium-99m-sulfur colloid, which is retained by both organs, and ^{99m}Tc-HIDA, which is retained only by the liver but not by the spleen, produce curves whose shape is different from each other and also from those agents (^{99m}Tc-labeled MDP, albumin, or pertechnetate) not retained by either organ. The choice of agent does not usually affect the values of arterial vs venous blood flow, because the first pass study is independent of the biokinetic behavior of the radiotracer [5].

Normal median portal venous blood flow is 78% and the median hepatic artery flow 22%. The median portal venous blood flow decreases to 68% in mild liver disease, and remains below 49% in severe liver disease. The median portal venous blood flow falls below 4% in patients with portal vein thrombosis. The scintigraphic technique is shown to be 90% sensitive and 100% specific in patients with portal vein thrombosis when portal blood flow falls below 20% [4]. Perfusion changes and indices of hepatic

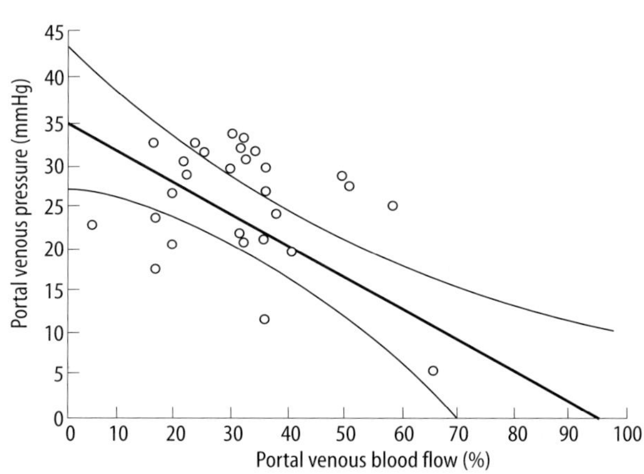

Fig. 5.2.5. Relationship between portal venous blood flow and portal venous pressure. There is an inverse relationship between the two; as the portal venous pressure increases, the portal venous blood flow decreases [7]

arterial blood flow in patients with cirrhosis can be measured by comparison with the renal or splenic arterial peak, thus avoiding the influence of portal venous reduction on the hepatic arterial peak [6]. Calculation of the hepatic arterial to portal venous ratio provides a non-invasive method to evaluate objectively the benefits of transjugular intrahepatic portosystemic shunt (TIPS) therapy. In a study involving 28 patients, the mean (SD) portal venous pressure of 25.5±4.6 mmHg before TIPS decreased to 18.5±3.9 mmHg after TIPS. The portal venous blood flow of 29.2±11.1% before, increased to 38.2±13.4% after TIPS, indicating its therapeutic benefits. Portal venous flow shows an inverse relationship with the portal venous pressure; portal venous blood flow decreases as the portal venous pressure increases. The relationship between portal venous flow and pressure tends to normalize after a successful TIPS procedure [7, 8].

References

1. Sarper R, Tarcan YA. An improved method of estimating the portal venous fraction of total hepatic blood flow from computerized radionuclide angiography. Radiology 1983;147:559–562
2. O'Connor MK, MacMathuna P, Keeling PWN. Hepatic arterial and portal venous components of liver blood flow. a dynamic scintigraphic study. J Nucl Med 1988;29:466–472
3. Biersack HJ, Torres J, Thelen M, Monzon O, Winkler C. Determination of liver and spleen perfusion by quantitative sequential scintigraphy: results in normal subjects and in patients with portal hypertension. Clin Nucl Med 1981;6:218–220
4. McMathuna P, O'Connor MK, Weir DG, Keeling PWN. Non-invasive diagnosis of portal vein occlusion by radionuclide angiography. Gut 1992;33:1671–1674
5. O'Connor MK, Krom RF, Carton EG, Sanchez-Urdazpal L, Juni JE, Ferguson DM, Wiesner RF. Ratio of hepatic arterial-to-portal venous blood flow – validation of radionuclide techniques in an animal model. J Nucl Med 1992;33:239–245
6. Koranda P, Myslivecek M, Erban J, Seidlova V, Husak V. Hepatic perfusion changes in patients with cirrhosis. Indices of hepatic arterial blood flow. Clin Nucl Med 1999;24:507–510
7. Menzel J, Schober O, Reimer P, Domschke W. Scintigraphic evaluation of hepatic blood flow after intrahepatic portosystemic shunt (TIPS). Eur J Nucl Med 1997;24:635–641
8. Ganger DR, Klapman JB, McDonald V, Matolon JA, Kaur S, Rosenblate H, Kave R, Saker M, Jensen DM. Transjugular intrahepatic portosystemic shunt (TIPS) for Budd-Chiary syndrome and portal vein thrombosis. Am J Gastroenterol 1999;94:603–608

5.3 Hepatopulmonary Syndrome

The functional relationship between the liver and lung originally recognized in 1935 is now called hepatopulmonary syndrome (HPS). The syndrome consists of a triad of: (1) liver disease, (2) increased alveolar-arterial oxygen gradient, and (3) intrapulmonary vasodilatation [1, 2].

Clinical Presentation

Patients usually present with a combination of symptoms indicative of both liver and lung disease: esophageal varices, gastrointestinal bleeding, spider nevi, ascites, and splenomegaly indicative of liver disease; and dyspnea, clubbing, platypnea, and orthodeoxia indicative of lung disease [3, 4]. Platypnea is dyspnea in an upright position which is relieved by assuming a supine position [5]. Orthodeoxia is arterial deoxygenation, exaggerated in the upright position and relieved by recumbency. Platypnea and orthodeoxia, which are found only in a small percentage of patients with cirrhosis (5%), are much more frequent and severe in intensity in patients with HPS, often reaching as high as 88–100% [6]. Spider nevi of the palms and around the umbilicus are considered the cutaneous markers of HPS [7]. As the liver reaches its end stage the patients develop ascites, generalized edema, pleural effusion, and interstitial fluid accumulation in the lungs. Chest X-ray changes consists of either finely diffuse spidery infiltrates or discrete, focal arteriovenous malformations [8].

Pathophysiology

Arterial deoxygenation due to intrapulmonary shunt is the hallmark of HPS. Pulmonary artery pressure remains normal or slightly low [6]. Severe hypoxemia (PaO_2 <60 mmHg), in the absence of primary lung disease, in combination with liver disease clinically should raise the suspicion of HPS. The pulmonary capillaries, which normally measure 8–15 µm, dilate up to 100 µm in diameter, often forming spider nevi on the pleural surface [9]. Radiolabeled macroaggregates of albumin (MAA) of 15–150 µm in diameter normally become trapped almost completely within the pulmonary capillary bed after intravenous injection. These radiolabeled ^{99m}Tc-MAA particles readily pass through the dilated pulmonary capillaries in patients with HPS and enter the systemic circulation to be trapped in normal size capillaries of the brain, liver, kidney, and other organs, in proportion to their blood supply [10–12]. Normally less than 6% of ^{99m}Tc-MAA particles bypass the lung to lodge in other organs [11, 13]. It is theorized that the liver in HPS either produces vasodilators or is incapable of inactivating vasodilators produced elsewhere. Incriminated vasodilators include prostaglandins, vasoactive intestinal polypeptide, calcitonin, glucagon, nitric oxide, and atrial natriuretic factor [6].

Diagnosis

Arterial blood gases are obtained to document hypoxemia (Table 5.3.1). Contrast 2D echocardiography (2D echo) with indocyanine green or agitated saline is the most preferred initial diagnostic imaging procedure [14, 15]. Saline agitation creates microbubbles of 60–90 µm size which opacify the right heart chambers within one to three cardiac cycles after injection into an antecubital vein. The left heart chambers are not opacified due to filtration of all bubbles by the normal lung capillaries [16]. The bubbles pass through dilated intrapulmonary capillaries in HPS to enter the pulmonary veins and left heart chambers. A confirmatory diagnosis of HPS requires documentation of arterial hypoxemia (PaO_2 less than 70 mmHg), normal pulmonary function tests, typical chest X-ray findings, and opacification of left heart chambers in the absence of a right to left cardiac shunt. Right to left cardiac shunt is suggested on a 2D echo when both right and left ventricular chambers are opacified simultaneously, within one to three cardiac cycles after intravenous injection of agitated saline [17].

Scintigraphic Quantification

A mild form of HPS is found in as many as 4–17% of patients with varieties of chronic liver diseases [18]. Despite being very sensitive, 2D echo lacks the specificity and ability to quantify the degree of shunt. A perfusion scintigraphy supplements 2D echo by providing both quantification and specificity for a definitive diagnosis of HPS.

Table 5.3.1. Diagnostic workup for hepatopulmonary syndrome (modified from ref. [18])

Cirrhosis with hypoxemia

Chest X-ray

↓ Normal ↓ Abnormal (treat, if hypoxemia persists)

↓

Contrast echo (EC) and pulmonary function tests (PFTs)

(–) CE and normal PFT	(+) CE and normal PFTs	(+) CE and abnormal PFTs	
↓	↓	↓	
No HPS	HPS	^{99m}Tc MAA scan	
		Shunt >6%	Shunt <6%
		↓	↓
		HPS	No HPS

Procedure. The patient is made to sit upright for 5 min to maximize the degree of intrapulmonary shunt. Macroaggregates of ^{99m}Tc-albumin particles are prepared carefully as per instructions provided in the package insert. A drop of the prepared material is fed into a hemocytometer chamber and examined under the light microscope to ascertain that at least 90% of the particles are in the 15- to 90-μm size range. A radiochromatogram is obtained to confirm that there is better than 90% radiolabeling. About 2–3 mCi ^{99m}Tc-MAA is injected into an antecubital vein while the patient is seated. After injection, the patient is made to lay supine. A large field of view dual head gamma camera, fitted with a low energy, all purpose, parallel hole collimator, is positioned laterally on each side, or in front and behind the head. The spectrometer is set for 140 keV photon peak energy with a 20% symmetrical window. The camera heads are positioned above the shoulders to avoid counts below the neck. The counts are taken for a preset time of 5 min with each head and recorded on a 64×64 computer matrix. After taking 5-min head counts, the detectors are moved over to the chest to the anterior and posterior position. Preset 5-min counts are taken again in the anterior and posterior view simultaneously and recorded on a 64×64 computer matrix.

Data Analysis. On the lateral or anterior and posterior views of the head, regions of interest are drawn to cover the entire brain, excluding the scalp and superior sagittal sinus when they are visible. On the anterior and posterior view chest images, regions of interest are drawn to cover both lungs. Care is taken to avoid the liver or kidneys in the lung ROI (Fig. 5.3.1). Geometric mean counts are calculated using the following formula:

$$\text{Geometric mean brain counts (GMBC)} = \sqrt{\text{Right lateral or anterior view brain counts} \times \text{left lateral or posterior view brain counts}}$$

$$= \sqrt{1022 \times 1262} = 1135$$

$$\text{Geometric mean lung counts (GMLC)} = \sqrt{\text{anterior view lung counts} \times \text{posterior view lung counts}}$$

$$= \sqrt{637{,}417 \times 970{,}115} = 786{,}363$$

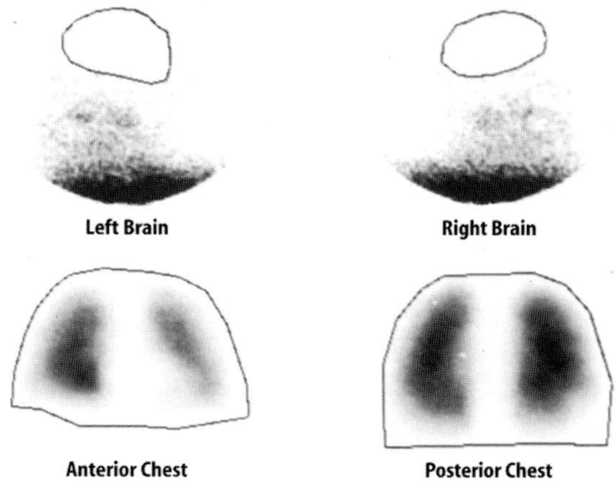

Fig. 5.3.1. Quantification of hepatopulmonary shunt: Regions of interest are drawn over the brain in two lateral views of the head and over the lungs in the anterior and posterior views of the chest. Total counts in 5 min are noted in each view. The geometric mean counts are obtained by using the equation given in the text. Hepatopulmonary shunt ratio is obtained by dividing geometric mean brain counts by the sum of geometric mean brain count and lung counts

An assumption is made that about 13% of the cardiac output is delivered to the brain [19]. By applying this correction factor, the hepatopulmonary shunt is calculated by the following equation:

$$\text{Hepatopulmonary shunt} = \frac{\frac{\text{GMBC (Brain)}}{0.13}}{\frac{\text{GMBC (Brain)}}{0.13} + \text{GMLC (Lung)}}$$

$$= \frac{1{,}135 / 0.13}{1{,}135 / 0.13 + 786{,}363}$$

$$= 8730 / 795{,}093 = 0.02 = 2\%$$

In normal subjects and in patients with intrinsic lung disease or with cirrhosis but without shunt, the hepatopulmonary shunt ratio varies from 3% to 6% [11, 17]. A value higher than 6% is considered indicative of HPS [17, 18]. Patients with Child's class A, B, or C liver disease without HPS generally show values below 5%. A shunt value of 37% was found in an 8-year-old child (Fig. 5.3.2) waiting for liver transplantation [20].

Standardization. The technique of measuring hepatopulmonary shunt is very simple and often there may be room for complacency. It is necessary to check rigidly for ^{99m}Tc-MAA particle size and percent labeling. Greater than 90% of the particles should be between 15 and 90 μm in size, and labeling efficiency better than 90%. A preparation not meeting these two requirements is discarded. Injection of too many small particles (below 15 μm) overestimates the degree of the shunt, and the shunt is underestimated when too many particles are much larger than 90 μm in size.

Treatment

Treatment is medical in early liver failure and surgical for end stage liver disease. Patients are treated medically with indomethacin [21], almitrine bismesylate [22], octreotide, or other drugs [6]. Surgical treatment involves liver transplantation for end

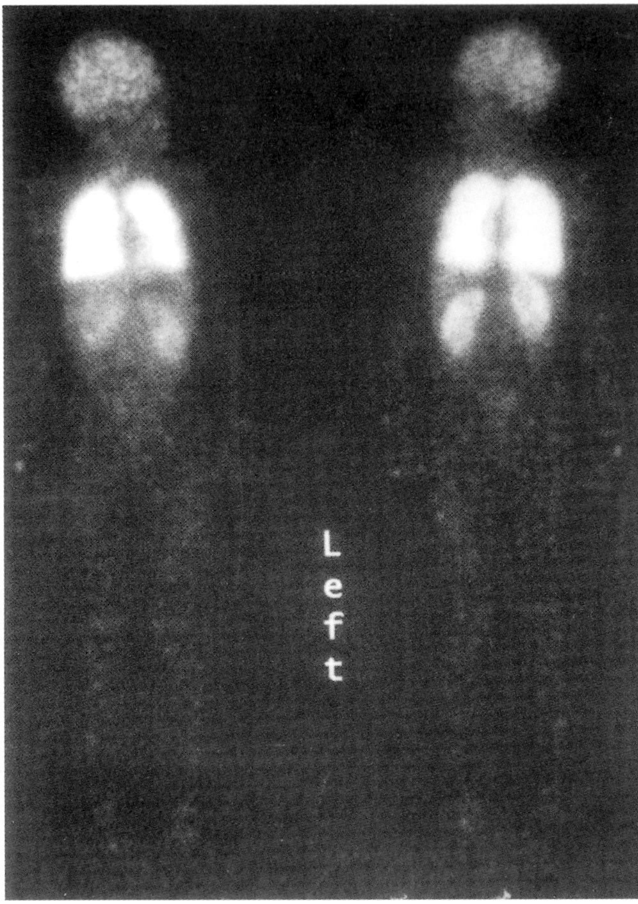

Fig. 5.3.2. Hepatopulmonary shunt. An 8-year-old boy waiting for liver transplantation has 37% right to left shunt due to intrapulmonary vasodilatation. In addition to brain, kidneys and liver are seen in a ^{99m}Tc-MAA scan [20]

stage liver disease. Liver transplantation, once listed as a clear contraindication, is now considered an optimal therapy for HPS and is shown to improve both liver and pulmonary functions [23]. In the Cleveland Clinic study, the mean ratio of 18.7% in HPS patients decreased to 4.5% after liver transplantation with a marked improvement of pulmonary blood gases [24].

References

1. Snell AM. The effect of chronic disease of the liver on composition and physiochemical properties of blood: changes in the serum proteins; reduction in the oxygen saturation of the arterial blood. Ann Intern Med 1935;9:690–711
2. Kennedy TC, Knudson RJ. Exercise aggravated hypoxemia and orthodeoxia in cirrhosis. Chest 1977;72:305–309
3. Krowka MJ, Cortese DA. Hepatopulmonary syndrome: an evolving perspective in the era of liver transplantation. Hepatology 1990;11:138–142
4. Robin ED, Laman D, Horn BR, Theodore J. Platypnea related to orthodeoxia caused by true vascular lung shunts. N Engl J Med 1976;294:941–943

5. Altman M, Robin ED. Platypnea (diffuse zone 1 phenomenon?) N Engl J Med 1969;281:1347–1348
6. Lange PA, Stoller JK. The hepatopulmonary syndrome. Ann Intern Med 1995;122:521–529
7. Sherlock S. Liver-lung interface. Semin in Respiratory Medicine 1988;9:247–253
8. Krawka MJ, Dickson ER, Cortese DA. Hepatopulmonary syndrome. Clinical observation and lack of therapeutic response to somatostatin analogue. Chest 1993;104:515–521
9. Berthalot P, Walker JG, Sherlock S, Reid L. Arterial changes in the lungs in cirrhosis of the liver – lung spider nevi. N Engl J Med 1966;274:291–298
10. Genovesi MG, Tierney DF, Taplin GV, Eisenberg H. An intravenous radionuclide method to evaluate hypoxemia caused by abnormal alveolar vessels. Limitation of conventional technique. Am Rev Respir Dis 1976; 114:59–65
11. Wolfe JD, Tashkin DP, Holly FE, Brachman MB, Genovesi MG. Hypoxemia of cirrhosis: detection of abnormal small pulmonary vascular channels by a quantitative radionuclide method. Am J Med 1977,63:746–754
12. Gates GF, Orme HW, Dore EK. Cardiac shunt assessment in children with macroaggragated albumin technetium-99m. Radiology 1974;112:649–653
13. Robin ED, Horn B, Goris ML, Theodore J, Kessel AV, Mazoub J, et al. Detection, quantitation, and pathophysiology of lung spiders. Trans Assoc Am Physicians 1975;88:202–216
14. Hind CR, Wong CM. Detection of pulmonary arteriovenous fistulas in patients with cirrhosis by contrast 2D echocardiography. Gut 1981;22:1042–1045
15. Shub C, Tajik AJ, Seward JB, Dines DE. Detecting intrapulmonary right-to-left shunt with contrast echocardiography. Observation in patients with diffuse pulmonary arteriovenous fistulas. Mayo Clin Proc 1976;51:81–84
16. Krowka MJ, Tajik AJ, Dickson ER, Wiesner RH, Cortese DA. Intrapulmonary vascular disorders (IPVD) in liver transplant candidates. Screening by two-dimensional contrast-enhanced echocardiography. Chest 1990:97:1165–1170
17. Abrams GA, Jaffe CC, Hoffer PB, Binder HJ, Fallon MB. Diagnostic utility of contrast echocardiography and lung perfusion scan in patients with hepatopulmonary syndrome. Gastroenterology 1995;109:1283–1288
18. Abrams GA, Nanda NC, Dubovsky EV, Krowka MJ, Fallon MB. Use of macroaggregated albumin lung perfusion scan to diagnose hepatopulmonary syndrome: a new approach. Gastroenterology 1998;114:305–310
19. Wade OL, Bishop JM. Cardiac output and regional blood flow. Blackwell Scientific, Oxford, 1962
20. Murakami JW, Rosenbaum DM. Right-to-left pulmonary shunting in pediatric hepatopulmonary syndrome. Clin Nucl Med 1999;24:897
21. Andrivet P, Cadranel J, Housset B, Harigault R, Harf A, Anot S. Mechanism of impaired arterial oxygenation in patient liver cirrhosis and severe respiratory insufficiency. Effect of indomethacin. Chest 1993;103:500–507
22. Krowka MJ, Cortese DA. Severe hypoxemia associated with liver disease. Mayo Clin experience and the experimental use of almitrine bismesylate. Mayo Clin Proc 1987;62:164–173
23. Scott VL, Dodson F, Kang Y. The hepatopulmonary syndrome. Surg Clin North Am 1999;79:23–41
24. Lange PA, Vogt DA, Carey WB, Stroller JK. Prevalence and reversibility of hepatopulmonary syndrome following liver transplantation. Am Rev Respir Dis 1993;147:540A (abstract)

5.4 Duodenogastric Bile Reflux

Gastrointestinal peristalsis begins at the gastric pacemaker located near the gastroesophageal junction and travels antegrade towards the gastric fundus, body, and pylorus, and progresses further along the small and large intestine. Peristaltic waves move the gastrointestinal intraluminal contents in an antegrade fashion. Duodenal contents are thus prevented from entering the stomach by the dual action of the antegrade peristalsis and contraction of pyloric sphincter [1]. Patients with atrophic gastritis, gastric ulcer, and esophagitis are often found to have bile in the stomach (duodenogastric bile reflux) raising an etiological relationship between dyspepsia and bile reflux [2].

Detection of bile by chemical analysis in the gastric juice aspirated through a nasogastric tube has been used over the years as a test for duodenogastric bile reflux. Chemical analysis is not only cumbersome but also the mere presence of bile in the aspirated gastric juice cannot be used as a reliable test for reflux, because the duodenal regurgitation may be induced by the act of insertion of the nasogastric tube itself. Counting or imaging of radiolabeled bile in the stomach makes the test technically much simpler and avoids the necessity of chemical analysis and intubation [3]. Gamma camera imaging with an online computer not only enables detection but also provides a means of quantifying the degree of duodenogastric bile reflux (DGBR). Gamma camera imaging avoids the necessity of gastric juice aspiration through the N-G tube and makes the test readily acceptable by both children and adults [4].

Rationale

After its secretion by the liver, the hepatic bile enters the gallbladder or duodenum, or both. During fasting, about 70% of the hepatic bile enters the gallbladder and the remaining 30% enters the duodenum directly [5]. Facilitated by the peristaltic waves, bile entering the duodenum moves forward with the rest of the duodenal contents received from the stomach. Since only the amount of bile entering the duodenum is available for reflux into the stomach, a technique that enables quantitative measurement of bile entry into the duodenum will be ideal for measuring bile flow forward into the jejunum or backward into the stomach (DGBR). Bile entering the gastrointestinal tract is quantified by selecting two regions of interest, one over the stomach, and the other over the intestinal tract (excluding liver, gallbladder, and bile ducts). Duodenogastric bile reflux is calculated by dividing stomach counts by total bile counts in the stomach plus intestine. The technique allows measurement of DGBR both during fasting and after administration of cholecystokinin or after feeding.

Data Collection and Analysis

Hepatic phase imaging data are used for calculation of D-G bile reflux during fasting, and gallbladder phase imaging data for calculation of postcholecystokinin or postprandial D-G bile reflux. Data are collected as outlined in Table 5.1.1. By 60 min postinjection, most ^{99m}Tc-HIDA clears from the liver, leaving the nearby gastric region free of interference by cross-talk counts from the left lobe of the liver (Fig. 5.4.1). All 60-min data are carefully reviewed in a cine display for any overlap of intestinal radioactivity onto gastric ROI [6]. A frame between 50 and 60 min (usually the 60-min frame) that does not contain any superimposition of intestinal loops onto the gastric bed is chosen for selection of gastric and intestinal ROI. Gastric ROI includes the traditional gastric bed, below the left lobe of the liver and to the left side of the distal common bile duct, and extending laterally up to the splenic bed. The intestinal ROI includes the rest of the upper abdomen, excluding the liver, gallbladder, and common bile duct. Urinary bladder is excluded from intestinal ROI (Fig. 5.4.2). Time/activity curves are generated from two ROIs. By 60 min postinjection, most radioactivity clears from the cardiac blood pool and kidneys. Sometimes the DGBR may occur early and empty in the late hepatic phase imaging. In such circumstances the frame with the peak DGBR is chosen for ROI selection. The counts are corrected for physical decay.

$$\text{Duodeno-gastric bile reflux (\%) (DGBR)} = \frac{\text{Total counts in gastric ROI} \times 100}{\text{Total counts in gastric ROI} + \text{Total counts in intestinal ROI}}$$

$$= \frac{54{,}173 \times 100}{54{,}173 + 74{,}066}$$

$$= 42\%$$

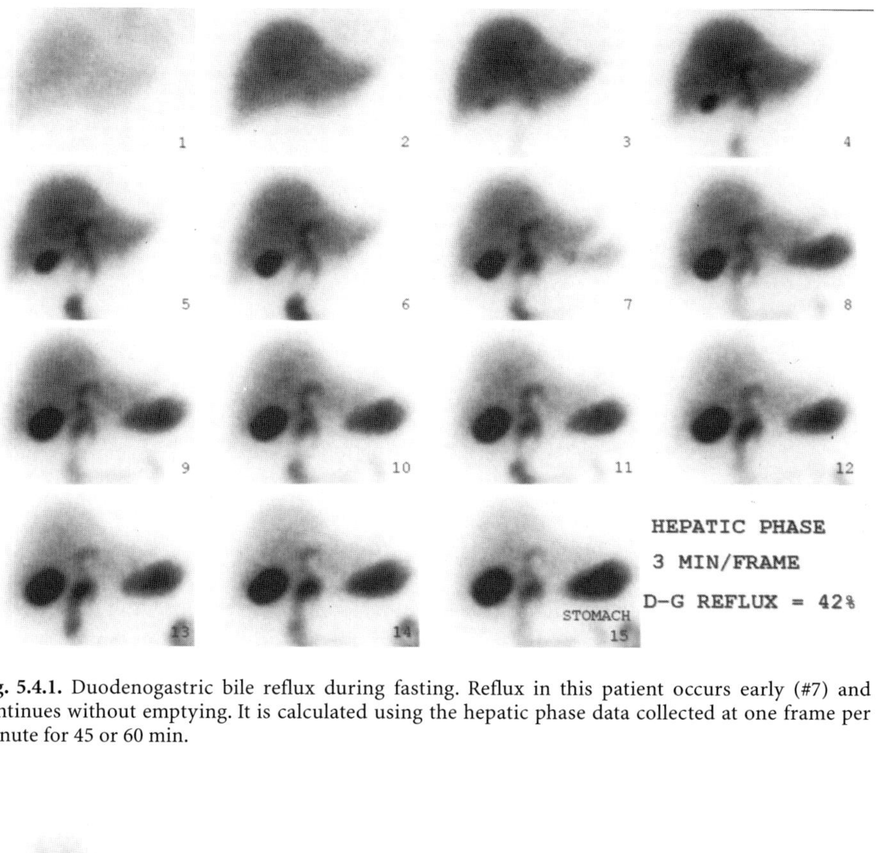

Fig. 5.4.1. Duodenogastric bile reflux during fasting. Reflux in this patient occurs early (#7) and continues without emptying. It is calculated using the hepatic phase data collected at one frame per minute for 45 or 60 min.

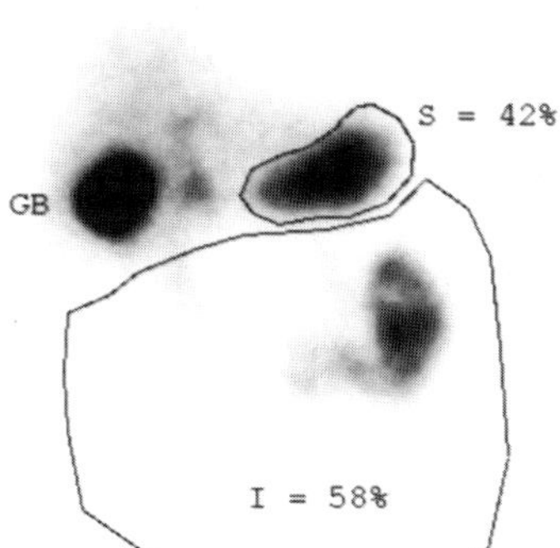

Fig. 5.4.2. Measurement of duodenogastric bile reflux. The gastric ROI (*S*) is drawn below the left lobe of the liver, on the left side of the distal common bile duct extending laterally to the splenic region. The intestinal ROI (*I*) encompasses the rest of the abdomen (excluding the liver, gallbladder, bile ducts, and urinary bladder). Note DGBR of 42% during fasting in this patient

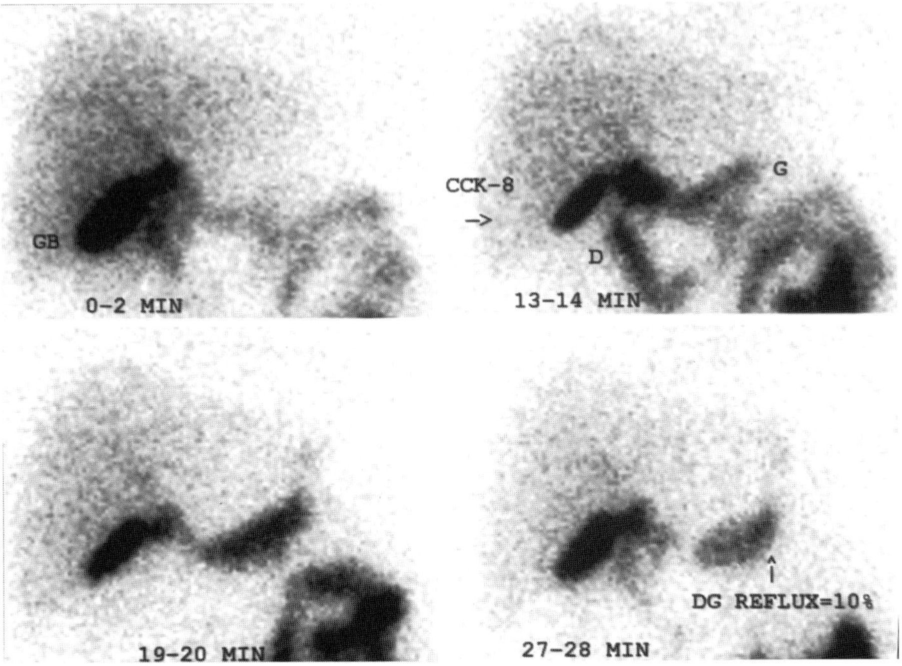

Fig. 5.4.3. Duodenogastric bile reflux after CCK-8. This is calculated using the gallbladder phase data. There is no DGBR during fasting (0–2 min). Bile reflux of 10% occurs after CCK-8 administration. *G*, stomach

Bile reflux after CCK-8 is similarly calculated using data obtained during the gallbladder phase. Cholecystokinin normally induces the contraction and emptying of the gallbladder, stimulates contraction of the pyloric sphincter, and simultaneously increases small intestinal peristalsis, facilitating rapid antegrade bile movement through the small bowel. Contraction of the pyloric sphincter, therefore, normally prevents DGBR. Post-CCK images are checked in the cine display to ascertain that there is no movement of bile radioactivity beyond the field of view of the gamma camera. If there is, then the gamma camera position is adjusted to include all bile regions and an additional view over the lower abdomen is taken. A cine display of all frames is essential to ascertain that no intestinal loop encroaches upon the gastric region, and when found such frames are excluded for ROI selection [7]. Often there is no D-G bile reflux during fasting, but may occur after CCK-8 (Fig. 5.4.3).

Table 5.4.1. Bile flow into stomach vs small intestine in 20 normal subjects

#	Subject	Total stomach counts	Total intestinal counts	% stomach	% intestine
1	HC	93,729	3,830,883	2.3	97.7
2	H	71,380	3,012,831	2.3	97.7
3	CC	36,521	2,684,925	1.3	98.7
4	E	51,226	1,483,318	3.3	97.3
5	EJ	103,127	3,651,893	2.7	97.3
6	GE	43,555	1,091,999	3.8	96.2
7	AP	67,967	2,661,020	2.5	97.5
8	B	42,169	1,309,127	3.1	96.9
9	BB	85,603	2,063,219	3.9	96.1
10	WD	20,095	616,171	3.2	96.8
11	HR	40,526	1,169,047	3.3	96.4
12	LC	23,421	3,343,890	0.7	99.3
13	KD	19,204	731,084	2.5	97.5
14	KJ	15,746	2,107,383	0.7	99.3
15	KC	26,342	2,259,335	1.1	99.9
16	MV	16,093	459,163	3.4	96.6
17	MK	20,084	1,299,986	1.5	98.5
18	NL	27,480	680,653	3.8	96.2
19	O	28,626	1,847,370	1.5	98.5
20	PJ	24,585	1,545,024	1.6	98.4
			Mean ± SD	2.4±1.05	97.6±1.05
			SE	0.23	0.23

Note: No background subtraction was made from either stomach or intestine

Bile Reflux in Health and Disease

The data shown in Table 5.4.1 were collected in 20 patients without gallstones, who were referred for measurement of gallbladder ejection fraction. They did not have any symptoms of gastric dyspepsia. Mean DGBR in these subjects was 2.4% (95% CI = 0.4–4.4%). DGBR during fasting or after CCK-8 administration is rare and usually does not exceed 5%. When significant bile reflux is found it may suggest bile gastritis being responsible for patient symptoms. Prokinetic agents are prescribed for patients with large volume D-G reflux.

References

1. Fisher RS, Cohen S. Physiological characteristics of the human pyloric sphincter. Gastroenterology 1973;64:67–75
2. Capper WM, Airth GR, Kilby JO. A test for pyloric regurgitation. Lancet 1966;2:621–623
3. Rokkjaer M, Marqversen J, Kraglund K, Peterson J. Quantitative determination of pyloric regurgitation in response to intraduodenal bolus injection. Scand J Gastroent 1977;12:827–832
4. Nicolai JJ, Silberbusch J, vanRoon F, Schopman W, Berg JWO. A simple method for quantification of biliary reflux. Scand J Gastroent 1980;15:775–780
5. Krishnamurthy GT, Bobba VR, McConnell D, Turner FE, Mesgarzadeh M, Kingston E. Quantitative biliary dynamics: introduction of a new non-invasive scintigraphic technique. J Nucl Med 1983;24:217–223
6. Sorgi M, Causer D, Wolverson RL, Mosimann F, Tulley N, Ghosh SK, Donovan IA, Alexander-Williams J, Harding LK. Quantification and the elimination of errors in bile reflux tests using a gamma camera. Scand J Gastroent 1984;19:33–35
7. Thomas WEG, Jackson PC, Cooper MJ, Davies ER. The problems associated with scintigraphic assessment of duodenogastric reflux. Scand J Gastroenterol 1984;19 (Suppl 92):36–40

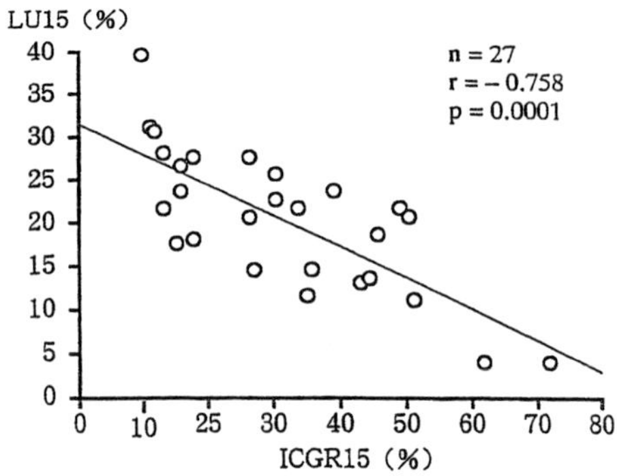

Fig. 5.5.1. Correlation between ^{99m}Tc-GSA uptake (LU15, %) and indocyanine green blood retention. There is a good inverse relationship between ^{99m}Tc-GSA uptake by the liver with plasma clearance of indocyanine green at 15 min [2]

5.5 Imaging and Quantification of Hepatocyte Asialoglycoprotein Receptors

Hepatocyte plasma membrane is rich in asialoglycoprotein (ASGP) receptors which are not found on any other cell in the body. The receptors are located along the basolateral and lateral domain, but not along the canalicular domain [1]. Technetium-99m-DTPA-galactosyl-human-serum albumin (^{99m}Tc-GSA) binds to these receptors and the amount bound varies inversely with the severity of liver disease [2–4]. ^{99m}Tc-GSA is not taken up by the spleen, and like radiocolloid not secreted into bile. Asialoglycoprotein receptor density on the membrane reflects the functional integrity of the hepatocyte accurately, much like the serum level of indocyanine green, cholinesterase, serum albumin, or hepaplastin [3]. The quantity of ^{99m}Tc-GSA uptake correlates well with blood clearance of indocyanine green (Fig. 5.5.1). Technetium-99m-GSA uptake decreases in patients with varieties of liver diseases including chronic hepatitis, cirrhosis, cholangiocarcinoma, hepatocellular cancer, metastasis, fulminant hepatic failure, and space occupying benign lesions of the liver [2–4].

Almost all of the injected radiotracer clears from blood and is taken up exclusively by the liver normally within 15 min. Several parameters are developed to express the hepatocyte function, the most common one being the extraction index at 15 min. It represents the percentage of the integral of the cumulative counts in the liver for 1 min between 15 and 16 min to the total injected dose [2].

Data Collection and Analysis

After 4–6 h of fasting, with the patient in the supine position, a gamma camera (single, double, or triple head) fitted with a low-energy, high-resolution, parallel hole collimator is positioned anterior to the liver. Sequential anterior planar images (128×128) at one frame per 30 s for 20 min are obtained immediately after a bolus injection of 5 mCi ^{99m}Tc-GSA (185 MBq) into the antecubital vein. Immediately after the planar images, SPECT data are acquired on a 128×128×16 matrix computer for 64 stops at 10 s per stop at a 5.6° interval [2]. The spectrometer is set for 140 keV at a 20% window. Liver uptake at 15 min is calculated by using the following formula:

$$\text{Liver uptake at 15 minute (LU15)} = \frac{\int_{15}^{16} C(t)dt \times 100\%}{\text{Total injected dose}}$$

Whole liver counts and residual liver counts are obtained by measuring organ volume from SPECT images. Whole organ volume is determined by detecting the edge for each slice and then adding all of the slices. Volume of each lobe is obtained by selecting the gallbladder fossa-inferior vena cava plane (plane of Sérégé-Cantlie), which divides the liver into physiologic right and left lobes, or by referring to the CT, or MRI references [2]. After obtaining the volume, each lobe is divided into its physiologic segments, the right lobe into anterior and posterior segments, and the left lobe into medial and lateral segments [2–4]. The ratio of the counts in each lobe to the whole liver counts provides the LU15 for the lobe.

Residual count ratio (RCR) is determined by the following formula:

$$\text{RCR} = \frac{\text{RC}}{\text{WC}}$$

where RC = residual count from SPECT images (counts from region of the liver not to be resected) and WC = whole liver count calculated from SPECT images.

Index of residual liver function (RLU15) = LU15×RCR

Some authors express uptake as hepatic GSA clearance using the Patlak plot method and generate functional images of clearance (Ku). This method is powerful but some may raise issue with the chosen terminology "clearance" for an agent that does not clear from the liver [3, 4]. The uptake shows an excellent correlation with indocyanine green plasma clearance. Estimation of predicted postoperative residual function after resection of the liver for hepatocellular carcinoma, cholangiocarcinoma, and metastatic liver tumors shows good correlation with postoperative liver function. This functional parameter may be ideal for predicting end stage liver disease and timing of liver transplantation.

References

1. Steer CJ. Receptor-mediated endocytosis: mechanisms, biologic function, and molecular properties. In: Zakim D, Boyer TD (editors). Hepatology. A textbook of liver disease. WB Saunders Company, Philadelphia, 1996, pp 149–214
2. Uetake M, Koizumi K, Yagawa A, Nogata H, Tezuka T, Kono H, Ozawa T, Kusano T, Miyaburuko M, Hosaka M. Use of Tc-99m DTPA galactosyl human serum albumin to predict postoperative residual liver function. Clin Nucl Med 1999;24:428–434
3. Hwang E, Taki J, Shuke N, Nakajima K, Kinuya S, Konishi S, Michigishi T, Aburano T, Tonami N. Preoperative assessment of residual hepatic functional reserve using Tc-99m-DTPA-galactosyl-human-serum albumin dynamic SPECT. J Nucl Med 1999;40:1644–1651
4. Sasaki N, Shiomi S, Iwata Y, Nishiguchi S, Kuroki T, Kawabe J, Oci H. Clinical usefulness of scintigraphy with Tc-99m-galactosyl-human serum albumin for prognosis of cirrhosis of the liver. J Nucl Med 1999;1652–1656

Gallbladder, Sphincter of Oddi, Cholecystokinin, and Opioid Inter-Relationship

The bile, essential for digestion and absorption of nutrients, is secreted by the liver continuously, stored in the gallbladder during fasting, and discharged into the duodenum intermittently after each meal. The bile salts, which are an important component of bile, promote efficient digestion and absorption of essential nutrients from the intestine. The gallbladder has a unique mechanism to sequester almost all of the bile salts during fasting and release them into the duodenum after the arrival of food. Food stimulates the release of endogenous cholecystokinin into the circulation from the endocrine cells lining the mucosa of the duodenum, jejunum, and upper ileum. Cholecystokinin acts on its receptors located in the smooth muscle and initiates the contraction and emptying of concentrated bile from the gallbladder, and simultaneously relaxes the sphincter of Oddi to allow smooth passage of bile into the duodenum. During the evolutionary process it appears as though nature has placed these three organs very close to each other anatomically to obtain the maximum efficiency of the biologic system (Fig. 6.1.1).

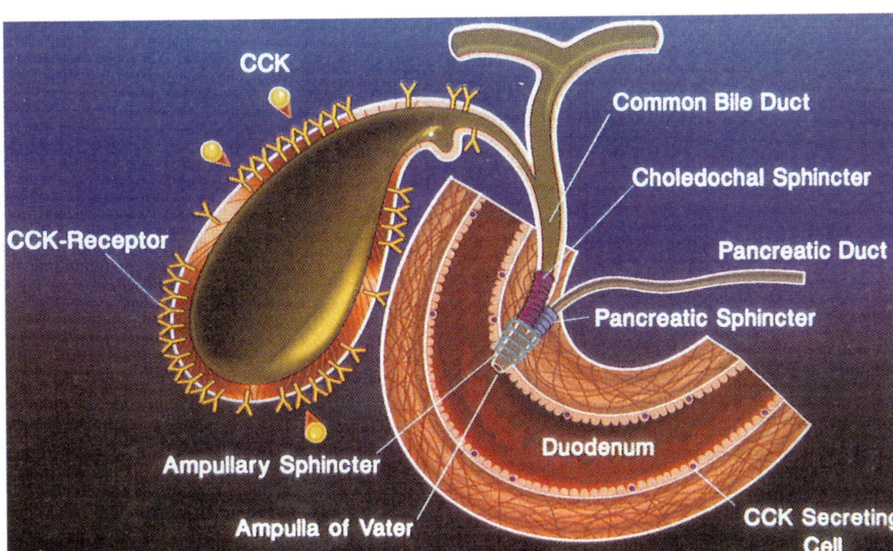

Fig. 6.1.1. Relationship among the sphincter of Oddi, gallbladder, and cholecystokinin. The sphincter of Oddi consists of three components: choledochal sphincter, pancreatic sphincter, and ampullary sphincter. The gallbladder wall contains mainly stimulatory (contraction) and the sphincter of Oddi inhibitory (relaxation) receptors for cholecystokinin. CCK secreting endocrine cells are distributed densely in the mucosa of the duodenum [44]

6.1 Effect of Cholecystokinin on the Gallbladder and Sphincter of Oddi

Cholecystokinin

A hormone mechanism responsible for contraction and emptying of the gallbladder was proposed first by Ivy and Oldberg in 1928 [1]. A year later, Ivy and associates identified the hormone and named it "cholecystokinin" [2].

Source

Cholecystokinin (CCK) is found in various organs of the body including the gastrointestinal, endocrine, genitourinary, and nervous systems [3]. The highest concentration is found in the upper intestinal tract, cerebral cortex, and anterior pituitary gland [4, 5]. In the gastrointestinal tract, the cells secreting cholecystokinin are distributed primarily in the mucosa of the duodenum, jejunum, and upper ileum (Fig. 6.1.2). There are about 40 million (1.3 million/cm) CCK secreting cells in the duodenum, 80 million (0.55 million/cm) in the jejunum, and about 5 million in the entire ileum [4]. There are no CCK secreting cells in the esophagus, stomach, distal ileum, colon, and rectum. The cerebellum and posterior pituitary gland do not contain any CCK secreting cells. Two types of hormone secreting cells are found in the intestinal mucosa: open endocrine cells and closed endocrine cells. Open endocrine cells are tall and flask shaped with microvilli along the free border, which enable direct contact with the digested nutrients passing through the intestinal lumen. Closed endocrine cells are basket shaped without any microvilli and do not reach the mucosal surface; hence they have no direct contact with the nutrients passing through the intestinal lumen [6].

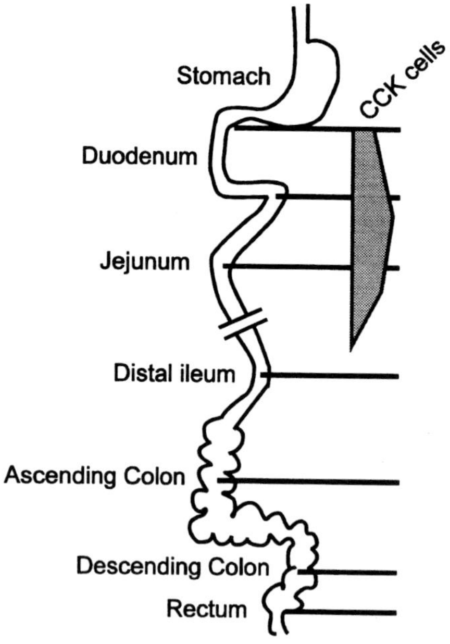

Fig. 6.1.2. Regional distribution of cholecystokinin secreting cells in the alimentary canal. The hormone secreting cells are concentrated mainly in the duodenum, jejunum, and proximal ileum. There are no CCK secreting cells in the esophagus, stomach, and intestinal tract beyond the proximal ileum. Modified from Sjolung et al: Gastroenterology 1983; 85: 1120–30 [4]

Structure

At least five molecular forms of cholecystokinin have been identified. All five are linear chain polypeptides, each with a varying number of amino acids in its molecule [3, 7]. The longer hormones with 33–58 amino acids can be cleaved at different locations to yield hormones of shorter molecular length. The component which retains the carboxyl-terminal tetrapeptide exhibits most of the biologic function of the parent molecule (Fig. 6.1.3). Component I with more than 40 and component II with 33–39 amino acids in the molecule are the most abundant forms. Component III contains 12, component eight (octa-peptide or CCK-8), and component-V four amino acids in the molecule. Component V with four amino acids is the shortest biologically active form.

Hormone CCK-8 has been synthesized and is available for clinical use as sincalide (Kinevac). The terminal amino acid, phenylalanine, is amidated and the seventh amino acid, tyrosine, is sulfated. Sulfation of tyrosine is essential for retention of the biological potency of the hormone (Fig 6.1.4). To be biologically active, each component must possess the carboxy-terminal tetrapeptide. When the amino acids are numbered serially beginning at the carboxyl-terminal ($CO\text{-}NH_2$) end, the hormonal fragments are called CCK-4, CCK-8, CCK-12, CCK-33, CCK-39, etc. The molecular weight of CCK-8 is 1143. Because of its shorter length and lesser mass, CCK-8, on a molar basis, is 4–5 times biologically more potent than CCK-33. All five components of CCK are found in the small intestinal mucosa and the central nervous system. Currently it is believed that each component is secreted, in vivo, by a specific group of CCK secreting cell. The concentration of larger components (CCK-33, CCK-39) is higher in the central nervous system and the gastrointestinal tract, whereas the concentration of smaller components (CCK-8) is higher in the anterior pituitary gland [5].

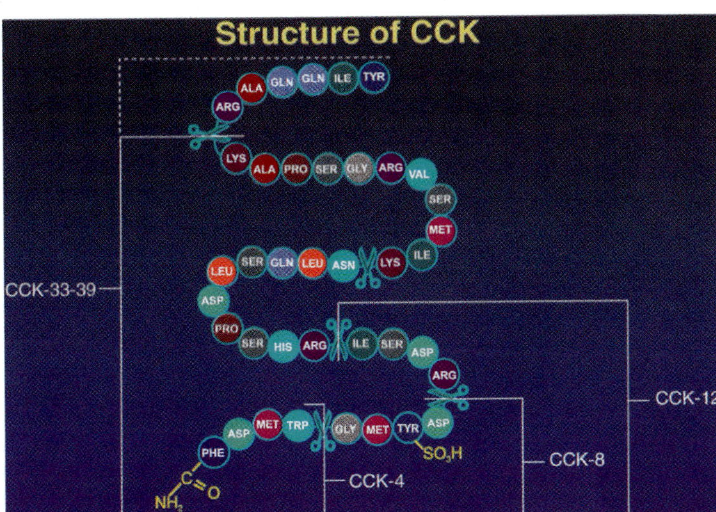

Fig. 6.1.3. Molecular structure of cholecystokinin. It consists of 33–39 amino acids which can be cleaved (scissors) at several locations to produce shorter fragments. Amino-terminal tetrapeptide (CCK-4) is necessary for biological actions of the fragments [44]

Cerulein

Other peptides with a carboxyl-terminal tetrapeptide identical to that of CCK also possess a cholecystokinetic effect. Gastrin and cerulein are two such peptides with an identical carboxy-terminal tetrapeptide and both exhibit a cholecystokinetic effect. Cerulein, isolated first from the skin of an Australian frog, is not found in humans. It resembles CCK-8 structure closely and consists of ten amino acids (decapeptide), two more than CCK-8. The seventh amino acid, tyrosine, is sulfated. The sixth amino acid is threonine in cerulein, and methionine in CCK-8 (Fig. 6.1.4). Biologically, cerulein is ten times more potent than CCK-33 on a molar basis, and 47 times more potent on the basis of its net weight. The molecular weight is 1352 [8].

Release of CCK

Cholecystokinin is released into the circulation soon after the arrival of food into the duodenum. Fat is the most potent stimulant of all nutrients. Serum CCK level begins to rise 8–10 min after a meal, and reaches its peak level by 30–60 min [9, 10]. The serum level remains above the basal level for 2–4 h postmeal, depending upon the nature of food ingested. The serum half-life of CCK is 2.5 min [11].

CCK Receptors

Two types of cholecystokinin receptors have been identified, CCK-A and CCK-B [12]. The gallbladder contains only CCK-A and the pancreas, mostly CCK-B type receptors [13]. These receptors are located on the surface of the cell and provide an easy access to cholecystokinin. Cholecystokinin binds to CCK-A receptors in the gallbladder smooth muscle and initiates its contraction and bile emptying immediately. By binding to CCK-B type receptors, cholecystokinin stimulates pancreatic enzyme and bicarbonate secretion. Cholecystokinin antagonists (loxiglumide, devazepide, and TP-680) either block or reverse its actions by competitively binding to CCK receptors. These antago-

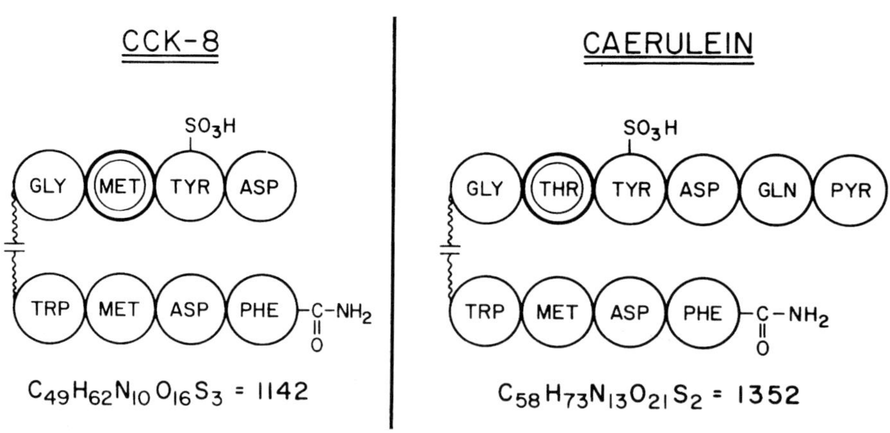

Fig. 6.1.4. Structure of CCK-8 and cerulein. Both contain an identical N-terminal tetrapeptide. The sixth amino acid is methionine in CCK-8 and threonine in cerulein. Both are sulfated on the seventh amino acid, tyrosine. Cerulein has two amino acids (decapeptide) more than CCK-8. Molecular weight of CCK-8 = 1142 and cerulein = 1352 [32]

nists increase appetite, food intake, and weight gain in the animals by blocking CCK receptors [14, 15].

Actions of CCK

The stimulation of the gallbladder contraction and subsequent bile emptying is one of the most important and the best known actions of cholecystokinin. Cholecystokinin simultaneously relaxes the sphincter of Oddi and facilitates smooth passage of bile through it into the duodenum [16]. Cholecystokinin also exhibits other biological actions listed in Table 6.1.1. It increases both the volume and flow of hepatic bile by increasing water secretion by bile canaliculi and bile ducts. For a short while it was thought that a separate hormone (pancreozymin), different from CCK, acted on the pancreas to increase its enzyme and bicarbonate secretion [17]. It is now well recognized that a single hormone, cholecystokinin, possesses both actions: induction of gallbladder contraction and stimulation of pancreatic enzyme secretion [18]. In the pancreas, both cholecystokinin and secretin bind to the same receptor and increase enzyme and bicarbonate secretion [19]. Cholecystokinin increases intestinal peristalsis and promotes antegrade flow of bile and nutrients through the lumen. By inducing contraction of the pyloric sphincter, CCK prevents duodenogastric bile reflux.

Table 6.1.1. Actions of cholecystokinin

1.	Contracts and empties gallbladder
2.	Increases pancreatic enzyme and bicarbonate secretion
3.	Relaxes sphincter of Oddi and lower esophageal junction
4.	Increases secretion of insulin, glucagon, and somatostatin by islet cells
5.	Contracts pyloric sphincter, preventing duodenogastric bile reflux
6.	Increases hepatic bile secretion
7.	Increases intestinal peristalsis
8.	Increases intestinal blood flow
9.	Suppresses appetite
10.	Relaxes lower esophageal sphincter
11.	Protects of gastric mucosa through release of somatostatin
12.	Decreases systolic blood pressure

Cholecystokinin binds to stimulatory CCK-A receptors in the gallbladder smooth muscle and initiates its contraction [13]. Simultaneously, it binds to inhibitory receptors in the sphincter of Oddi smooth muscle and promotes its dilatation. These combined, but paradoxical, actions promote smooth passage of bile from the gallbladder into the duodenum [20]. CCK-A receptor rich smooth muscle is distributed mostly in the fundus and body of the gallbladder. Very few receptors are found in the smooth muscle of the neck and the cystic duct. When serum CCK level rises above the threshold, the fundus contracts first, followed by the body. The relaxation of the sphincter of Oddi occurs at the same time, allowing smooth passage of bile through it [21, 22].

Cholecystokinin and cerulein both act on the same receptors [23–26]. The cystic duct smooth muscle, which has only few CCK receptors, does not usually contract, because its threshold for contraction is set at a much higher level than the threshold for contraction of the smooth muscle in body and fundus. When a large bolus dose of CCK-8 is injected, however, the cystic duct often contracts and prevents gallbladder emptying [27]. In cystic duct syndrome (acalculous chronic cholecystitis), not only is there a decrease in the total number of CCK receptors in the body and fundus, but also the cystic duct smooth muscle threshold is lowered, allowing contraction of the body, fundus, and cystic duct, all at the same time, resulting in non-emptying of the gallbladder [28].

Due to the low serum concentration of cholecystokinin during fasting, most CCK receptors in the smooth muscle are free, facilitating maximum relaxation of the gallbladder wall and a maximum increase in the tonus of the sphincter of Oddi. Both of these factors acting together promote preferential hepatic bile entry into the gallbladder during fasting. Upon CCK release postmeal, these receptors become saturated, initiating contraction of the gallbladder (stimulatory receptors) with simultaneous relaxation (inhibitory receptors) of the sphincter of Oddi. The degree of gallbladder bile emptying (ejection fraction) correlates directly with the total number of CCK receptors in the gallbladder smooth muscle [29].

Dose Response

The degree of gallbladder emptying is dependent both upon the dose rate and duration of infusion of cholecystokinin or cerulein [30]. The higher the dose, the greater the degree of emptying, as long as the administered dose is within the physiologic range (Fig. 6.1.5). The threshold for beginning of gallbladder contraction and emptying lies between 0.5 and 1.0 ng/kg/min CCK-8 or cerulein. Peak emptying is noted between 3 and 5 ng/kg/min dose [31, 32]. A further increase in CCK-8 dose actually decreases gallbladder emptying. An infusion of 0.02 µg/kg (20 ng/kg) or 0.04 µg/kg (40 ng/kg) over a 3-min period results in an ejection fraction which is much lower than that obtained with 0.01 µg/kg over 3 min (Fig. 6.1.6). The CCK-8 doses listed in Table 6.1.2

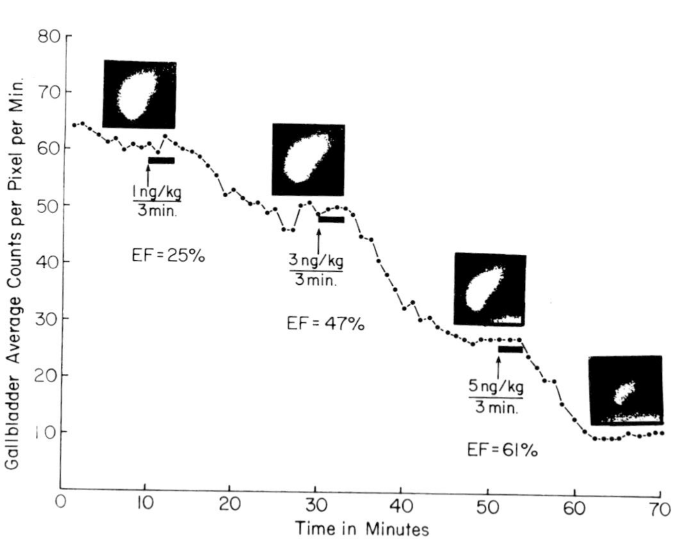

Fig. 6.1.5. Dose response curve: the gallbladder ejection fraction increases as the dose of ceruletide (or CCK-8) increases [32]

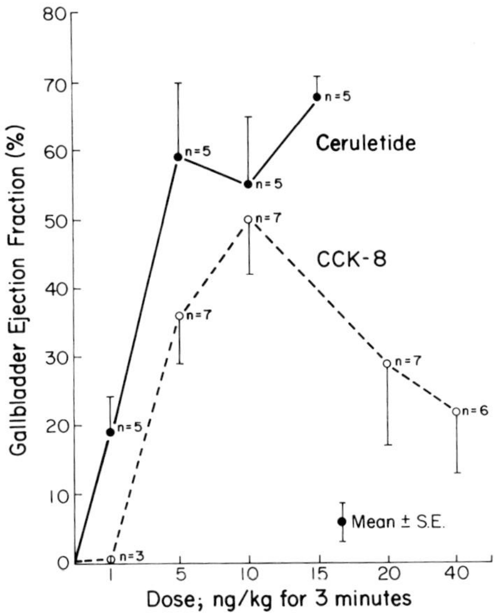

Fig. 6.1.6. Effect of non-physiologic CCK-8 or ceruletide dose on gallbladder emptying. After the peak response at 5 ng/kg/3 min for ceruletide and 10 ng/kg/3 min for CCK-8, the gallbladder ejection fraction begins to decrease for any further increase in dose [31]

are shown to be within the physiologic range and promote smooth contraction and emptying of the gallbladder. For an identical dose, dose rate, and duration, it appears that ceruletide may be more potent than CCK-8. For a 3-min infusion of 5 ng/kg, the gallbladder mean ejection fraction is 61% with ceruletide and 38% with CCK-8 (Fig. 6.1.6).

Table 6.1.2. Cholecystokinin-33 (CCK-33), octa-peptide of cholecystokinin (CCK-8) and ceruletide dose for measurement of gallbladder ejection fraction

Hormone [ref.]	Route	Dose rate	Trade name	Manufacturer	GBEF (%)
CCK-33 (PI)	i.v.	1 IDU/kg/min	CCK-33/Kabi	Pharmacia Lab, Piscataway, NJ	–
CCK-8 [31]	i.v.	10 ng/kg/3 min	Kinevac	Bracco Diagnostics, Princeton, NJ	>35%
Ceruletide [32]	i.v.	5 ng/kg/3 min	Tymtran	Adria Lab., Columbus, OH	>40%
Ceruletide (PI)	i.m.	300 ng/kg	Tymtran	Adria Lab., Columbus, OH	–

IDU = Ivy dog unit; PI = package insert

Effect of a Large Bonus Dose of CCK-8

The dose required during quantitative cholescintigraphy, in general, is found to be much lower than the hormonal dose recommended in the package insert (Kinevac) by the vendor. The package insert dose originally was developed for the oral cholecystogram or for stimulating pancreatic enzyme secretion [30]. The recommended dose in the package insert (0.02 μg/kg or 20 ng/kg) often produces abdominal pain and low ejection fraction (Fig. 6.1.7) when used in control subjects [33–35]. A low ejection fraction response obtained with a larger dose of CCK-8 is attributed to reaching the cystic duct smooth muscle threshold for contraction, with the resultant effect of non-emptying of the gallbladder [27]. Cholecystokinin dual action of antegrade intestinal peristalsis and simultaneous contraction of the pyloric sphincter normally produces forward bile flow through the intestinal lumen and prevents duodenogastric bile reflux [36, 37].

Sequential CCK Doses

The gallbladder ejection fraction remains constant for a fixed dose of cholecystokinin or ceruletide, given on two separate occasions (Fig. 6.1.7). A second identical dose of CCK-8 or ceruletide given 20–30 min after the first dose produces an ejection fraction similar to that of the first dose. There is neither potentiation nor inhibition effect from the first dose, when a period of 20–30 min is allowed between doses. A short serum half-life of 2.5 min does not seem to leave any significant residual CCK activity from the first dose to influence the effect of the second dose [38, 39]. This unique feature enables cholescintigraphy to be used to study the effect of various drugs on the sphincter of Oddi and the gallbladder, after a single dose of ^{99m}Tc-HIDA. The dose of CCK-8 (Kinevac, Bracco Lab., Princeton, NJ) and ceruletide (Tymtran, Adria Lab., Columbus, OH) is measured in microgram units, and cholecystokinin-33 (CCK, Pharmacia Lab., Piscataway, NJ) in Ivy dog units. One Ivy dog unit is defined as the amount of CCK-33 which, when injected intravenously over 10–15 s, increases the pressure within the gallbladder by 1 cmH_2O [40].

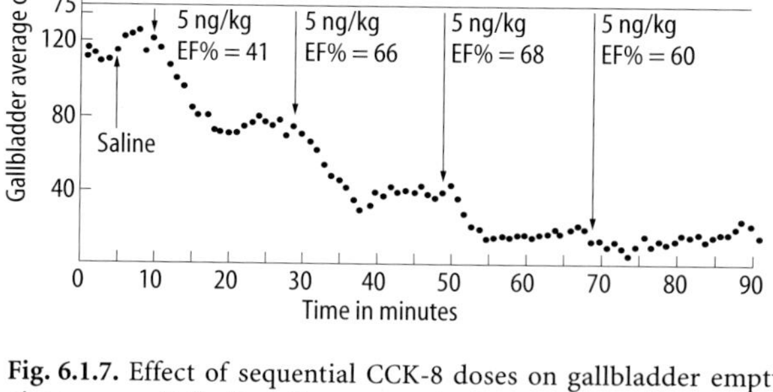

Fig. 6.1.7. Effect of sequential CCK-8 doses on gallbladder emptying. A 5-ng/kg/3 min CCK-8 dose given sequentially four times on a single occasion, with 30 min between doses, produces a similar ejection fraction. Note that a 20-ng/kg/3 min CCK-8 dose given on a different day produces a lower ejection fraction [38]

Sphincter of Oddi

Rugero Oddi in 1887 first proposed a sphincter mechanism at the distal end of the common bile duct which today bears his name [41]. The existence of the sphincter remained controversial for many years, until Boyden in 1937 put an end to the controversy by showing both macroscopic and microscopic details of the sphincter in both animals and humans [42, 43].

Structure and Function

The human sphincter of Oddi is about 10–15 mm in length, situated within the muscular layer of the media of the duodenum (Fig. 6.1.1). It consists of three distinct segments: (1) sphincter choledochus, (2) sphincter pancreaticus, and (3) ampullary sphincter. The choledochal sphincter covers the distal end of the intraduodenal part of the common bile duct, before it joins with the pancreatic duct (duct of Wirsung). The pancreatic sphincter is located at the distal end of the pancreatic duct. The ampullary sphincter covers the distal end of both ducts after they unite to form a single common channel which opens into the duodenal lumen at an elevation called the ampulla of Vater [44]. The title "sphincter of Oddi" refers to all three sphincters.

The main function of the sphincter of Oddi is regulation of bile flow through it and to prevent reflux of duodenal contents into the common bile duct and pancreatic duct. Internally, it prevents bile reflux into the pancreatic duct and reflux of pancreatic enzymes into the common bile duct. In the majority of humans (86%), the distal common bile duct and the distal pancreatic duct join together, forming a common channel of 10–12 mm length which opens into the duodenum at the papilla of Vater. In 6% of patients, the two ducts join together just before opening into the duodenum with a common channel. In the remaining 8% of patients, the two ducts open separately into the duodenal lumen at the ampulla of Vater [45]. The sphincter consists of a circular and a longitudinal layer of muscle. In humans, the entire sphincter is located within the duodenal wall and the wall has to be cut open to expose the sphincter of Oddi for clinical and experimental studies. In the American and Australian opossums, on the other hand, the entire sphincter is situated outside of the duodenal wall, making it easy to study its function, without any need to cut open the duodenal wall.

Sphincter Pressure

The basal pressure within the sphincter Oddi is 15–18 mmHg and rises with the arrival of periodic phasic waves. Phasic waves occur at an average of four waves/min, and each wave lasts for 10–15 s (Fig. 6.1.8). During the passage of a phasic wave, the pressure within the sphincter of Oddi rises sharply, reaching a peak amplitude as high as 90–140 mmHg [46, 47]. Normally, 80% of phasic waves progress antegrade (towards the duodenum), 9% retrograde (towards the liver), and 13% occur simultaneously (Table 6.1.3) at the proximal, middle, and distal segments of the sphincter [48]. The wave normally begins proximally and travels distally within the sphincter. The sphincter of Oddi basal pressure, phasic wave frequency, and direction of propagation remain unchanged after cholecystectomy. Wide variations in normal sphincter of Oddi pressures reported in the literature are often due to technical differences among the studies and

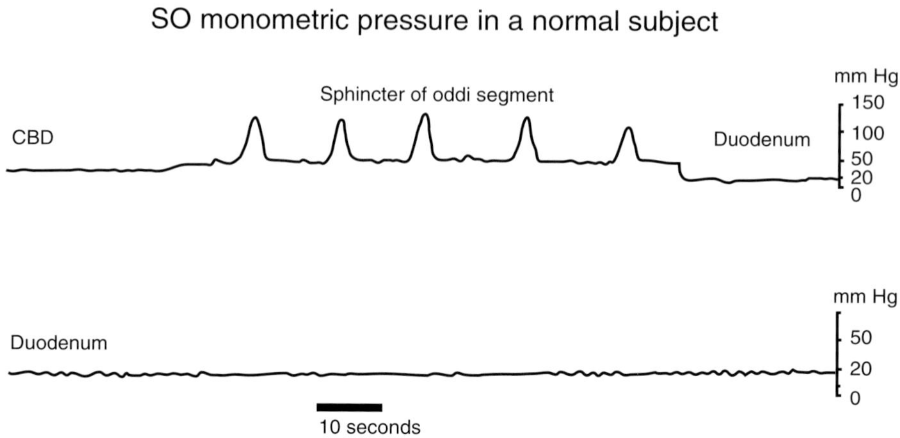

Fig. 6.1.8. Manometric pressure changes in the normal common bile duct and sphincter of Oddi. Sphincter of Oddi basal pressure of 15 mmHg raises to as high as 100–150 mmHg at the peak of a phasic wave. Pressure within the common bile duct remains at 15–20 mmHg [46]

should be taken into account when comparing the results of one study with another. Pressure changes within a sphincter of Oddi remain constant between repeat studies when a standardized technique is applied [49].

Table 6.1.3. Pressure and wave frequency, sequence and amplitude changes in a normal sphincter of Oddi [48]

Parameter	Median	Range
Basal pressure (mmHg)	15	5–35
Wave amplitude (mmHg)	135	95–195
Wave frequency (no./min)	4	2–6
Wave sequence (%):		
Antegrade	80	12–100
Simultaneous	13	0–50
Retrograde	9	0–50

Action of Cholecystokinin on the Sphincter of Oddi

Cholecystokinin acts on the sphincter of Oddi smooth muscle and abolishes immediately the phasic wave activity (Fig. 6.1.9). The hormone reduces the sphincter of Oddi wave amplitude and pressure from a peak of 130–140 mmHg to less than 10 mmHg pressure and reduces the wave frequency from 4 to less than 1. Abolition of waves and reduction in wave amplitude decrease pressure inside and simultaneously promote dilatation of the sphincter orifice [49, 50]. Reduction in wave amplitude and frequency reach a nadir within 2–4 min after a single bolus injection of CCK-8, and the basal state is reestablished after 8–10 min, reflecting the effect of a short serum half-life (2.5 min) of the hormone [11]. The effect on the sphincter is maintained throughout the duration of infusion of the hormone. The sphincter remains open for 2–3 h postmeal due to a longer duration of endogenous CCK release.

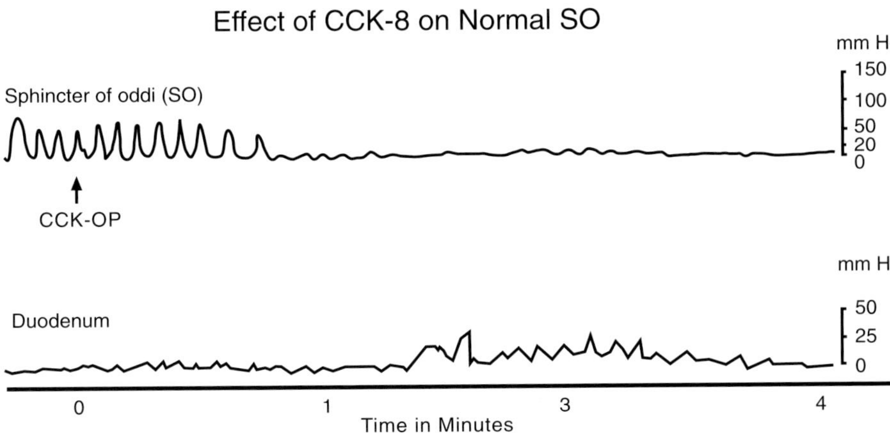

Fig. 6.1.9. Action of CCK-8 on normal sphincter of Oddi. CCK-8 abolishes the phasic waves in the sphincter of Oddi and increases the number of waves and pressure in the duodenum [46]

Gallbladder

The main function of the gallbladder is to store and concentrate bile during fasting and discharge into the duodenum soon after the arrival of food from the stomach. A normal gallbladder holds about 50 ml and empties almost completely following a fatty meal. Since bile salts are essential for efficient digestion and absorption of nutrients, the gallbladder sequesters almost all of them by selectively absorbing water and electrolytes through the wall during fasting. Absorption of water takes place through widely open lateral intercellular spaces between columnar epithelial cells lining the mucosa. (Fig 2.1.4, Chapter 2)

Cholecystokinin Receptors

The gallbladder contraction and emptying is induced by binding of cholecystokinin to CCK-A receptors in its smooth muscle [22]. Degree of gallbladder emptying is related directly to the total number of CCK-A receptors. Emptying decreases as the number of receptors decreases [29]. Cholecystokinin receptors, which are scattered sparsely in the neck and cystic duct smooth muscle, show a much higher threshold for contraction than the receptors distributed densely in the fundus and body. The smooth muscle receptors in neck and cystic duct do not respond (contract) when the CCK dose is within the physiological range. However, the receptors in the neck and cystic duct often respond when a large bolus dose of CCK is administered; and often produce abdominal pain and low ejection fraction in normal subjects [31, 35, 40].

Reduction in gallbladder ejection fraction in patients with biliary dyskinesia is attributed to either a decrease in total number of receptors in the body and fundus or a decrease in threshold for contraction of the CCK receptors in the neck and cystic duct or both [44, 51]. Because of this phenomenon, it is essential to keep CCK-8 dose within the physiological range during quantitative cholescintigraphy in the diagnosis of biliary dyskinesia. Cholecystokinin antagonists like loxiglumide, devazepide, and TP-680 decrease gallbladder emptying by competitively occupying CCK-A receptor in the gallbladder smooth muscle. Animals given CCK antagonists show a reduction in gallbladder emptying and an increase in appetite and weight gain [14, 15]. Cholecystokinin has been shown recently to protect gastric mucosal integrity through release of somatostatin. It relaxes the lower esophageal sphincter through activation of CCK-A receptors at the distal end of the esophagus [52, 53].

References

1. Ivy AC, Oldberg E. A hormone mechanism for gallbladder contraction and evacuation. Am J Physiol 1928;86:599–613
2. Ivy AC, Kloster Gl, Lueth HC, Drewyer GE. On the preparation of "cholecystokinin". Am J Physiol 1929;91:336–344
3. Rehfeld JF. Four basic characteristics of the gastrin-cholecystokinin system. Am J Physiol 1981;240:G255–G266
4. Sjolund K, Sanden G, Hakanson R, Sundler F. Endocrine cells in human intestine: an immunocytochemical study. Gastroenterology 1983;85:1120–1130
5. Rehfeld JF, Lindholm J, Andersen BN, Bardram L, Cantor P, Fenger M, Ludecke DK. Pituitary tumors containing cholecystokinin. N Engl J Med 1987;316:1244–1247
6. Wilding PPH, Ghatei MA, Bloom SR. Hormones of the gastrointestinal tract. In: DeGroot LJ, Ed. Endocrinology. W.B. Saunders Co, Philadelphia 1995, Volume 3, pp 2870–2894
7. Elyseelein VE, Reeve JR Jr, Shively JE, Hawke D, Walsh JH. Partial structure of a large canine cholecystokinin (CCK58): amino acid sequence. Peptides 1982;3:687–691
8. Basso N, Bagarani M, Materia A, Gizzonio D, DePaolis C, Praga C, Speranza V. Effect of caerulein in patients with biliary colic. Gastroenterology 1985;89:605–609
9. Low-Beer TS, Harvey RF, Davies ER, Read AF. Abnormalities of serum cholecystokinin and gallbladder emptying in celiac disease. N Engl J Med 1975;292:961–963
10. Wiener I, Inoue K, Fagan CJ, Lilja P, Watson LC, Thompson JC. Release of cholecystokinin in man: correlation of blood levels with gallbladder contraction. Ann Surg 1981;194:321–327
11. Thompson JC, Fender HR, Ramus NI, Villar HV, Rayford PL. Cholecystokinin metabolism in man and dogs. Ann Surg 1975;182:496–504
12. Wank SA, Pisegna JR, deWeerth A. Brain and gastrointestinal cholecystokinin receptor family: structure and functional expression. Proc Natl Acad Sci 1992;89:8691–8695
13. Tang C, Biemond I, Lamers CB. Cholecystokinin receptors in human pancreas and gallbladder muscle: a comparative study. Gastroenterology 1996;111:1621–1626
14. Hewson G, Leighton GE, Hill RG, Hughes J. The cholecystokinin receptor antagonist L364,718 increases food intake in the rat by attenuation of the action of endogenous cholecystokinin. Br J Pharmacol 1988;93:79–84
15. Tachibana I, Kanagawa K, Yamamoto Y, Otsuki M. Pharmacological profile of a new serine derivative cholecystokinin receptor antagonist TP-680 on pancreatic, biliary and gastric function. J Pharmacol Exp Ther 1996;279:1404–1412
16. Mutt V. Cholecystokinin: Isolation, structure, and function. In: Glass GBJ. ed, Gastrointestinal hormones. Raven Press, New York 1980: pp 169–221
17. Harper AA, Raper HS. Pancreozymin, a stimulant of the secretion of pancreatic enzymes in extracts of the small intestine. J Physiology 1943;103:115–125
18. Jorpes E, Mutt V. Cholecystokinin and pancreozymin, one single hormone? Acta Physiol Scand 1966;66:196–202
19. Grossman MI. Gastrin, Cholecystokinin and Secretin act on one receptor (hypothesis). Lancet 1970;1 (7656):1088–1089
20. Behar J, Biancani P. Pharmacologic characterization of excitatory and inhibitory cholecystokinin receptors of the cat gallbladder and sphincter of Oddi. Gastroenterology 1987;92:764–770
21. Ivy AC, Drewyer GE, Orndoff BH. The effects of cholecystokinin on the human gallbladder. Endocrinology 1930;14:343–348
22. Steigerwalt RW, Goldfine ID, Williams JA. Characterization of cholecystokinin receptors on bovine gallbladder membranes. Am J Physiol 1984;247:G709–G714

23. Behar J, Biancani P. Effects of cholecystokinin and the octapeptide of cholecystokinin on the feline sphincter of Oddi and gallbladder. Mechanisms of action. J Clin Invest 1980;66:1231–1239
24. Sarles JC, Bidart JM, Devaux MA, Echinard C, Castagnini A. Action of cholecystokinin and caerulein on the rabbit sphincter of Oddi. Digestion 1976;14:415–423
25. Wetzner SM, Vincent ME, Robbins AH. Ceruletide-assisted cholecystography: a clinical assessment. Radiology 1979;131:23–26
26. Hedner P, Rorsman G. On the mechanism of action for the effect of cholecystokinin on the choledochoduodenal junction in the cat. Acta Physiol Scand 1969;76:248–254
27. Courtney DF, Clanachan AS, Scott GW. Cholecystokinin constricts the canine cystic duct. Gastroenterology 1983;85:1154–1159
28. Torsoli A, Romarino ML, Alessandrini A. Motility of the biliary tract. Rendic R Gastroenterol 1970;2:67
29. Upp JR Jr, Nealon WH, Singh P, Fagan CJ, Jonas AS, Greeley GH Jr, Thompson JC. Correlation of cholecystokinin receptors with gallbladder contractility in patients with gallstones. Ann Surg 1987;205:641–648
30. Sturdevant RA, Stern DH, Resin H, Isenberg JI. Effect of graded doses of octapeptide of cholecystokinin on gallbladder size in man. Gastroenterology 1973;64:452–456
31. Krishnamurthy GT, Bobba VR, Kingston E. Optimization of octapeptide of cholecystokinin (OP-CCK) dose for gallbladder emptying. In: Raynaud C. ed; Proceedings of the IIIrd world congress of nuclear medicine and biology. Paris, France. Pergamon Press 1982, pp 2244–2247
32. Krishnamurthy GT, Turner FE, Mangham D, Bobba VR, White SA, Langrell K. Ceruletide intravenous dose-response study by a simplified scintigraphic technique. Am J Roentgenol 1985;144:733–737
33. Krishnamurthy S, Krishnamurthy GT. Gallbladder ejection fraction: a decade of progress and future promise (editorial). J Nucl Med 1991;32:542–544
34. Zeissman HA. Cholecystokinin Cholescintigraphy: Victim of its own Success? J Nucl Med 1999;40:2038–2042
35. Toftdahl DB, Hojgaard L, Winkler K. Dynamic cholescintigraphy: induction and description of gallbladder emptying. J Nucl Med 1996;37:261–266
36. Valenzuela JE, Defilippi C. Inhibition of gastric emptying in humans by secretin, the octapeptide of cholecystokinin, and intraduodenal fat. Gastroenterology 1981;81:898–902
37. Fraser R, Fone D, Horowitz M, Dent J. Cholecystokinin octapeptide stimulates phasic and tonic pyloric motility in healthy humans. Gut 1993;34:33–37
38. Krishnamurthy GT, Bobba VR, Kingston E, Turner FE. Measurement of gallbladder emptying sequentially using a single dose of 99mTc-labeled hepatobiliary agent. Gastroenterology 1982,83:773–776
39. Sostre S, Canto MI, Kalloo AN. Gallbladder response to a second dose of cholecystokinin during the same imaging study. Eur J Nucl Med 1992;19:964–965
40. Torsoli A, Romarino ML, Colagrande C, Demaio G. Experiments with cholecystokinin. Acta Radiologica 1961;55:193–206
41. Oddi R. D'une disposition a sphincter speciale del'ouverture du canal cholique. Arch Ital Biol 1887;8:317–322
42. Boyden EA. The sphincter of Oddi in man and certain representative mammals. Surgery 1937;1:25–37
43. Boyden EA. The anatomy of the choledochoduodenal junction in man. Surg Gynecol Obstet 1957;104:641–652
44. Krishnamurthy S, Krishnamurthy GT. Biliary dyskinesia: role of the sphincter of Oddi, gallbladder, and cholecystokinin. J Nucl Med 1997;38:1824–1830
45. Hess W. Surgical Anatomy. In: Surgery of the biliary passages and the pancreas. D Von Nostrand Co, Inc, Princeton, NJ, 1965, pp 3–32
46. Geenen JE, Hogan WJ, Dodds WJ, Stewart ET, Arndorfer RC. Intraluminal pressure recording from the human sphincter of Oddi. Gastroenterology 1980;78:317–324
47. Carr-Locke DL, Gregg JA. Endoscopic manometry of pancreatic and biliary sphincter zones in man. Basal results in healthy volunteers. Dig Dis Sci 1981;26:7–15
48. Thune A, Scicchitano J, Roberts-Thomson IC, Toouli J. Reproducibility of endoscopic sphincter of Oddi manometry. Dig Dis Sci 1991;36:1401–1405
49. Toouli J, Roberts-Thompson C, Dent J, Lee J. Manometric disorders in patients with suspected sphincter of Oddi dysfunction. Gastroenterology 1985;88:1243–1250
50. Toouli J, Hogan WJ, Geenen JE, Dodds WJ, Arndorfer RC. Action of cholecystokinin-octapeptide on sphincter of Oddi basal pressure and phasic wave activity in humans. Surgery 1982;92:497–503
51. Hogan WJ, Geenen JE. Biliary dyskinesia. Endoscopy 1988;20:179–183
52. Konturek JW, Hengst K, Konturek SJ, Sito E, Stachura J, Domschke W. Physiological role of cholecystokinin in gastroprotection in humans. Am J Gastroenterol 1998;93:2385–2390

53. Boeckxstaens GE, Hirsch DP, Fakhry N, Holloway RH, D'Amato M, Tytgat GNJ. Involvement of cholecystokinin-A receptors in transient lower esophageal sphincter relaxations triggered by gastric distension. Am J Gastroenterol 1998, 93:1823–1828

6.2 Opioids

Opioids are the mainstay in the management of moderate to severe intensity pain of diverse etiology. They are the drugs of first choice for the treatment of postoperative pain. Opioids are often mixed with other pain medications including many non-steroidal anti-inflammatory drugs, such as aspirin and acetaminophen. The opioids raise the sphincter of Oddi pressure by acting on its smooth muscle and thus interfere with cholecystokinin or fatty meal stimulated gallbladder ejection fraction. Action of many opioids on the sphincter lasts much longer than their serum half-life would indicate, suggesting that drug metabolites may also possess a constrictive action on the sphincter of Oddi. The interaction between the opioids and the sphincter of Oddi calls for their careful scrutiny during quantitative cholescintigraphy.

History of Opioids

"Opioid" is a generic name that refers to both natural and synthetic compounds with a "morphine-like action." They are derived from opium, which in Greek means juice. The juice comes from the capsule of the unripe seed of *Papaver somniferum*. The milky juice from the seed is dried and made into opium powder, which contains more than 20 alkaloids. Serturner first isolated a pure substance from this powder in 1806, which produced somnolence first, followed by a state of dreaming. He called it morphine after the Greek god of dreams, Morpheus. Codeine was isolated from opium powder in 1832 and papaverine in 1848 [1]. The analgesic action of all opioids is graded with reference to morphine, which serves as the gold standard for pain control. Table 6.2.1 shows different opioids available for pain control and their effect on the sphincter of Oddi.

Biokinetics of Morphine

Morphine consists of an OH group at positions 3 and 6 and a CH_3 group at 17 (Fig. 6.2.1). Other opioids differ structurally from morphine by having different chemical substitutions at the 3, 6, and 17 positions. Morphine is administered by oral, subcutaneous, intramuscular, or intravenous routes. Many dermal patches are now available for long-term continuous application. Intravenous injections are preferred for hospital patients, especially during the immediate postoperative period. Upon intravenous injection, morphine is distributed in an initial volume of 71.8 l/kg and clears from the plasma with two components: component I with a half-time of 0.16 h and component II with a half-time of 2.5 h (Table 6.2.2). Morphine is metabolized in the liver and converted into morphine glucuronide, which clears from plasma much more slowly than the parent molecule. About 60% of injected morphine is excreted in urine in 24 h, and 73% in 3 days. Excretion rate does not change in patients with cirrhosis of the liver [2].

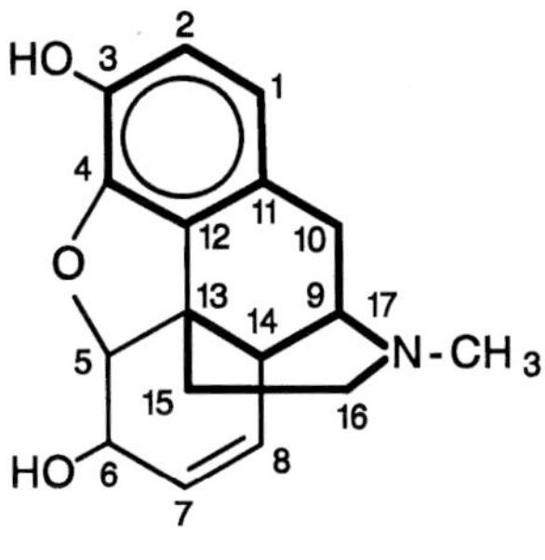

Fig. 6.2.1. Structure of morphine. Note OH group at positions 3 and 6 and CH_3 at position 17. The structure of other opioids differs mainly in having different chemical substitution at these positions

Table 6.2.1. Effect of opioids on the sphincter of Oddi. The drugs are grouped under four major categories into marked, moderate, mild, and no effect based on the extent of sphincter of Oddi pressure rise

Effect	Generic name	Proprietary name
Marked rise in sphincter pressure	Morphine	Morphine
	Levorphanol	Dromoran
	Meperidine (pethidine)	Demerol
Moderate rise in sphincter pressure	Dextromoramide	Palfium
	Diacetyl morphine	Heroin
	Codeine	Codeine
	Fentanyl	Sublimaze
	Butorphanol	Stadol
	Nalbuphine	Nubain
	Hydrocodone	Hycodon
	Oxycodone	Roxicodone
	Propoxyphene	Darvon
	Bupremorphine	Buprenex
Mild rise in sphincter pressure	Dextropropoxyphene HCl	Doloxene
	Pentazocine	Talwin
	Phenazocine	Norphen
	Phenoperidine	Operidine
No effect on sphincter	Hydroxyzine	Hydroxyzine

Table 6.2.2. Pharmacokinetics of morphine [2]

Initial volume of distribution (l/kg)	71.8±65.2
Clearance half-time of fast component (h)	0.16±0.1
Clearance half-time of slow component (h)	2.5±1.5
Plasma protein binding (%)	19.8±6.1
Urinary excretion in 72 h (% dose)	72.9±10.0

Morphine Dose

A minimum of 0.04 mg/kg intravenous morphine is recommended during ^{99m}Tc-HIDA cholescintigraphy [3]. Intravenous doses as large as 15 mg are well tolerated [4]. In adults, a total intravenous dose of 3–4 mg morphine sulfate is usually adequate for confirmation of acute cholecystitis with cholescintigraphy. Liver extracts 60–80% of morphine on first pass and converts rapidly into a glucuronide form. Because of high extraction and rapid metabolism in the liver, oral morphine is not as effective as an intravenous dose.

Action of Morphine on the Sphincter of Oddi

Morphine acts on the sphincter of Oddi within 2–3 min after an intravenous injection and increases the sphincter basal wave frequency from 4 to 10–12/min and the wave amplitude from 70 to 136 mmHg (Fig. 6.2.2). The common bile duct basal pressure increases from 10 to 29 mmHg [4]. A low dose increases only the rate and amplitude whereas higher doses increase basal pressure as well [5]. During a ^{99m}Tc-HIDA study, most gallbladders with a patent cystic duct are visualized within 5–15 min after an intravenous dose of morphine. The effect of morphine on the sphincter of Oddi is mediated by all types of opioid receptors. Naloxone and atropine slightly modify, but do not completely abolish, the effect of morphine on the sphincter.

Morphine is the most potent of all opioids. The effect of other opioids on the sphincter of Oddi is a function of their structural configuration (Table 6.2.1). The effect of levorphonol, dextromoramide, and meperidine on the sphincter of Oddi is equivalent to that of morphine [6, 7]. Fentanyl, nolbuphine, hydrocodon, propoxyphene, and bupremorphine show a moderate spasmodic effect on the sphincter. Pentazocine, phenozocine, and phenoperidine show a mild effect and hydroxyzine has no effect on the sphincter of Oddi [8].

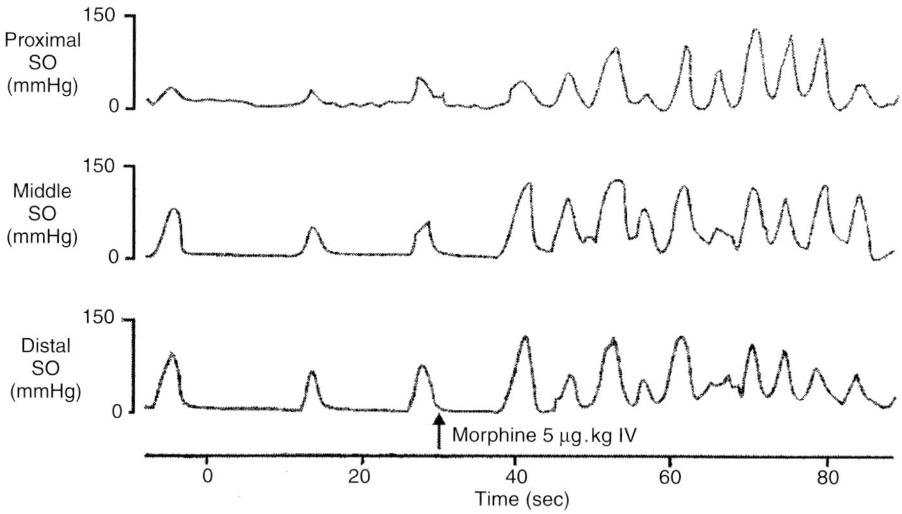

Fig. 6.2.2. Effect of morphine on the sphincter of Oddi. Morphine increases both the number and the amplitude of wave pressure throughout the sphincter of Oddi and forces hepatic bile entry into gallbladder when the cystic duct is patent [4]

Screening for Opioid Intake

Quantitative cholescintigraphy is frequently used in the diagnosis of biliary dyskinesia, which consists of two disease entities: cystic duct syndrome (CDS) and sphincter of Oddi spasm (SOS). The most consistent quantitative functional abnormality in patients with biliary dyskinesia is a reduction in gallbladder ejection fraction in the case of cystic duct syndrome, and bile reflux into hepatic duct followed by a rapid refilling of the gallbladder in the case of sphincter of Oddi spasm [9]. Because of the spasmodic effect on the sphincter of Oddi, it is critical to ensure that the patient is not on any opioids prior to performing a quantitative cholescintigraphy [10]. This issue becomes even more complex in outpatients, where many patients are unaware that a non-steroidal anti-inflammatory drug they take for a variety of indications (arthritis, headache, peptic ulcer, or primary or metastatic cancer) may contain an opioid. This problem is relatively easy to recognize in hospitalized patients by careful review of the chart for the list of current medication.

As only about 60–75% of the administered dose of morphine is excreted in 24–72 h urine, a safe rule is to allow a minimum of 24 h for inpatients and 48 h for outpatients off opioids before performing a quantitative cholescintigraphy for the diagnosis of biliary dyskinesia [2]. If the ejection fraction is within the normal range in a patient who has received an opioid, then there is no need to repeat the test. The test should be repeated if the ejection fraction is low and the patient has received an opioid within the previous 48 h. The ejection fraction measured after discontinuation of an opioid for longer than 48 h often shows a dramatic increase in value when compared to the value before discontinuation (Fig. 6.2.3).

Morphine or Cholecystokinin; One, Neither, or Both?

Varieties of protocols are used in the performance of a ^{99m}Tc-HIDA study. The clinical indication for a ^{99m}Tc-HIDA study is established first in order to determine when to give or not to give morphine or cholecystokinin [11, 12]. In patients with suspected acute cholecystitis, giving morphine before or during cholescintigraphy is appropriate, espe-

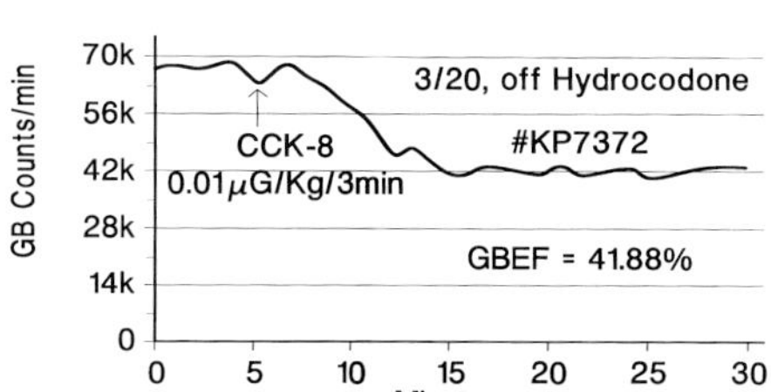

Fig. 6.2.3. Effect of CCK-8 on gallbladder ejection fraction with and without opioids. Note an ejection fraction of 21.16% while on hydrocodone and a value of 41.88% while off hydrocodone

cially when the gallbladder is not seen by 60 min. In a patient with suspected biliary dyskinesia, however, it is inappropriate to give morphine or cholecystokinin prior to cholescintigraphy. In suspected biliary dyskinesia, it is better to wait and take delayed images at 2–4 h after injection of ^{99m}Tc-HIDA. Cholecystokinin is given later to measure the gallbladder ejection fraction. Poor emptying of the gallbladder is a characteristic feature of biliary dyskinesia. The gallbladder also empties poorly in patients given an opioid (Fig. 6.2.3). When the gallbladder is not seen by 60 min in a patient with suspected acute cholecystitis, it is appropriate to administer 0.04 mg/kg morphine intravenously at 60 min and take images for an additional 30 min. When the gallbladder appears after 0.04 mg/kg intravenous morphine, CCK-8 (0.02 μg/kg or 20 ng/kg) infused slowly over 30 min is shown to elicit gallbladder emptying in some patients up to 50% [13]. It is important, however, to find out first the ejection fraction in normal subjects after infusing CCK-8 slowly over 30 min for comparison with patients.

References

1. Jaffe JH, Martin WR. Opioid analgesics and antagonists. In: Gilman AG, Rall TW, Niles AJ, Taylor P. eds. Goodman and Gilman's The pharmacological basis of therapeutics. Eighth edition, Pergamon Press, New York, 1990, pp 485–521
2. Patwardhan RV, Johnson RF, Hoyumpa A Jr, Sheehan JJ, Desmond PV, Wilkinson GR, Branch RA, Schenker S. Normal metabolism of morphine in cirrhosis. Gastroenterology 1981;81:1006–1011
3. Choy D, Shi EC, McLean RG, Hoschl R, Murray IPC, Ham JM. Cholescintigraphy in acute cholecystitis: use of intravenous morphine. Radiology 1984;151:203–207
4. Helm JF, Venu RP, Geenen JE, Hogan WJ, Dodds WJ, Toouli J, Arndorfer RC. Effects of morphine on the human sphincter of Oddi. Gut 1988;29:1402–1407
5. Venu R, Toouli J, Geenen JE, Hogan WJ, Helm J, Dodds WJ, Arndorfer RC. Effect of morphine on motor activity of the human sphincter of Oddi. Gastroenterology 1982;84:1342 (Abs)
6. Jones RM, Fiddian-Green R, Knight PR. Narcotic induced choledochoduodenal sphincter spasm reversed by glucagon. Anesth Analg 1980;59:946–947
7. Hopton DS, Torrance HB. Action of various new analgesic drugs on the human common bile duct. Gut 1967;8:296–300
8. Chessick KC, Black S, Hoye SJ. Spasm and operative cholangiography. Arch Surg 1975;110:53–57
9. Krishnamurthy S, Krishnamurthy GT. Biliary dyskinesia: role of the sphincter of Oddi, gallbladder, and cholecystokinin. J Nucl Med 1997;38:1824–1830
10. Joehl RJ, Koch KL, Nahrwold DL. Opioid drugs cause bile duct obstruction during hepatobiliary scans. Am J Surg 1984;147:134–138
11. Westlake PJ, Hershfield NB, Kelly JK, Kloiber R, Lui R, Sutherland LR, Shaffer EA. Chronic right upper quadrant pain without gallstones: does HIDA scan predict outcome after cholecystectomy? Am J Gastroenterol 1990;85:986–990
12. Krishnamurthy S, Krishnamurthy GT. Cholecystokinin and morphine pharmacological intervention during 99mTc-HIDA cholescintigraphy: a rational approach. Semin Nucl Med 1996;26:16–24
13. Achong DM, Oates E. Normal gallbladder ejection fraction after morphine augmentation. Clin Nucl Med 1999;24:837–841

Intrahepatic Cholestasis

Cholestasis is retention of bile within the hepatobiliary system resulting in an accumulation of bile products in the body fluids. It is divided into intrahepatic and extrahepatic types, depending upon the location of pathology. Intrahepatic cholestasis is defined traditionally as bile retention within the hepatocytes, bile canaliculi, cholangioles, and small or large bile ducts down to and including the proximal two-thirds of the right hepatic and left hepatic ducts. Extrahepatic cholestasis is bile stasis due to a pathology located at the distal one-third of the right hepatic and left hepatic ducts and beyond, down to and including the sphincter of Oddi. The previous classification into obstructive and non-obstructive jaundice is no longer popular clinically [1].

Bile Secretion

Formation of bile is an osmotic pressure dependent uptake and secretory process that occurs along the basolateral and canalicular domains of the hepatocyte, respectively. Of a total of approximately 600 ml bile produced by the liver per day, 450 ml is secreted by the hepatocytes and the remaining 150 ml by cells lining the bile canaliculi and bile ducts (Chap. 2, Fig. 1). About 50% of bile secreted by the hepatocytes (225 ml) is bile acid dependent and the remaining 50% (225 ml) is independent of bile acid secretion. The uptake of bile acids, non-bile acid organic anions, cations, and other solutes by the hepatocytes from blood in the space of Disse occurs along the basolateral border. Of the several mechanisms utilized for the solute uptake, Na^{+}-K^{+} ATPase pump, Na^{+}-BS^{-} (bile salt) co-transport, sodium-hydrogen exchange, Na-HCO_3^- symporter, and organic anion endocytosis play the major roles [2]. Bile salts (taurocholate) are the most important and abundant solutes in bile. Transport of bile salts from blood into hepatocytes is mediated by the sodium taurocholate co-transporter (NTCP) system [3]. AT-Pase of the basolateral border regulates the extracellular and intracellular ion concentration gradient [4].

Active transport of solutes across the canalicular membrane is the rate limiting step in the amount of bile produced per day. The tight junction between the two adjacent hepatocytes is functionally leaky (a leaky tight junction) and allows passage of water and electrolytes from blood into the canalicular lumen. The canalicular lumen situated between two adjacent hepatocytes is about 0.75 μm in diameter and the wall contains microvilli of 500–1000 nm in length, and 100 nm in diameter. The canaliculi and their microvilli contract and propel bile towards larger bile ducts. Secretion of large lipophilic cations (anticancer drugs, calcium-channel blockers, cyclosporin A, and other drugs) is mediated by a transporter protein called multidrug-resistance-1 P-glycoprotein (MDR1). Secretion of phosphatidylcholine is facilitated by another protein called multidrug-resistance-3 P-glycoprotein called MDR3.

7.1 Imaging with ^{99m}Tc-HIDA

Transport of organic anions, including Bromosulphalein, glucuronides, and possibly ^{99m}Tc-HIDA, across the canalicular membrane is attributed to multidrug resistance protein 2 (MRP2). Endotoxin lipopolysaccharide induces cholestasis by an early retrieval followed by downregulation of MRP2, which moves from the canalicular membrane to the interior of the cell [5]. Inhibition of contraction of the canalicular wall and microvilli results in atony and dilatation of the canaliculi leading to intrahepatic cholestasis (Fig. 7.1.1). ^{99m}Tc-HIDA is secreted into canalicular bile in free form, without undergoing any biotransformation during its intracellular transit. This free status can be confirmed by reinjecting ^{99m}Tc-HIDA labeled gallbladder bile intravenously into the same animal, reproducing the original biokinetic parameters [6]. Reduction in uptake and slow transit through the hepatocytes, and collection in the dilated canaliculi, produces a low hepatic extraction fraction and prolongation of excretion half-time in a ^{99m}Tc-HIDA study.

Etiology of Intrahepatic Cholestasis

Three types of injury are recognized as being responsible for cholestasis: (1) direct injury, (2) immunologic, and (3) cholestatic. These injuries are caused by microorganisms, poisons, drugs, and metabolic, granulomatous, veno-occlusive, ischemic, and other diseases (Fig. 7.1.2). The injury may involve the endoplasmic reticulum, lysosomes, mitochondria of the hepatocytes or the canalicular cells. In the case of drugs, the injury may be caused directly by the offending agent or by one of its metabolic products [7].

Viral Hepatitis. All types of viral hepatitis (A, B, C, D, E, and G) cause intrahepatic cholestasis and all produce an identical image pattern. The diagnosis is usually made

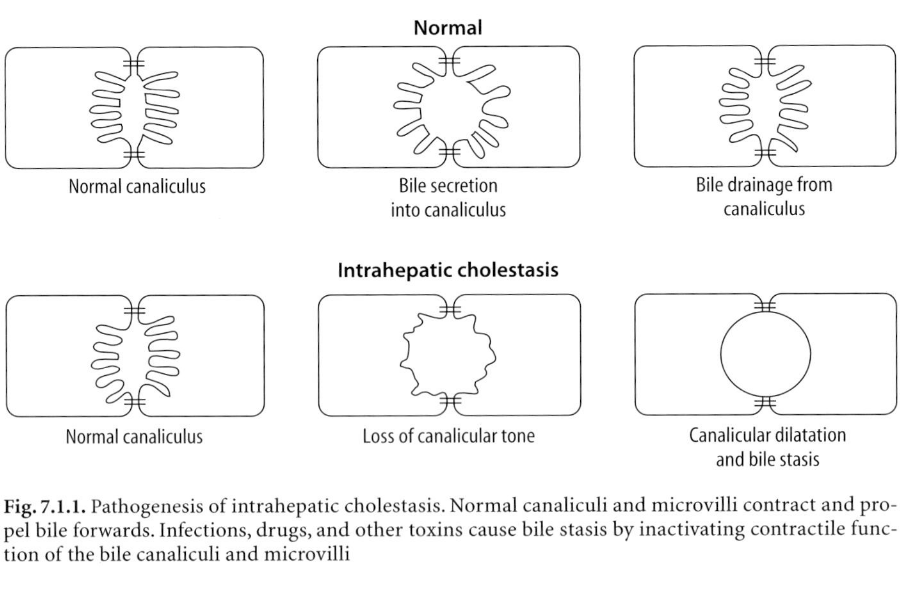

Fig. 7.1.1. Pathogenesis of intrahepatic cholestasis. Normal canaliculi and microvilli contract and propel bile forwards. Infections, drugs, and other toxins cause bile stasis by inactivating contractile function of the bile canaliculi and microvilli

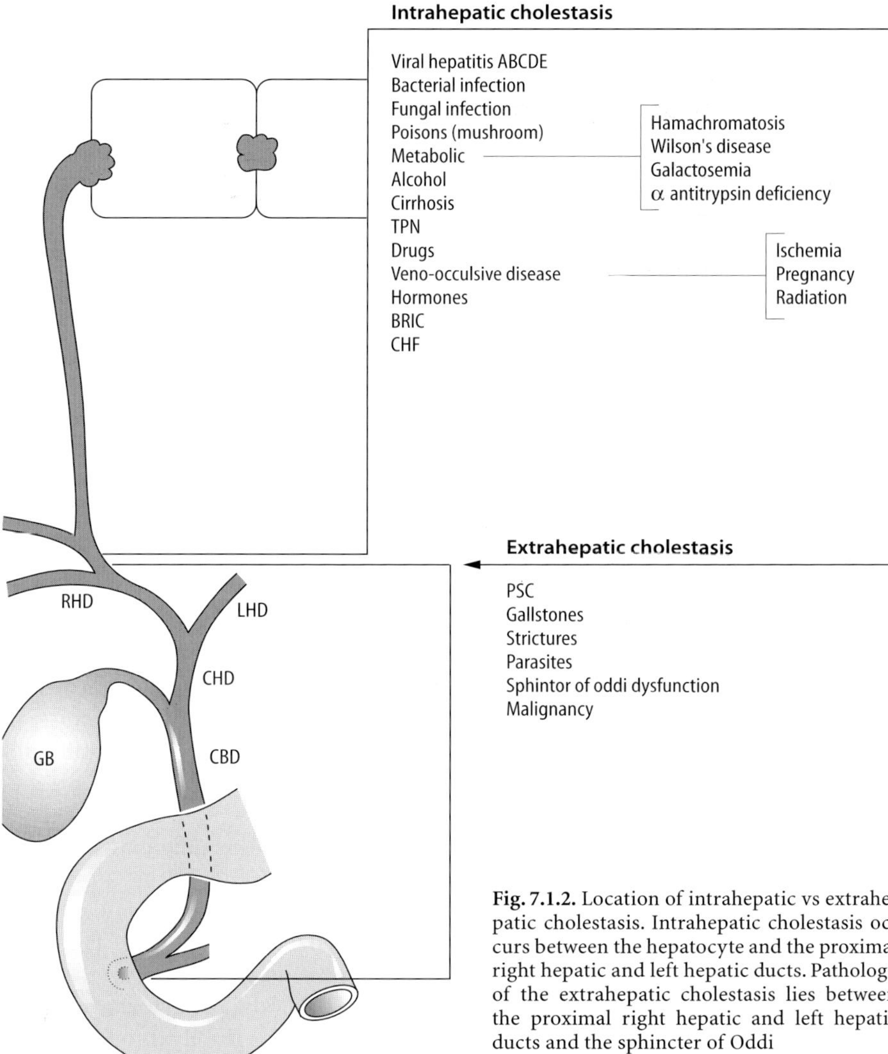

Fig. 7.1.2. Location of intrahepatic vs extrahepatic cholestasis. Intrahepatic cholestasis occurs between the hepatocyte and the proximal right hepatic and left hepatic ducts. Pathology of the extrahepatic cholestasis lies between the proximal right hepatic and left hepatic ducts and the sphincter of Oddi

by a getting a detailed clinical history and by obtaining a serum hepatitis profile. Bacterial and fungal infections and toxins (mushroom poisoning) also cause intrahepatic cholestasis primarily by affecting the hepatocytes and cholangioles. Bile secretion rate is reduced; hence bile ducts and the gallbladder appear late in a ^{99m}Tc-HIDA study (Fig. 7.1.3).

Drugs. Drugs are the most common cause of intrahepatic cholestasis, which is classified into two major types [8]: (1) hypersensitive (exudative) and (2) canalicular. The hypersensitive type is characterized by fever, anorexia, marked eosinophilia, and increased levels of serum cholesterol and alkaline phosphatase. The canalicular type is

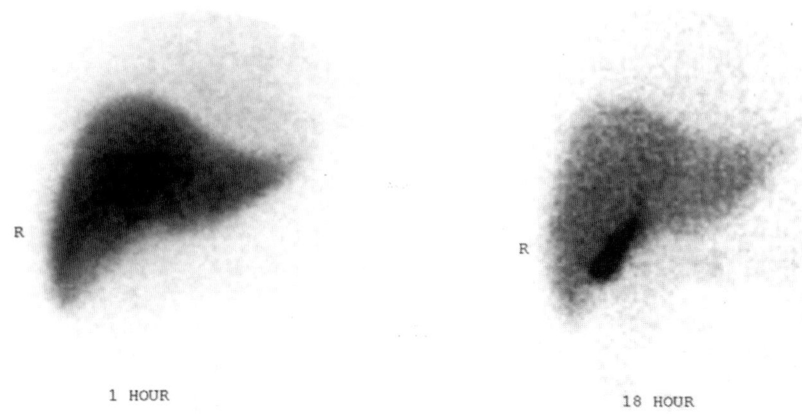

Fig. 7.1.3. Hepatitis A. Diffuse radiotracer retention with no bile secretion for 1 h in a patient with hepatitis A. Gallbladder is seen at 18 h and the intestinal activity has moved away from the field of view of the gamma camera

characterized by intense pruritus, associated with a normal eosinophil count and serum alkaline phosphatase level [9]. Sulfonamides, quinidine, and allopurinol are incriminated in the hypersensitivity type of intrahepatic cholestasis. Sex hormones, phenothiazines, antibiotics (erythromycin), and nitrofurantoin are common causes of the canalicular type of intrahepatic cholestasis. The drug or one of its metabolites secreted into bile canaliculi interferes with canalicular contraction, causing intrahepatic cholestasis [10].

It is estimated that about 2% of hospitalized patients in the United States suffer from some form of intrahepatic cholestasis related to a prescription drug. As many as 1% of patients receiving chlorpromazine develop intrahepatic cholestasis [9]. Various drugs that cause intrahepatic cholestasis are listed in Table 7.1.1. Most of the drugs react with cytochrome p450 and undergo conjugation with glucuronic acid, sulfate, amino acids, or glutathione prior to elimination from the body. The cytochrome p450 system is under genetic control and produces cytotoxic effects mainly through formation of electrophiles and free radicles [11, 12]. A detailed drug history aids in identifying the offending agent responsible for intrahepatic cholestasis. The cholescintigraphic image pattern remains non-specific in intrahepatic cholestasis [13].

Metabolic Causes. Hemochromatosis due to iron overload, Wilson's disease due to copper overload, and fatty infiltration, and deficiency of several enzymes are known metabolic causes of intrahepatic cholestasis [14, 15].

Alcoholic Hepatitis. Alcohol is metabolized primarily in the liver and converted into acetaldehyde through the enzyme alcohol dehydrogenase. Acetaldehyde in turn is converted into acetate by the enzyme aldehyde dehydrogenase. Each gram of alcohol produces seven calories of energy. Most of the liver injury from alcohol occurs primarily due to its metabolite, acetaldehyde, whose accumulation exerts a toxic effect on the plasma membrane, tubulin, and the other cytoskeleton of the hepatocyte [16]. When alcohol intake continues for many years, other toxic effects are manifested in the form of fatty infiltration, fibrosis, and ultimately cirrhosis of the liver and portal hypertension.

Table 7.1.1. Localization of drug induced intrahepatic cholestasis [9].

Hepatocyte	Canaliculus	Hepatocyte and canaliculus	Bile Ducts
Carbon tetrachloride	Estrogens	Phenytoin	Benoxyprofen
Halothane	Testosterone	Quinidine	Ascending cholangitis
Chloroform	Phenothiazine	Allopurinol	Floxuridine
Amiodarone	Erythromycin	Butazolidine	–
Methyldopa	Nitrofurantoin	Thiobendozole	–
Isoniazid	Azathioprine	Furosemide	–
Ketoconazole	Cyclosporin A	Sulfonamide	–
Acetaminophen	Tranquilizers	–	
Rifampin	Antipsychotic agents	–	–
Indomethacin	–	–	–
Tetracycline	–	–	–
Valproic acid			
Flexin			
Novobiocin			
Cocaine			
Flutamide			

Primary Biliary Cirrhosis (PBC). Primary biliary cirrhosis is a disease of unknown etiology and affects primarily the canaliculi, cholangioles, and small bile ducts. Clinically, PBC presents with pruritus and malaise accompanied by elevation of serum liver enzymes and lipoproteins. It is more common in middle aged women than men. Serum antimitochondrial antibody is found in almost 100% of patients [17]. Both planar and SPECT cholescintigraphy with ^{99m}Tc-HIDA show diffuse parenchymal retention with uniform prolongation of excretion half-time from all regions of the liver. The extrahepatic biliary tree remains normal, a common feature for all intrahepatic cholestasis. Cholescintigraphic features enable differentiation of PBC from primary sclerosing cholangitis, where the parenchymal retention is non-uniform [18]. The gallbladder remains normal in size but shows a reduction of CCK-8 stimulated ejection fraction. In a middle aged woman with a positive serum antimitochondrial antibody who clinically presents with pruritus and malaise, a ^{99m}Tc-HIDA study is confirmatory for PBC if it shows a diffuse prolongation of excretion half-time and no obstruction of the extrahepatic biliary tree. A normal extrahepatic biliary tree may even preclude the need for a contrast cholangiogram to exclude primary sclerosing cholangitis, which PBC often clinically mimics [18]. Characteristic cholescintigraphic features of primary sclerosing cholangitis and primary biliary cirrhosis enable differentiation between two relatively rare conditions [18, 19].

Benign Recurrent Intrahepatic Cholestasis (BRIC). BRIC is a rare disorder affecting patients in their 30s and often found in several members of the same family. Intense pruritus with elevation of liver enzymes, accompanied by spontaneous recovery, are its characteristic features. The extrahepatic biliary tree is normal [20]. There are no identifiable serum markers for BRIC. The hepatocytes are unable to get rid off bile acids and other organic anions from the body [21]. Uptake of ^{99m}Tc-HIDA by the hepatocyte is normal, but secretion into bile is delayed or absent, resulting in nondelineation of the entire biliary system, often mimicking total acute common bile duct obstruction. The image pattern appears much like a radiocolloid scan without the spleen.

Total Parenteral Nutrition (TPN). The major liver enzyme abnormalities in patients with TPN are elevation of gamma glutamyl transferase, Alaline aminotransferase (ALT), and alkaline phosphatase. Peak enzyme elevation occurs 1–4 weeks after initiation of TPN. Early pathological changes include fatty infiltration in adults and intrahepatic cholestasis in children. When TPN is continued for many years, fibrosis and cirrhosis set in [22]. Uptake of ^{99m}Tc-HIDA by the hepatocyte is maintained but secretion is markedly delayed or even absent, mimicking total CBD obstruction. The gallbladder is often non-visualized [23].

Ischemic Hepatitis. This condition is often due to an acute reversible hypotension or cardiac failure. Following the ischemic episode there is a rapid rise in aspartate amino transferase and lactic dehydrogenase, and mild elevation of bilirubin and glucose. Liver enzyme abnormality returns to normal, usually within 8–10 days [24]. Functional abnormalities tend to be much more severe in intrahepatic cholestasis than in patients with early partial obstruction of the common bile duct [25].

Acute Cholangitis. Acute cholangitis clinically presents as a "Charcot triad," which consists of fever with chills, jaundice, and abdominal pain, as described originally by Charcot in 1877 [26]. Obstruction of the common bile duct first initiates the process and then sustains acute cholangitis. Obstruction leads to bacterial overgrowth and reflux of infected bile from the liver into the blood stream. As many as 90% of patients may remain asymptomatic when the obstruction of the common bile duct is not critical or complete [27, 28]. The Charcot triad sets in mostly when the obstruction becomes complete. Both gram-positive and gram-negative organisms are found with equal frequency. Serum bilirubin rises above 5 mg% in more than 50% of patients. Leukocytosis is`frequent (63%) and elevation of serum amylase occurs in 30% of patients [29]. Elevation of serum bilirubin above 5 mg% is a common feature of acute cholangitis, but not of acute cholecystitis (Table 7.1.2).

In the past, choledocholithiasis and postoperative stricture were the most common causes of acute cholangitis. In series reported prior to 1980, stone or postoperative stricture accounted for almost 90% of acute cholangitis; now they account for only 26%. Instrumentation (ERCP) of the biliary tract is now the most common cause of acute cholangitis (35%), indicating a shift in etiology of acute cholangitis in more recent years [29].

Scintigraphic Features of Intrahepatic Cholestasis

Injury to the hepatocyte, bile canaliculi, and small bile ducts produces a non-specific image pattern in a ^{99m}Tc-HIDA study. The exact site of injury among these three locations cannot be determined from the images. An etiologic diagnosis, therefore, requires a thorough knowledge of clinical presentation, liver function tests, and a serum viral profile for hepatitis. The diseases that combine the features of both intrahepatic and extrahepatic cholestasis (e.g., sclerosing cholangitis) have a very characteristic image presentation and often enable an etiologic diagnosis to be made [18, 19].

The dose of ^{99m}Tc-HIDA for imaging is increased to 5 and 10 mCi to compensate for a decrease in hepatocyte uptake secondary to a high serum bilirubin, which competes with ^{99m}Tc-HIDA. The hepatic extraction fraction decreases and excretion half-time increases, in direct proportion to an elevation of serum bilirubin (Fig. 7.1.4). Delayed images at 4 or 24 h are necessary to show intestinal activity, which establishes patency of the bile duct. In a patient who presents clinically with a Charcot triad, non-visualization of the gallbladder with features of intrahepatic cholestasis in a ^{99m}Tc-HIDA study suggests acute cholangitis (Fig. 7.1.5).

Table 7.1.2. Clinical and laboratory findings in acute cholangitis vs acute cholecystitis [29]

Parameter	Acute cholangitis	Acute cholecystitis
Clinical features		
Mean age (years)	60	50
Male:female	1:1	3:2
Fever (%)	90	90
Chills (%)	75	50
Jaundice (%)	95	30
RUQ pain (%)	80	95
RUQ tenderness (%)	80	95
Laboratory findings		
WBC >10,000 (%)	70	70
WBC >20,000 (%)	10	5
Bilirubin >1.5 mg (%)	95	30
Bilirubin >5.0 mg (%)	55	5
Elevation of alkaline phosphatase (%)	90	40
Increase in SGOT and SGPT (%)	95	50
Increase in serum amylase (%)	35	15

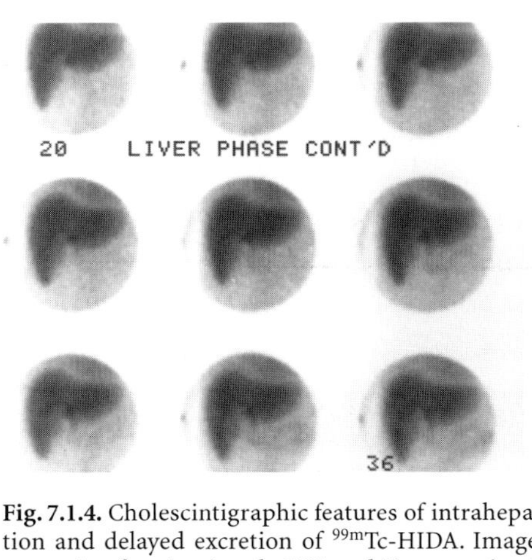

A

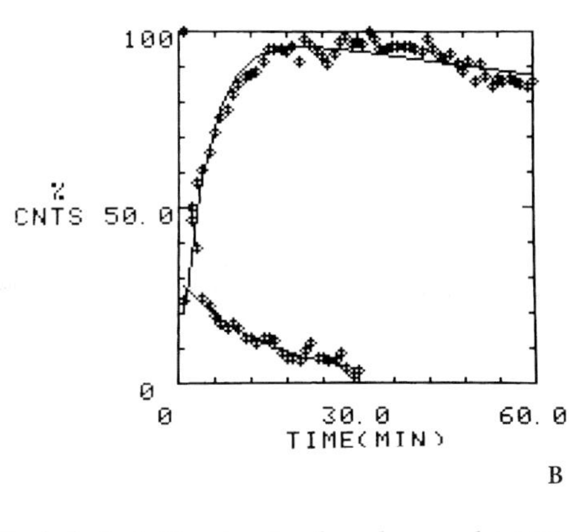

B

Fig. 7.1.4. Cholescintigraphic features of intrahepatic cholestasis. Hepatocytes show decreased extraction and delayed excretion of ^{99m}Tc-HIDA. Images are shown between 20 and 36 min (**A**). Hepatic extraction fraction is only 28% and $T_{1/2}$ excretion is 278 min (**B**)

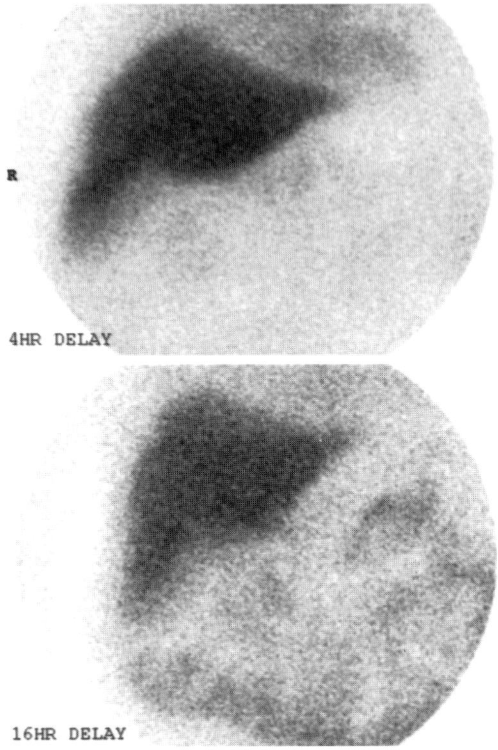

Fig. 7.1.5. Acute cholangitis secondary to acute cholecystitis. The gallbladder is non-visualized due to obstruction of the cystic duct and the there is diffuse retention at 4 and 16 h. Common bile duct is patent and allows bile entry into small intestine

References

1. Sherlock S, Dooley J (1997). Cholestasis. In: Diseases of the liver and biliary system. 10th edition. Blackwell Science, Malden, MA, pp 217–237
2. Trauner M, Meier PJ, Boyer JL. Molecular pathogenesis of cholestasis. N Eng J Med 1998;339:1217–1227
3. Hagenbuch B, Meier PJ. Sinusoidal (basolateral) bile salt uptake system of hepatocytes. Semin Liver Dis 1996;16:129–136
4. Sellinger M, Barrett C, Malle P, Gordon ER, Boyer JL. Cryptic Na^+, K ($^+$)-ATPase activity in rat liver canalicular plasma membrane: evidence for its basolateral origin. Hepatology 1990;11:223–229
5. Kubitz R, Wettstein M, Warskulat U, Haussinger D. Regulation of the multidrug resistance protein 2 in the rat liver by lipopolysaccharide and dexamethasone. Gastroenterology 1999;116:401–410
6. Loberg MD, Cooper M, Harvey E, Callery P, Faith W. Development of new radiopharmaceuticals based on N-substitution of iminodiacetic acid. J Nucl Med 1976;17:633–638
7. Sherlock S. Patterns of hepatic injury in man. Lancet 1982;1 (8275):782–786
8. Lee WM. Drug-induced hepatotoxicity. N Engl J Med 1995;333:1118–1128
9. Sherlock S, Dooley J (1997). Drugs and the liver. In: Diseases of the liver and biliary system. 10th edition, Blackwell Science, Malden, MA, pp 337–369
10. Corcoran GB, Racz WJ, Smith CV, Mitchell JR. Effects of N-acetylcysteine on acetaminophen covalent binding and hepatic necrosis in mice. J Pharmacology Exp Ther 1985;232:864–872
11. Smith CV, Hughes H, Mitchell JR. Free radicals in-vivo. Covalent binding to lipids. Mol Pharmacol 1984;26:112–116

12. Seeff LB, Cuccherini BA, Zimmerman HJ, Adler E, Benjamin SB. Acetaminophen hepatotoxicity in alcoholics. Ann Intern Med 1986;104:399–404
13. Lieberman DA, Krishnamurthy GT. Intrahepatic versus extrahepatic cholestasis. Discrimination with biliary scintigraphy combined with ultrasound. Gastroenterology 1986;90:734–743
14. Powell LW, Halliday JW, Cowlishaw JL. Relationship between serum ferritin and total body iron stores in idiopathic hemochromatosis. Gut 1978;19:538–542
15. Bearn AG. Wilson's disease. An inborn error of metabolism with multiple manifestations. Am J Med 1957;22:747–753
16. Lauterburg BH, Bilzer H. Mechanisms of acetaldehyde hepatotoxicity. J Hepatol 1988;7:384–390
17. Walker JG, Doniach D, Roitt IM, Sherlock S. Serological tests in diagnosis of primary biliary cirrhosis. Lancet 1965;1:827–831
18. Keeffe EB, Lieberman DA, Krishnamurthy S, Krishnamurthy GT, Gilbert SA. Primary biliary cirrhosis: Tc-99m-HIDA planar and SPECT scanning. Radiology 1988;166:143–148
19. Rodman CA, Keeffe EB, Lieberman DA, Krishnamurthy S, Krishnamurthy GT, Gilbert SA, Eklem MJ. Diagnosis of sclerosing cholangitis with Tc-99m labeled iminodiacetic acid planar and single photon emission computed tomographic scintigraphy. Gastroenterology 1987;92:777–785
20. Lesser PB. Benign familial recurrent intrahepatic cholestasis. Am J Dig Dis 1973;18:259–264
21. Minuk GY, Shaffer EA. Benign recurrent intrahepatic cholestasis. Evidence for an intrinsic abnormality in hepatocyte secretion. Gastroenterology 1987;93:1187–1193
22. Quigley EM, Marsh MN, Shaffer JL, Markin RS. Hepatobiliary complications of total parenteral nutrition. Gastroenterology 1993;104:286–301
23. Shuman WP, Gibbs P, Rudd TG, Mack LA. PIPIDA scintigraphy for cholecystitis: False-positives in alcoholism and total parenteral nutrition. Rm J Roentgenol 1982;138:1–5
24. Gitlin N, Serio KM. Ischemic hepatitis: Widening horizons. Am J Gastroenterol 1992;87:831–836
25. Lima J, Brown R, Krishnamurthy S, Krishnamurthy GT. Reliability of quantitative Tc-99m-Mebrofenin scintigraphy (QMS) in the diagnosis of intrahepatic cholestasis (IHC). J Nucl Med 1991;32:976–977
26 Charcot JM: Lecons surles maladies du foie des voies biliaires at des veins. Paris Faculte' de medecine. Recueilleies et publices Bournelle et Senestre. 1877
27. Flemma RJ, Flint LM, Osterhout S. Bacterologic studies of biliary tract infection. Ann Surg 1967;166:563–572
28. Pitt HA, Postier RG, Cameron JL. Biliary bacteria: significance and alterations after antibiotic therapy. Arch Surg 1982;117:445–450
29. Pitt HA, Cameron JL. Acute cholangitis. In: Way LW, Pelligrini CA, eds. Surgery of the gallbladder and bile ducts. WB Saunders, 1987. pp 295–313

7.2 Imaging with ^{99m}Tc-Galactosyl Human Serum Albumin (GSA)

Identification of unique asialoglycoprotein (ASGP) receptors on the plasma membrane of the hepatocyte [1], and introduction of ^{99m}Tc-DTPA-galactosyl-human serum albumin (^{99m}Tc-GSA), which binds to it, allows non-invasive functional imaging and quantification. Asialoglycoprotein receptor concentration on the plasma membrane is an indicator of the functional integrity of the hepatocyte. The quantity of ^{99m}Tc-GSA uptake correlates inversely with blood retention of indocyanine green [2]. Liver uptake of ^{99m}Tc-GSA decreases in patients with chronic hepatitis, cirrhosis, cholangiocarcinoma, hepatocellular cancer, metastasis, fulminant hepatic failure, and space occupying benign lesions of the liver [2–5].

Data Collection and Analysis

Most of the clinical studies reported in the literature are from Japan and the agent is not available in most other countries including the United States. Functional imaging and quantification requires standardization to keep the variables to a minimum. Patient fasting, which is not necessary during imaging with ^{99m}Tc-S-colloid, is essential for imaging with ^{99m}Tc-GSA, because the uptake may be variable due to postprandial hyperperfusion of the GI tract. After 4–6 h of fasting, the patient is positioned supine underneath a gamma camera (single, double, or triple head) fitted with a low-energy, high-resolution, parallel hole collimator positioned anterior to the liver. Sequential anterior planar images (128×128) at one frame per 30 s for 20 min are obtained immediately after a bolus injection of 5 mCi ^{99m}Tc-GSA (185 MBq) into the antecubital vein. Immediately after the planar images, SPECT data are acquired on a 128×128×16 computer matrix for 64 stops at 10 s per stop at 5.6° intervals [2]. The spectrometer is set at 140 keV at a 20% window. Liver uptake index at 15 min is calculated as described in Chap. 5.

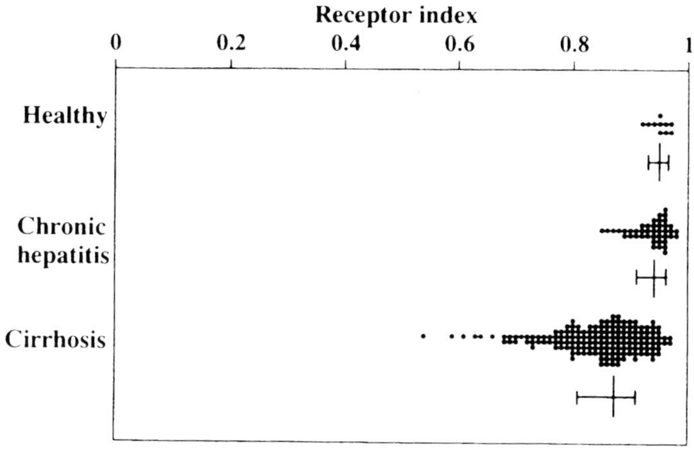

Fig. 7.2.1. Relationship between ^{99m}Tc-GSA receptor index and liver disease. Normal hepatocytes rich in ASGP receptors show a high index. Reduction of ^{99m}Tc-GSA receptor index occurs in patients with chronic hepatitis and cirrhosis of the liver [4]. *GSA*, galactosyl human serum albumin

Some authors express uptake as hepatic GSA clearance using the Patlak plot method and generate functional images of clearance [3, 4]. The receptor index decreases in patients with chronic hepatitis and cirrhosis (Fig. 7.2.1). Since the cells other than the hepatocytes do not take up any ^{99m}Tc-GSA, preoperative imaging allows accurate measurement and prediction of residual liver function postoperatively after resection of hepatocellular carcinoma, cholangiocarcinoma, and metastatic liver tumors (Fig. 7.2.2). It is not known at this time if this functional parameter may serve as an ideal marker for end stage liver disease and timing of liver transplantation.

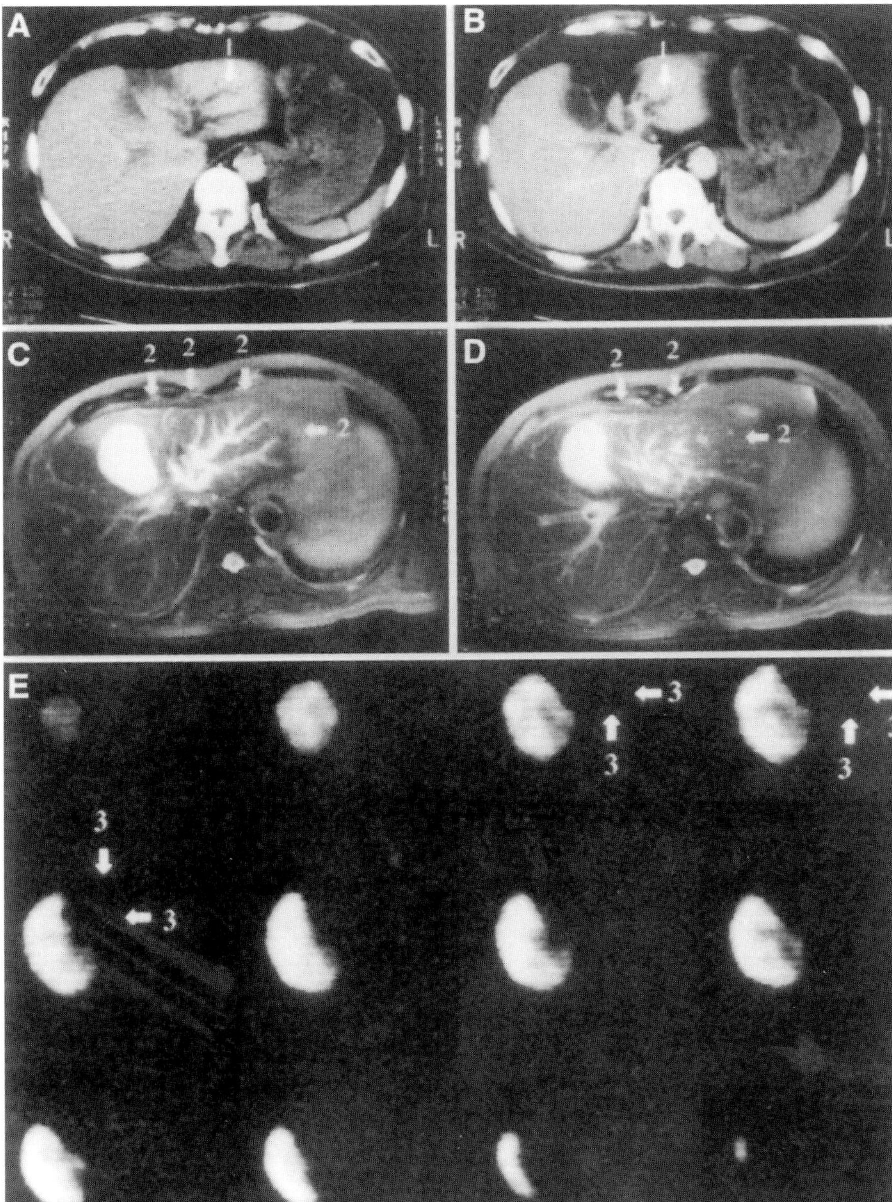

Fig. 7.2.2. Absence of ^{99m}Tc-GSA uptake by tumor. CT with contrast shows dilatation of bile ducts in the left lobe (**A,B** *arrow*) of a patient with cholangiocarcinoma. T2-weighted MR image shows hyperintensity of left lobe bile ducts (**C,D** *arrow*). Liver SPECT shows no uptake of ^{99m}Tc-GSA (**E**) by the left lobe. *GSA*, galactosyl human serum albumin [3]

References

1. Steer CJ. Receptor-mediated endocytosis: mechanisms, biologic function, and molecular properties. In: Zakim D, Boyer TD (editors). Hepatology. A textbook of liver disease. WB Saunders Company, Philadelphia, 1996, pp 149–214
2. Uetake M, Koizumi K, Yagawa A, Nogata H, Tezuka T, Kono H, Ozawa T, Kusano T, Miyaburuko M, Hosaka M. Use of Tc-99m DTPA galactosyl human serum albumin to predict postoperative residual liver function. Clin Nucl Med 1999;24:428–434
3. Hwang E, Taki J, Shuke N, Nakajima K, Kinuya S, Konishi S, Michigishi T, Aburano T, Tonami N. Preoperative assessment of residual hepatic functional reserve using Tc-99m-DTPA-galactosyl-human-serum albumin dynamic SPECT. J Nucl Med 1999;40:1644–1651
4. Sasaki N, Shiomi S, Iwata Y, Nishiguchi S, Kuroki T, Kawabe J, Ochi H. Clinical usefulness of scintigraphy with Tc-99m-galactosyl-human serum albumin for prognosis of cirrhosis of the liver. J Nucl

Extrahepatic Cholestasis

Extrahepatic cholestasis is retention of bile products within the body secondary to a pathology located outside of the liver parenchyma, usually beyond the middle one-third of the right and left hepatic ducts, including the common hepatic and common bile ducts (Fig. 7.1.2 of Chapter 7). Causes of extrahepatic cholestasis can be divided into four major categories depending upon the exact site of location of the pathologic process: (1) intraluminal, (2) wall thickening, (3) combined intrahepatic and extrahepatic causes, and (4) extrinsic compression (Table 8.1.1). The mode of clinical presentation depends very much upon the duration, degree of obstruction, and the exact site of pathology.

Normally the biliary structures appear in a sequential pattern in a ^{99m}Tc-HIDA study; the right and left hepatic ducts appear first, followed by the common hepatic duct, gallbladder, common bile duct, and duodenum. Quantitative parameters show normal hepatic extraction fraction and excretion half-time (Fig. 8.1.1). Ducts proximal to the right and left hepatic ducts are not usually seen clearly. They become prominent only when there is obstruction to bile flow distally.

8.1 Intraluminal Causes

Clinical Presentation

Intraluminal obstruction is usually caused by gallstones, inspissated bile, parasites, blood clots, or pedunculated tumors arising from the wall (Table 8.1.1). The onset of signs and symptoms depends upon the degree and duration of obstruction. A patient with acute complete obstruction of the common bile duct usually presents with sudden onset of epigastric or right upper quadrant pain, which often radiates to the chest, shoulder, or

Table 8.1.1. Intraluminal causes of extrahepatic cholestasis

a) Gallstones (choledocholithiasis)
b) Hemobilia (blood clots)
c) Parasites (roundworm)
d) Inspissated bile or concretions
e) Miscellaneous causes
   Tumor emboli
   Papilloma
   Adenomyoma
   Fibroma
   Cystadenoma

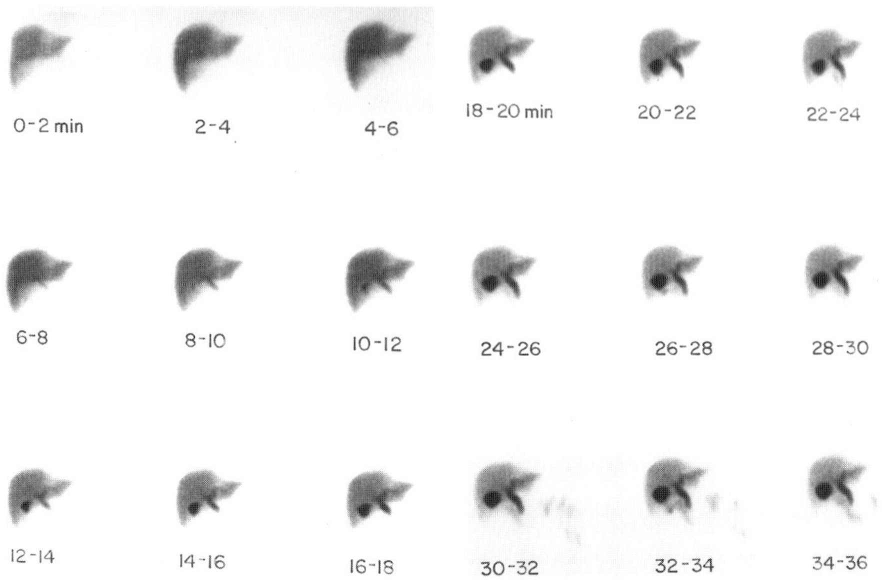

A B

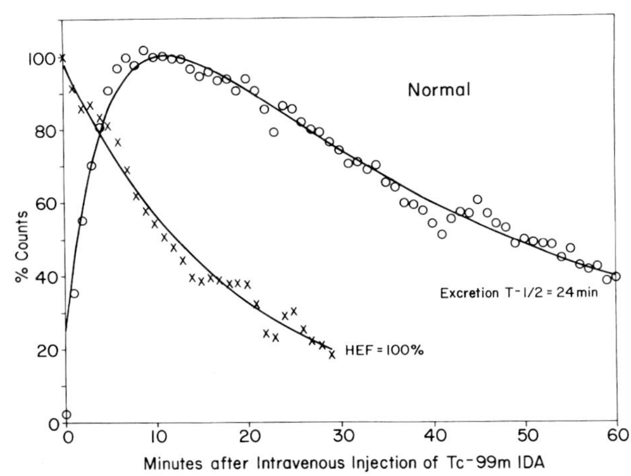

C

Fig. 8.1.1. Normal cholescintigraphy. Liver shows excellent uptake and excretion of ^{99m}Tc-HIDA. The right hepatic duct (*RHD*) and left hepatic ducts (*LHD*), common hepatic duct, and gallbladder are seen early (**A**), followed by the common bile duct and duodenum (**B**). Ducts proximal to RHD and LHD are not seen. Hepatic extraction fraction (*HEF*) and excretion values are normal (**C**)

interscapular region in the back. When complete obstruction persists for more than 3 days, acute cholangitis may set in with onset of the clinical "Charcot triad," which consists of fever with chills, jaundice, and biliary colic. The time for the serum liver function tests to become abnormal after the onset of obstruction depends upon the presence or absence of the gallbladder; in the absence of the gallbladder, the liver function tests become abnormal within 4–6 h, whereas they may take as long as 48–72 h with an intact gallbladder. In the presence of the gallbladder the liver function tests become abnormal much earlier when the level of obstruction lies proximal to the junction of the cystic duct with the common hepatic duct than when the obstruction lies distal to their junction. Patients with partial bile duct obstruction usually make a benign clinical presentation.

Choledocholithiasis

Formation of gallstones is initiated with secretion of a lithogenic bile, which is the first indication of a breakdown of normal mechanisms responsible for keeping bile solutes in solution [1]. The majority of gallstones are composed of cholesterol and few consist of bile pigments. The stone may form de novo within the common bile duct (primary stone) or it may originate in the gallbladder or liver and then move down into the common bile duct (secondary stone). About 85–90% of all stones are secondary and the rest are primary. Secondary stones are more common in western China, Hong Kong, and other Asian countries. In certain ethnic groups, as many as 50% of CBD stones are primary [2].

Pathophysiology of Bile Duct Obstruction

The pathophysiologic changes that follow bile duct obstruction depend upon several factors of which the mode of onset (sudden vs gradual) and severity (partial vs complete) are the most important. Much of our knowledge about postobstructive pathophysiologic changes is derived from ligation of the common bile duct in experimental animals. Following complete ligation of the common bile duct in the rat, the serum alkaline phosphatase and alanine aminotransferase (ALT) levels begin to rise rapidly within 5 h, reach peak levels by 20 h, and later begin to decline to reach a steady state by 4 days. Serum bilirubin begins to rise by 5 h, reaches peak levels by 4 days, and then begins to decline to reach a new steady state level, which is often set at a much lower level than the peak. Serum alkaline phosphatase level begins to rise and reach peak levels much earlier than serum bilirubin level. The number of bile canaliculi doubles in 5 h and then begins to decrease after 4 days. The hepatocytes shrink in size and reach a steady state by 2 days. Postobstructive shrinkage of the hepatocytes and swelling of bile canaliculi together lead to bile leak into the blood stream [3]. Bile flow decreases to 65% of the basal value when the pressure within the ducts exceeds 16–17 cm water and the bile secretion ceases completely when the pressure rises above 20–30 cm water [4, 5].

In piglets, the serum levels of aspartate aminotransferase (AST), ALT, alkaline phosphatase, total bilirubin, and direct bilirubin more than double by 24 h after ligation of the common bile duct. Elevation of bile duct pressure occurs much sooner than the dilatation of the common bile duct. Common bile duct pressure raises from a basal 7.2 cmH_2O to 19.0 cmH_2O, whereas the duct diameter increases from a basal 5.6 mm to 9.8 mm, and the bile concentration of ciprofloxacin reduces to one-seventh of the original concentration, emphasizing the importance of pressure changes on the rate of secretion of bile and bile components [6].

In dogs, the liver function tests may remain normal for up to 3 h, but become abnormal by 24 h following complete ligation of the common bile duct. The hepatocyte uptake and secretion into bile of ^{99m}Tc-HIDA continue for up to 3 h postligation, enabling cholescintigraphic delineation of the gallbladder and hepatobiliary tree, proximal to the site of obstruction. The hepatobiliary tree often simulates features seen in a physiologically tight sphincter of Oddi, where all of the hepatic bile may be diverted into the gallbladder, and none enters the duodenum. By 24 h, the hepatocytes continue to concentrate ^{99m}Tc-HIDA but are unable to secrete it into bile, which results in total non-visualization of the entire biliary tree [7]. Scintigraphy then appears much like a radiocolloid liver scan without the spleen.

Cholescintigraphic Features of Total Obstruction of the Common Bile Duct

The cholescintigraphic features merely reflect the pathophysiologic changes that follow obstruction of the common bile duct as described above in animals. The normal mean secretory pressure of hepatocytes in humans is about 35 cm water. Mean pressure in the gallbladder is 10 cm, in the common bile duct (CBD) 12 cm, and in the sphincter of Oddi 15 cm of water[8]. Bile secretion continues at a normal rate as long as all these normal pressure differentials are maintained. Bile secretion begins to decrease when CBD pressure begins to rise, and the secretion ceases completely when CBD pressure equals or exceeds the secretory pressure of the hepatocytes [9]. Normally about 30% of the hepatic bile that enters the duodenum during fasting enables cholescintigraphic visualization of the small intestine within 60 min in about 80% of subjects. In the remaining 20% of normal subjects, the duodenum is not seen due to entry of all the hepatic bile into the gallbladder [10–12]. The flow of entire hepatic bile into the gallbladder and none into the duodenum during fasting in normal subjects is simply a reflection of an increase in the tonus of the sphincter of Oddi.

After 6–8 h of fasting, a normal gallbladder is usually filled to its full capacity of 50 ml and its ability to accommodate a constant inflow of hepatic bile (about 0.3 ml/min) is due to absorption of an equal volume of water through the wall. When only the gallbladder is seen by 60 min, but not the duodenum, the reasons for non-visualization may include a physiologically tight sphincter of Oddi or a complete obstruction of the common bile duct. After CCK-8 infusion, the gallbladder contracts and empties bile normally into the duodenum in the case of a physiologically tight sphincter of Oddi [10], but no bile enters the duodenum in the case of complete obstruction of the CBD [13, 14].

Bile Duct Obstruction less than 48 h (Hyperacute). A gallstone dislodged from either the gallbladder or intrahepatic ducts or acute edematous pancreatitis is the most common cause of acute complete obstruction of the CBD. A dislodged gallstone usually becomes trapped just above or within the sphincter of Oddi, the narrowest part of the CBD. The time interval between the onset of acute CBD obstruction and cessation of hepatic bile secretion is variable, depending upon the level (below or above the entrance of the cystic duct into the common hepatic duct), degree (complete or partial), and presence or absence of the gallbladder. Following acute complete obstruction of the CBD, the liver continues to secrete bile slowly for 24–48 h. The uptake of ^{99m}Tc-HIDA remains relatively high (Fig. 8.1.2A), but the secretion slows, resulting in delayed visualization of biliary structures (Fig. 8.1.2B,C). The gallbladder and bile ducts (proximal to the level of obstruction) are seen, but not the duodenum. Quantitative parameters show a normal hepatic extraction fraction and prolongation of excretion half-time (Fig. 8.1.3). Administration of CCK-8 increases bile secretion and flow by the intrahepatic bile ducts and forces the hepatic bile to enter the gallbladder; and there is no bile entry into the duodenum. Due to high pressure in the common bile duct, the gallbladder fails to empty in response to CCK-8 infusion. Some patients show an immediate bile flow into the gallbladder, while others may take few more minutes after CCK-8 (Fig. 8.1.4). Filling of the gallbladder in response to CCK-8 is a physiological paradox and a confirmatory feature for acute total obstruction of the common bile duct. The only other condition which shows a similar feature is spasm of the sphincter of Oddi (Chap. 10).

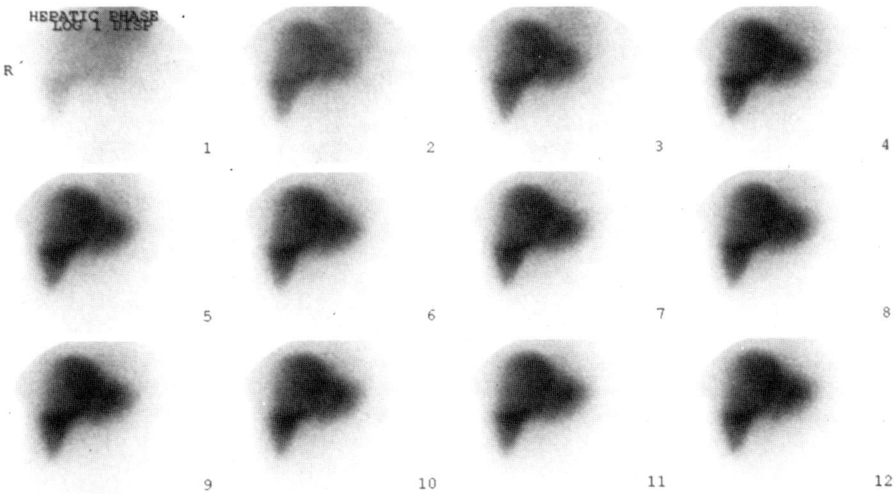

A

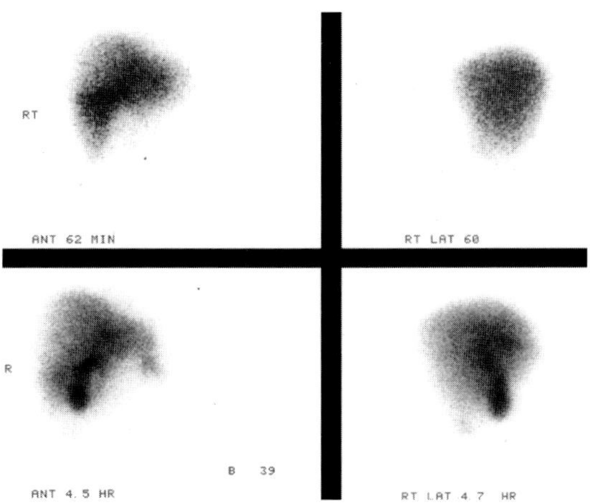

B

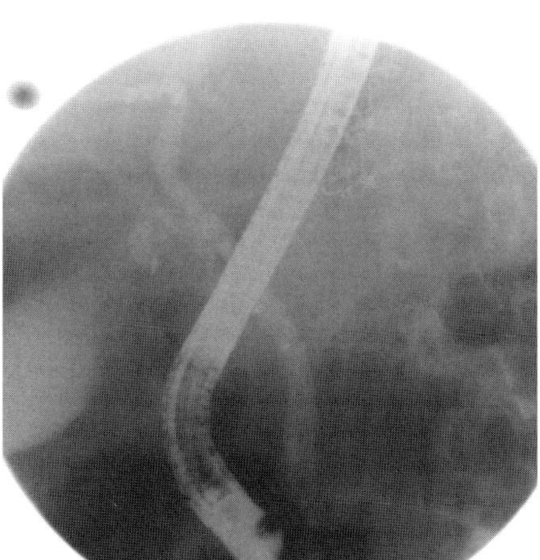

C

Fig. 8.1.2. Hyperacute CBD obstruction (less than 48 h). Obstruction shows excellent uptake of ^{99m}Tc-HIDA by the hepatocytes. Bile secretion is delayed (**A**). The gallbladder is seen at 4.5 h (**B**). The cholangiogram confirms obstruction due to a stone at the distal end of the non-dilated CBD (**C**)

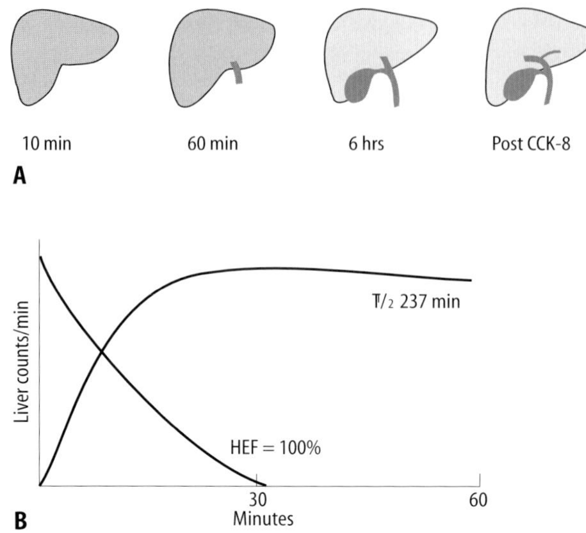

Fig. 8.1.3. Effect of acute complete duct obstruction on functional parameters. The gallbladder appears late and there is no bile entry into the duodenum (**A**). Hepatic extraction fraction (*HEF*) remains normal, but excretion half-time increases (**B**).

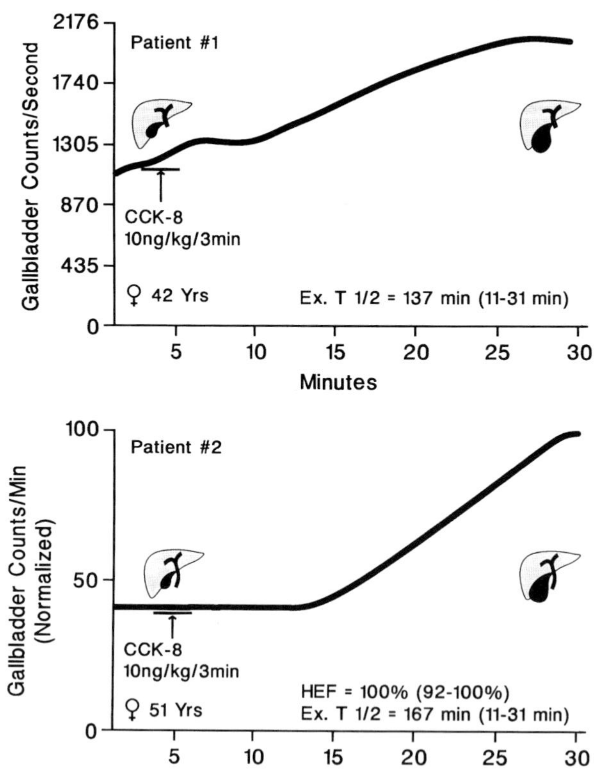

Fig. 8.1.4. Cholecystokinin induced paradoxical filling of the gallbladder. Cholecystokinin administration in patients with hyper acute complete CBD obstruction increases bile secretion by intrahepatic ducts and forces the hepatic bile to enter the gallbladder. In patient #1 (Top), gallbladder fills in immediately and it takes few more minutes to fill in patient #2 (Bottom). Gallbladder size and counts increase after CCK

Bile Duct obstruction for more than 48 h. Extraction of ^{99m}Tc-HIDA by the hepatocytes is maintained at a relatively high level, but the secretion into bile ceases completely. Cholescintigraphy obtained after 48 h of obstruction, therefore, shows good liver uptake without delineation of any of the biliary structures (Fig. 8.1.5A). Hepatic extraction fraction values in the range of 50–85% are common between 2 and 5 days, and the values fall below 50% when total obstruction persists for longer than 5 days (Fig. 8.1.5B). Cholescintigraphic images and quantitative parameters accurately reflect histopathologic changes of bile duct obstruction as described above in experimental animals. In the rat, for example, a mean HEF value of 97% before bile duct ligation falls to 70% by 2 h and 16% by 48 h, after complete ligation of the common bile duct. Long standing CBD

A

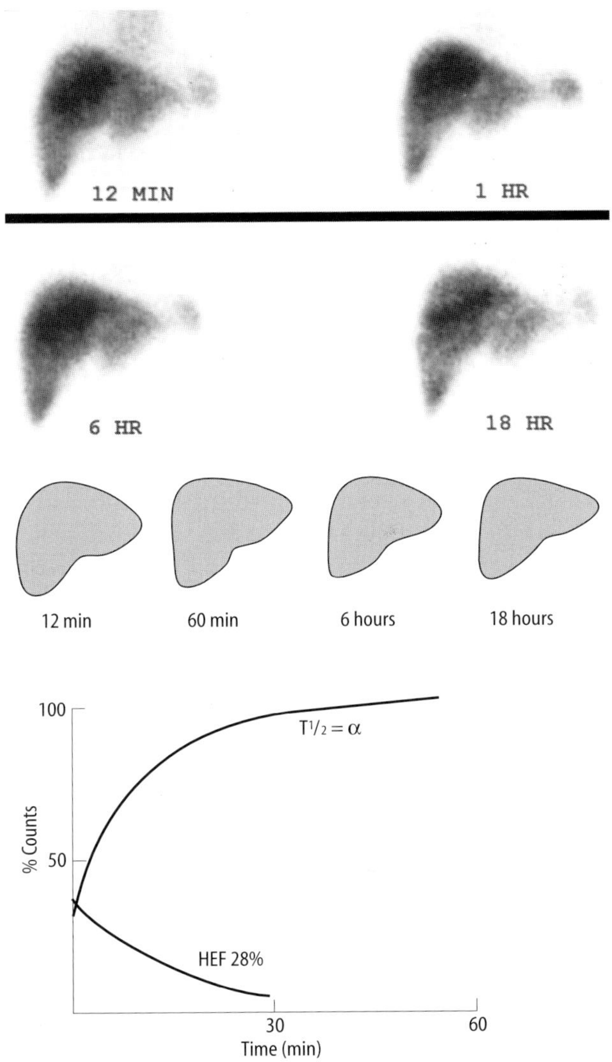

B

Fig. 8.1.5. Complete obstruction of the duct for more than 48 h. There is rapid uptake by the hepatocytes but no secretion of the radiotracer into bile. The entire biliary tree and the small intestine are non-visualized for 18 h (**A**). Hepatic extraction fraction (*HEF*) is reduced to 28% and excretion half-time shows infinity (**B**) obstruction ultimately compromises hepatocyte function and results in a low HEF value [15–17].

Both bilirubin and ^{99m}Tc-HIDA share a common organic anion receptor mediated endocytosis for uptake by the hepatocyte. When serum levels are high, bilirubin occupies most of the available receptor sites and blocks the uptake of ^{99m}Tc-HIDA by the hepatocytes and produces a low HEF value. Technetium-99m-mebrofenin competes with bilirubin for hepatocyte uptake much better than ^{99m}Tc-labeled diisopropyl IDA (DISIDA), diethyl IDA, para-isopropyl-IDA (PIPIDA), or para-butyl IDA. The reciprocal relationship between ^{99m}Tc-HIDA uptake and serum bilirubin level is well documented in both animal and human studies [17, 18]. In a patient with acute onset of biliary pain, an HEF value above 65% combined with cessation of bile secretion (non-visualization of the bile ducts and gallbladder) is a reliable indicator of pure biliary disease (complete CBD obstruction), whereas an HEF value below 50% under similar circumstances indicates accompanying severe hepatocellular damage [19, 20].

Partial Obstruction. Patients with a partial bile duct obstruction usually present with mid-abdominal or right upper quadrant pain. Elevation of serum alkaline phosphatase or gamma glutamyl transferase is the earliest biochemical abnormality. Cholescintigraphic features of partial CBD obstruction include normal hepatic extraction fraction, bile stasis in ducts proximal to obstruction, and prolongation of excretion half-time value (Fig. 8.1.6A). Intestinal activity may be seen within 60 min, or delayed slightly in a few of the patients. Diagnosis of obstruction of the common bile duct can neither be excluded nor confirmed solely on the basis of appearance or non-appearance of the duodenum, respectively.

Quantitative parameters indicate severity of the disease and an etiological diagnosis (biliary vs hepatocellular) is usually made in combination with the image pattern. A mean HEF value of 94% was obtained in 14 patients with isolated partial CBD obstruction, and a value of 96% in 13 patients with sclerosing cholangitis. In contrast, 14 patients with cirrhosis had a mean HEF of 60%. Hepatic extraction values below 30% are more common in patients with Child class C than class A and B cirrhosis [20]. Complete CBD obstruction of more than 5 days duration, however, compromises hepatocyte function and lowers HEF value to levels seen in patients with cirrhosis [15]. Excretion half-time values begin to increase immediately after onset of CBD obstruction and reach values as high as 200–300 min (Fig. 8.1.6B). Many patients with critical obstruction may show only an upslope to the curve with a $T_{1/2}$ value of infinity [15, 20]. Cholescintigraphic features of partial CBD obstruction are non-specific and an etiologic diagnosis (stone vs stricture) can be made only in a few of the patients based solely on an image pattern. A gallstone lodged in CBD may cause a filling defect with a convex superior border, enabling an etiologic diagnosis in a few of the patients [21].

Functional Recovery Pattern

The liver recovers its function rapidly after relief of CBD obstruction. Generally, serum bilirubin values decline much more rapidly than serum alkaline phosphatase levels, a feature opposite of what takes place during the onset of obstruction [3]. Serum bilirubin levels decline by 50% of the preoperation value within 2 days, reach 25% by 1

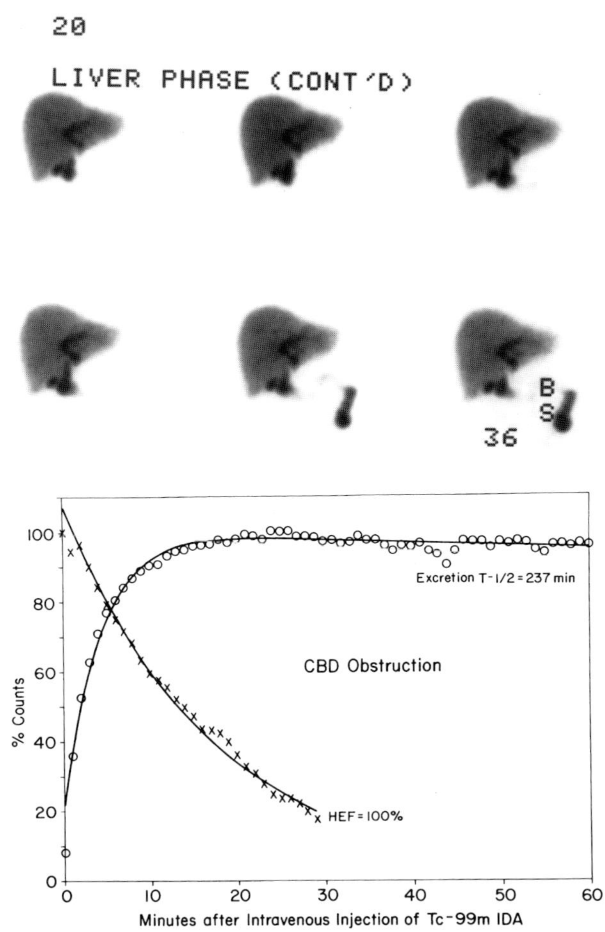

A

B

Fig. 8.1.6. Partial obstruction of the common bile duct. Uptake of the radiotracer remains normal but excretion is slowed. The common bile duct is poorly visualized. There is bile pooling in the intrahepatic ducts. The gallbladder and small intestine are seen **(A)**. Hepatic extraction fraction (*HEF*) remains normal but the excretion half-time increases to 237 min **(B)**

week, and 10% by 3 weeks (Fig. 8.1.7). By 10 days after the relief of obstruction, the serum bilirubin level declines to 25%, whereas the alkaline phosphatase level may decline only to 60% of the preoperation value [9].

Hemobilia

Hemobilia is a unique name that combines both Greek (*haima* meaning blood) and Latin (*bilis* meaning bile) to convey the exact meaning of the pathologic process: a mixture of blood and bile. Blunt and penetrating liver trauma are the most common current causes followed by iatrogenic factors secondary to instrumentation, or surgery on or around the biliary tract. Liver biopsy, endoscopic retrograde cholangiopancreatography (ERCP), and transhepatic cholangiography are the most common iatrogenic causes [22]. Gunshot injury is becoming a more common cause in recent years due to the rapid rise in gun related crimes. Penetrating injury may rupture an artery or a vein, with the accompanying bile duct establishing a direct communication between blood and bile.

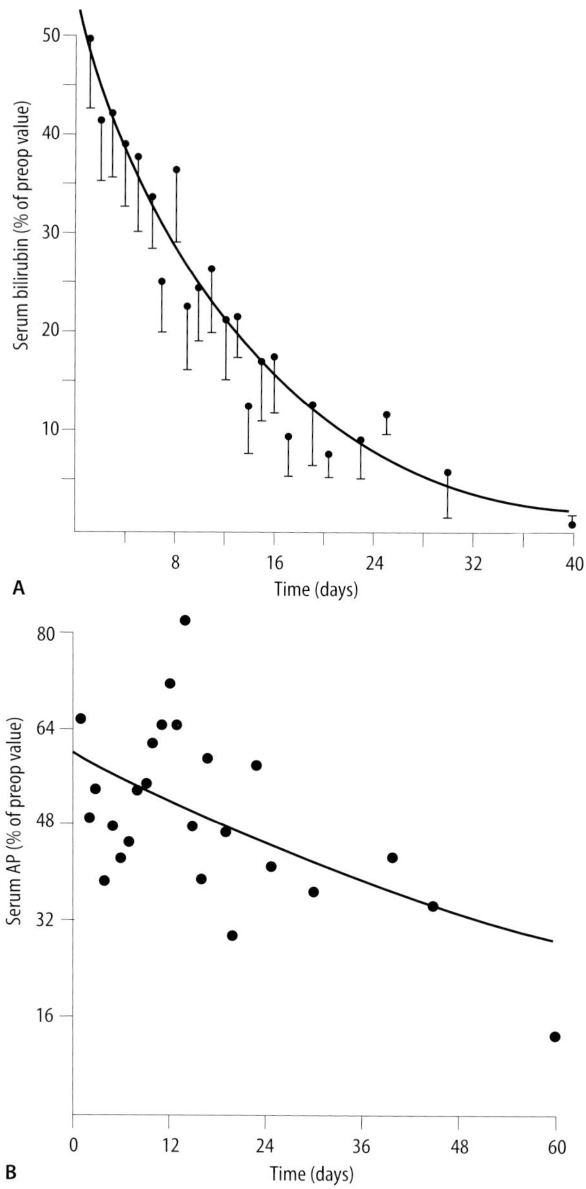

Fig. 8.1.7. Recovery of liver function. After relief of bile duct obstruction, bilirubin level declines much more rapidly than alkaline phosphatase. Serum bilirubin declines to 50% of preoperative value in 2 days, to 25% by 1 week, and to less than 10% by 3 weeks. Alkaline phosphatase level, however, remains above 50% of the preoperative value at the end of 1 week [9]

Parasites

Obstruction of the common bile duct due to parasites is usually caused by migration of the roundworm (*Ascaris lumbricoides*) through the sphincter of Oddi. A female roundworm is about 25–35 cm in length and 3–6 mm in diameter. A male worm is slightly smaller in size, measuring 15–30 in length and 2–4 mm in diameter. The upper small intestine is the usual habitat and often live worms are passed in the stool. When the worm migrates into the common bile duct, the usual symptoms of bile duct obstruction (right upper quadrant pain, vomiting, fever, and jaundice) occur. A history of passing the parasites in the stool is the most helpful diagnostic clue. Ova are found on the microscopic examination of the stool specimen [23]. An appearance of "a bulls eye" sign in an ultrasound study of the common bile duct suggests a roundworm, especially in countries with a high prevalence of ascariasis [24].

Miscellaneous Causes

Tumor emboli from cholangiocarcinoma (near the bifurcation), foreign bodies, inspissated bile, papilloma, adenomyoma, fibroma, cystadenoma, and giant cell tumors are some of the rare causes of intraluminal obstruction [25].

Segmental Biliary Obstruction

An intraluminal segmental or lobar bile duct obstruction produces a characteristic scintigraphic pattern. Obstruction due to a gallstone is more common in China, Hong Kong, and other Far Eastern countries than in the western hemisphere [26]. The scintigraphic pattern depends upon whether the obstruction is partial or complete. In the case of a partial segmental bile duct obstruction, the uptake and excretion of ^{99m}Tc-HIDA by the hepatocytes into hepatic bile continues manifesting bile pool within the duct, proximal to the level of obstruction [27]. A focal retention is seen over the involved segment, while the rest of the normal liver clears most of its radioactivity in the images obtained between 45 and 60 min after injection [28]. In the right lobe, where the segmental ducts are positioned anterior and posterior, a right lateral view is necessary to identify the obstructed duct. In the case of the left lobe, where the segmental ducts are positioned medial and lateral, an anterior view image alone will suffice to identify the obstructed duct. When the segmental or area duct obstruction is complete and persists for a longer duration, uptake of ^{99m}Tc-HIDA decrease or ceases completely, resulting in a filling defect.

Measurement of Duct Size on Cholescintigraphy

Measurement of actual duct size from the cholescintigraphic images is prone to inaccuracy due the effect of specific activity, scatter, and pooling of radiolabeled bile within the biliary system. An in vitro experiment (Fig. 8.1.8) clearly illustrates the effect of changing of the dose or intensity of image settings on duct size. A 4-mm-internal-diameter tube is measured in different sizes when the dose and/or intensity settings are changed. High specific activity hepatic bile in a normal subject or bile pooling within the duct in a patient with distal bile obstruction increases the photon scatter, depicting the duct as though it is dilated when in actuality it is not. Ultrasound is far superior for measurement of ductal dilatation.

Cholescintigraphy supplements contrast cholangiopancreatography (ERCP) when it fails to identify the intrahepatic segmental duct obstruction primarily due to lack of retrograde flow of the contrast [26, 29]. Magnetic resonance cholangiopancreatography (MRCP) is an emerging new technology which may eventually replace ERCP in some patients with obstruction of the extrahepatic biliary tree. Magnetic resonance does not require any contrast agent to visualize the bile ducts, but depends upon ductal dilatation to be able to detect the level of obstruction [30, 31].

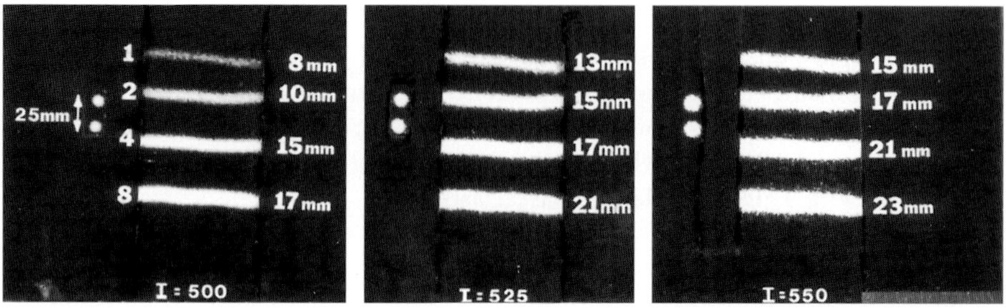

Fig. 8.1.8. Effect of bile pooling on duct size. Measurement of duct size from cholescintigraphy is subject to error due to the effect of the scatter and image intensity (*I*). *Numbers 1–4* denote increases in radioactivity. A 4-mm-internal-diameter tube appears at various sizes depending upon activity and *I* settings

References

1. Admirand WH, Small DM. The physiological basis of cholesterol gallstone formation in man. J Clin Invest 1968,47:1043–1052
2. Madden J. Common duct stones. Their origin and surgical management. Surg Clin North Am 1973;53:1095–1113
3. Vital A, Bioulac-Sage P, Iron A, Balabaud C. Morphologic structure of bile canaliculi after bile duct ligation in the rat. A time-course study. Arch Pathol Lab Med 1982;106:464–467
4. Accatino L, Contreras A, Fernandez S, Quintana C. The effect of complete biliary obstruction on bile flow and bile acid secretion: post-cholestatic choleresis in the rat. J Lab Clin Med 1979;93:706–717
5. Johnson G, Sundman L. Bile and dry matter output at elevated liver secretion pressure. Acta Clin Scand 1964;128:153
6. Chen C, Shiesh S, Wu M, Lin X. The effect of bile duct obstruction on the biliary secretion of ciprofloxacin in piglets. Am J Gastroenterol 1999;94:2408–2411
7. Klingensmith WC III, Whitney WP, Spitzer VM, Klintmalm GB, Koep LM, Kuni CC. Effect of complete biliary-tract obstruction on serial hepatobiliary imaging in an experimental model: concise communication. J Nucl Med 1981;22:866–868
8. Oster MJ, Csendes A, Funch-Jensen P, Skjoldborg H. Intra-operative pressure measurements of the choledocho-duodenal junction, common bile duct, cystico-choledochal junction, and gallbladder in humans. Surg Gynecol Obstet 1980;150:385–389
9. Pelligrini CA. Pathophysiology of biliary obstruction. In: Way LW, Pelligrini CA (eds) The surgery of the gallbladder and bile ducts. WB Saunders, Philadelphia, 1987. pp 103–117
10. Williams W, Krishnamurthy GT, Brar HS, Bobba VR. Scintigraphic variations of normal biliary physiology. J Nucl Med 1984;25:160–165
11. Krishnamurthy GT, Bobba VR, McConnell D, Turner F, Mesgarzadeh M, Kingston E. Quantitative biliary dynamics: introduction of a new non-invasive scintigraphic technique. J Nucl Med 1983;24:217–223
12. Doo E, Krishnamurthy GT, Eklem MJ, Gilbert S, Brown PH. Quantification of hepatobiliary function as an integral part of imaging with technetium-99m-mebrofenin in health and disease. J Nucl Med 1991;32:48–57
13. Blue PW. Hyperacute complete common bile duct obstruction demonstrated with Tc-99m-IDA cholescintigraphy. Nucl Med Commun 1985;6:275–279
14. Lee AW, Ram MD, Shin WJ, Murphy K. Technetium-99m BIDA biliary scintigraphy in the evaluation of the jaundiced patient. J Nucl Med 1986;27:1407–1412
15. Juni JE, Reichle R. Measurement of hepatocellular function with deconvolutional analysis: application in the differential diagnosis of acute jaundice. Radiology 1990;177:171–175
16. Lima J, Shankaran H, Krishnamurthy GT, et al. Evaluation of hepatocyte function following acute common bile duct obstruction (ACBDO) by Tc-99m-mebrofenin scintigraphy in rats. Eur J Nucl Med 1992;19:687 (abstract)
17. Lima J. Quantificaçáo em hepatologia nuclear. Thesis submitted to the University of Coimbra as partial fulfilment for a doctoral degree. University of Coimbra, Portugal. 1997
18. Krishnamurthy S, Krishnamurthy GT. Technetium-99m-iminodiacetic acid organic anion: Review of biokinetics and clinical application in hepatology. Hepatology 1989;9:139–153

19. Lecklitner ML, Austin AR, Benedetto AR, Growcock GW. Positive predictive value of cholescintigraphy in common bile duct obstruction. J Nucl Med 1986;27:1403–1406
20. Brown PH, Juni JE, Lieberman DA, Krishnamurthy GT. Hepatocyte versus biliary disease: a distinction by deconvolutional analysis of technetium-99m-IDA time-activity curve. J Nucl Med 1988;29:623–630
21. Krishnamurthy GT, Lieberman DA, Brar HS. Detection, localization and quantitation of degree of common bile duct obstruction by scintigraphy. J Nucl Med 1985;26:726–735
22. Sandblom P. Hemobilia. In: Way LW, Pelligrini CA. (Eds). Surgery of the gallbladder and bile ducts. Philadelphia, WB Saunders, 1987, pp 643–654
23. Louw JH, Rode H. Ascariasis. In: Way LW, Pelligrini CA (eds). Surgery of the gallbladder and bile duct. Philadelphia, WB Saunders, 1987, pp 539–555
24. Cremin BJ. Ultrasonic diagnosis of biliary ascariasis " a bull's eye in the triple O". Br J Radiol 1982;55:683–684
25. Sherlock S, Dooley J. Diseases of the liver and biliary system. Blackwell Science, Malden, MA. 10th edition, 1997. pp 641–649
26. Yeh SH, Liu OK, Huang MJ, Sequential scintigraphy with technetium-99m-pyridoxylideneglutamate in the detection of intrahepatic lithiasis: concise communication. J Nucl Med 1980;21:17–21
27. Zeman RK, Gold JA, Gluck L, Caride VJ, Burrell M, Hoffer PB. Tc-99m-HIDA scintigraphy in segmental biliary obstruction. J Nucl Med 1981;22:456–458
28. Gupta S, Owshalimpur D, Cohen G, Margules R, Herrera N. Scintigraphic detection of segmental bile-duct obstruction. J Nucl Med 1982;23:890–891
29. Gibney RG, Cooperberg PL, Scudamore CH, Nagy AG. Segmental biliary obstruction: false-negative diagnosis with direct cholangiography without US guidance. Radiology 1987;164:27–30
30. Lee MG, Lee HJ, Kim MH, Kang EM, Kim YH, Lee SG, Kim PN, Ha HK, Auh YH. Extrahepatic biliary diseases: 3D MR cholangiopancreatography compared with endoscopic retrograde cholangiopancreatography. Radiology 1997;202:663–669
31. Asselah T, Ernst O, Sergent G, L'herminé C, Paris JC. Caroli's disease: a magnetic resonance cholangiopancreatography diagnosis. Am J Gastroenterology 1998;93:109–110

8.2 Wall Thickening

Wall thickening occurs gradually over weeks or months before causing impedances to bile flow due to narrowing of the lumen. Wall thickening may have a benign or malignant cause.

Benign Causes

Stricture

Many conditions that cause benign stricture are listed in Table 8.2.1. Wall injury that leads to benign stricture occurs more commonly following a diagnostic or therapeutic instrumentation of the biliary tree. Most strictures occur at the middle of the common hepatic duct, which lies directly across the point of ligation of the cystic duct during an open or laparoscopic cholecystectomy and likely to sustain injury more frequently[1]. Laparoscopic cholecystectomy, which has almost replaced open surgical cholecystectomy, is now the most common cause of benign stricture [2]. Small gallstones migrating from either the gallbladder or liver may temporarily lodge in the common bile duct and cause constant irritation and subsequent stricture formation. Ischemia [3], infusion of chemotherapy agents [4], infection, radiation [5], chronic pancreatitis [6], and liver transplantation [7] are other well established causes of benign stricture.

Table 8.2.1. Causes of benign stricture of the bile duct

1.	Open cholecystectomy
2.	Laparoscopic cholecystectomy
3.	Migrating stones
4.	Ischemia
5.	Hepatic intraarterial chemotherapy
6.	Radiation
7.	Infection
8.	Chronic pancreatitis
9.	Liver transplantation
10.	Blunt or penetrating trauma

Pathophysiology

The pathophysiological changes that follow a benign stricture are quite different from those that occur after an intraluminal obstruction. In contrast to an intraluminal obstruction which occurs suddenly, stricture formation takes months or years after the initiating injury. Post-transplant CBD stricture occurs at or just above the anastomotic site in 10–20% of patients with liver transplantation. Duct ischemia prior to transplantation is responsible for the stricture [7]. The cause of benign stricture in non-transplant patients often remains unknown.

Clinical Features

The clinical presentation of benign stricture often remains vague for many weeks or months due to its slow progression. Intermittent upper abdominal pain is the most common presenting symptom. Elevation of serum alkaline phosphatase or transaminase is the earliest liver function abnormality, followed by elevation of serum bilirubin, especially when the stricture becomes critical with dilatation of the bile duct.

Cholescintigraphic Diagnosis

Early in the course of benign stricture, the uptake (HEF) and excretion of ^{99m}Tc-HIDA by the hepatocytes are maintained within a normal range, but the bile flow through the stricture is reduced (Fig. 8.2.1A). The reduction in bile flow leads to bile stasis within the intrahepatic ducts with delineation of the segmental and area ducts (Fig. 8.2.1B). There is an increase in excretion half-time, which serves as a quantitative measure of the degree of obstruction (Fig. 8.2.1C). The delay in gallbladder filling may indicate an increase in its intraluminal pressure. The distal common bile duct initially shows a smooth tapering towards the stricture but this appearance changes when the duct above the stricture dilates (Fig. 8.2.1D). The stricture of the common bile duct diverts most of the hepatic bile to enter the gallbladder and very little bile enters the duodenum [8]. The hepatic extraction fraction remains high in early stricture but begins to fall when the obstruction becomes severe and persists for a longer duration [9].

Low extraction fraction with complete cessation of bile secretion occurs in critical stenosis with serum bilirubin levels above 10 mg% (Fig. 8.2.2).

Ultrasound is used frequently for the diagnosis, and its accuracy depends very much upon the presence or absence of ductal dilatation [10]. A normal common bile duct usually measures up to 10 mm in diameter and the ultrasound is unable to detect

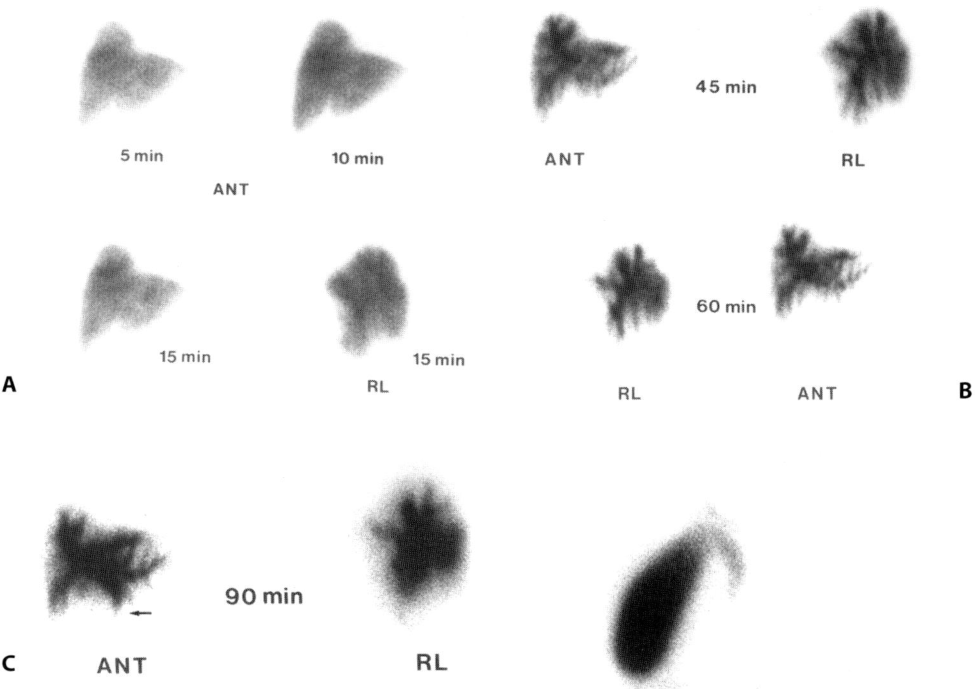

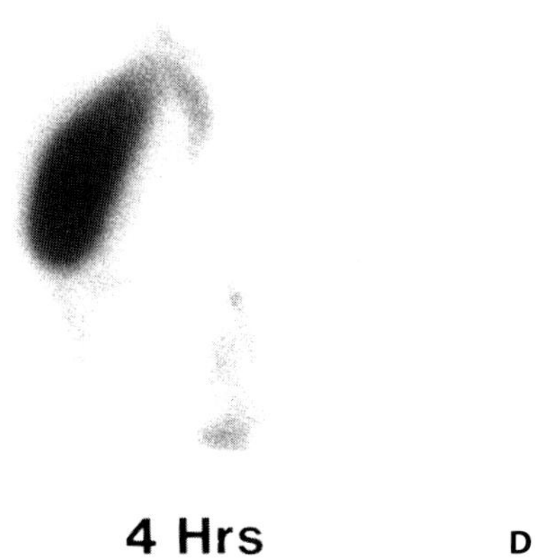

Fig. 8.2.1. Early benign stricture. Liver shows excellent uptake but slightly delayed secretion of ^{99m}Tc-HIDA into bile (**A**). Later, there is intense bile pooling within the intrahepatic ducts (**B, C**). Common bile duct and gallbladder appear late indicating high pressure within them. There is smooth tapering of the CBD towards the stricture (**D**)

the stricture when the duct size remains within the normal range (Fig. 8.2.3). Ultrasound accuracy, however, increases when the diameter of the common bile duct exceeds 10 mm, serum bilirubin level rises above 10 mg%, and jaundice persists for longer than 1 week [11]. Dilatation of extrahepatic ducts occurs much earlier than dilatation of the intrahepatic ducts, as dictated by the law of Laplace, which states that the stress is directly proportional to the internal diameter of the tubing [12]. Because of their larger internal diameter, the extrahepatic ducts sustain more stress and dilate much earlier than the intrahepatic ducts, which are much smaller in size.

Stricture impedes bile flow through and reduces gallbladder emptying in response to CCK-8 infusion. There may be prolongation of the latent period with a reduction in gallbladder ejection fraction [8]. The bile emptied from the gallbladder may reflux into the common hepatic duct and right and left hepatic ducts, instead of its forward flow into the duodenum. Bile reflux into the common hepatic and right and left hepatic ducts is one reliable sign of obstruction and is referred to as the Krishnamurthy-Bobba sign [13, 14]. Refluxed bile reenters the gallbladder immediately after cessation of CCK-8 infusion, and the gallbladder curve often shows a rapid refilling. In patients

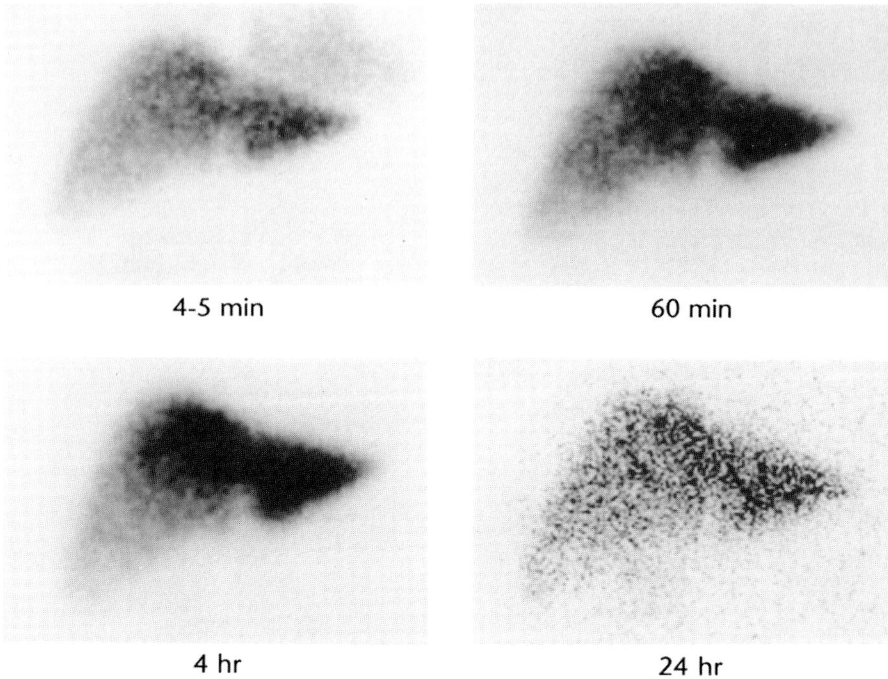

A

B

NORMALS:	HEPATIC EXTRACT. FRACTION (100%)	HEPATIC EXCRET. T-1/2 (11-31)	HEPATIC UPTAKE T-1/2 (1.1-9.0)
RU LOBE	59.2%	982.7MIN	3.4MIN
RL LOBE	68.2%	326.0MIN	4.0MIN
LT LOBE	61.1%	650.5MIN	3.3MIN

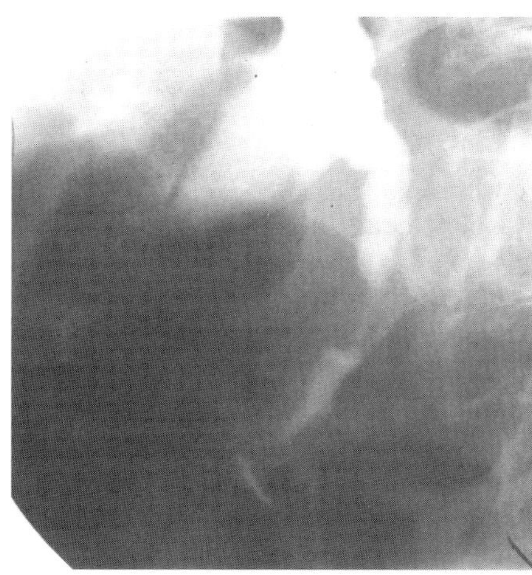

C

Fig. 8.2.2. Critical stricture. Bile secretion ceases (**A**) and the hepatic extraction fraction decreases (**B**). The bile ducts, gallbladder, and intestine are not seen even at 24 h. The cholangiogram confirms critical stenosis of the common bile duct (**C**)

with right upper quadrant pain, mild elevation of serum alkaline phosphatase, and normal bilirubin, cholescintigraphy maintains a much higher sensitivity for the detection of obstruction than ultrasound. Ultrasound, on the other hand, becomes a preferred modality for diagnosis in cases with high serum bilirubin and dilatation of ducts [11, 15, 16].

In normal subjects, the mean time of appearance of the common bile duct is 16 min, gallbladder 20 min, and duodenum 24 min. A gallbladder ejection fraction of 35% or

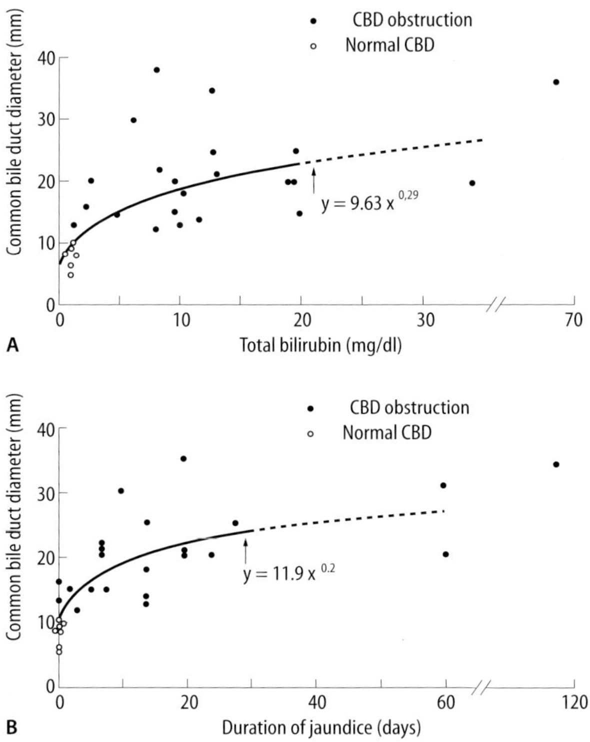

Fig. 8.2.3. Relationship of common bile duct size with serum bilirubin and duration of jaundice. There is usually no dilatation of the common bile duct (*CBD*) with bilirubin levels below 5 mg%; dilatation occurs when serum bilirubin rises above 10 mg%; dilatation is variable between 5 and 10 mg% (**A**). Diameter of the CBD increases (**B**) as the duration of jaundice increases [11]

higher is obtained in response to a 3-min infusion of 10 ng/kg (3.3 ng/min for 3 min) of CCK-8. The latent period is less than 3 min and the ejection period is between 8 and 12 min. The curve over the common bile duct may show a peak corresponding to the second half of the gallbladder ejection period. The common hepatic duct curve usually does not show any peak as the bile emptied from the gallbladder flows antegrade through the sphincter of Oddi and enters the duodenum [17–19]. Because of forward bile entry into the duodenum, there is no rapid refilling of the gallbladder.

During quantitative cholescintigraphy, patients with bile duct obstruction often experience a mild to moderate degree of abdominal pain due to either contraction of the gallbladder or distension of the common bile duct. Pain is experienced mostly during the gallbladder ejection period. Pain experienced after completion of the gallbladder ejection is considered non-biliary in origin. Since cholecystokinin increases intestinal peristalsis, late onset abdominal pain (after the gallbladder ejection period) is considered to indicate pain of intestinal origin due to increased peristalsis. A precise documentation of the temporal relationship between the onset of pain and the phase of gallbladder emptying is essential for defining the exact origin of abdominal pain [20, 21].

Cholescintigraphic Accuracy of Biliary Obstruction

Of a total of 214 patients with well documented biliary obstruction (Table 8.2.2), cholescintigraphy accurately detected obstruction in 200, with a sensitivity of 93% [12,

19, 22–28]. Differentiation between functional and anatomic obstruction is made by using either amyl nitrite or a calcium channel blocker, nifedipine. These drugs, which relieve functional but not anatomic obstruction, promote smooth passage of bile only in the case of a functional obstruction [29, 30]. The quantitative cholescintigraphic parameters are technically simple to measure, reliable, and easily reproducible within and between individuals and among institutions [31, 32]. Simultaneous quantification provides an objective parameter that may alter patient management strategy as to the timing of therapy, and also to test later whether or not the chosen therapy has achieved its intended goals. In most patients, nuclear hepatology studies supplement morphology imaging studies; however, in patients where functional alterations precede morphologic changes, one may have to depend mostly on the findings of cholescintigraphy [33]. An etiologic diagnosis of biliary obstruction, whether it is intraluminal, wall thickening, or extrinsic compression, often cannot be made from cholescintigraphy alone. Ultrasound, CT ERCP, or MRCP is required for an etiological diagnosis. ERCP may be ideal for confirmation of an intraluminal obstruction, ultrasound for wall thickening, and CT for an extrinsic compression.

Table 8.2.2. Sensitivity of ^{99m}Tc-HIDA cholescintigraphy in the detection of biliary obstruction

Author [ref.]	Number of patients with biliary obstruction	Obstruction identified with cholescintigraphy
Zeman [22]	60	59
Krishnamurthy [19]	14	13
Lecklitner [24]	25	23
Lieberman [26]	19	14
Darweesh [23]	15	10
Brown [12]	14	14
Juni [25]	10	10
Lieberman [27]	13	13
Lee [28]	44	44
Total	214	200 (93%)

Malignant Causes

Cholangiocarcinoma

Cholangiocarcinoma is the most common malignancy of the biliary system that causes wall thickening and obstruction to bile flow. Its incidence appears to have risen in recent years, which is partly related to the higher frequency of its detection by using more sophisticated diagnostic methods [34]. Cholangiocarcinoma occurs more commonly in the 6th decade of life, and affects men more frequently than women in the ratio of 1.2:1. The proximal common hepatic duct or one or both of its bifurcating branches are the most common locations [35]. About 58% of cholangiocarcinomas occur in the proximal one-third, 17% in the middle one-third, 18% in the distal one-third, and the remaining 7% are distributed diffusely throughout the common hepatic and common bile duct (Fig. 8.2.4). The site and frequency of occurrence of cholangiocarcinoma have changed in the more recent reports, probably reflecting early diagnosis by non-invasive imaging methods and early confirmation by cholangiopancreatography [36, 37].

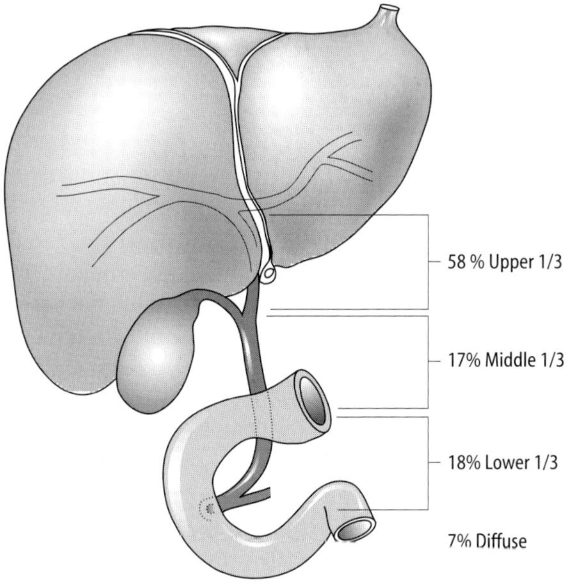

Fig. 8.2.4. Location of cholangiocarcinoma. Most occur in the common hepatic duct at its bifurcation [37]

Clinical Presentation

Presenting symptoms and signs include weight loss, jaundice, and pruritus. Serum bilirubin levels may fluctuate but the general trend is one of sustained increase. Patients usually seek medical attention late in the course of the disease, many after the onset of jaundice. By this time there is dilatation of bile duct proximal to the site of cancer which is readily detected on ultrasound or CT examination [38]. Bismuth classifies cholangiocarcinoma into four types based on its location and extent (Fig. 8.2.5). Type I involves the common bile duct or the distal common hepatic duct. The proximal common hepatic duct and right hepatic and left hepatic ducts are free of cancer. In type II, the carcinoma extends up to the level of the junction of the right and left hepatic ducts, but the proximal part of both the right and left hepatic ducts are free of

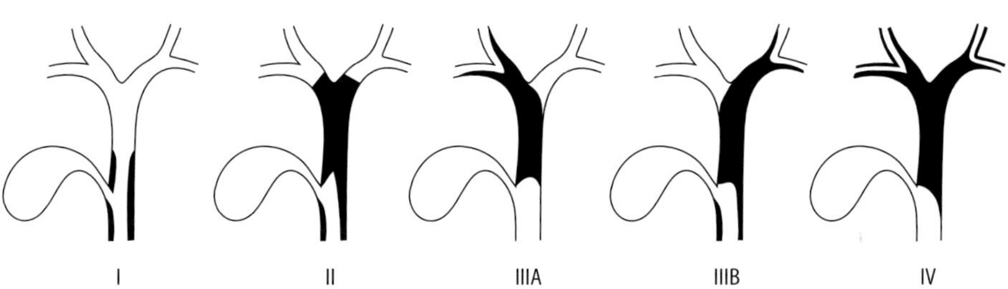

Fig. 8.2.5. Staging of cholangiocarcinoma. In stage I, only the common duct is involved; both right hepatic duct (*RHD*) and left hepatic duct (*LHD*) are free of cancer. In stage II, both proximal hepatic duct and distal RHD and LHD are involved. Stage III involves the common hepatic duct along with either the right hepatic duct (*IIIA*) and the left hepatic duct (*IIIB*). In stage IV, the entire extrahepatic biliary tree is involved including both right and left hepatic ducts along with their segmental branches

cancer. In type III, the cancer involves either the right hepatic (IIIa) or the left hepatic duct (IIIb). One of the lobar ducts is free of cancer. Type IV extends to both right and left hepatic ducts and their segmental branches, and the cancer is unresectable [39].

Carcinoma of the Ampulla of Vater

Of the 18% of the cholangiocarcinomas arising from the distal one-third of the common bile duct (Fig. 8.2.5), 75% are less than 4 mm from the ampulla of Vater [36]. The clinical presentation of the periampullary cholangiocarcinoma is distinctly different from those arising from the common hepatic duct and its bifurcation. Periampullary carcinoma presents more often as painless jaundice. Courvoisier first made the observation in 1890 that a palpable, painless gallbladder in a patient with jaundice has either a periampullary or a pancreatic cancer [40]. Periampullary cholangiocarcinoma accounts for less than 1–3% of obstructive jaundice. The common age group is between 55 and 65 years, with equal prevalence in men and women. There is frequent association with primary sclerosing cholangitis [41].

About 50% of patients with cholangiocarcinoma already have intraabdominal and intrahepatic metastasis at the time of their first presentation to a clinician [42]. Obstruction manifests two types of image pattern on ^{99m}Tc-HIDA study, depending upon the degree (partial vs complete obstruction) and duration of obstruction. Early segmental duct partial obstruction may show a normal or slightly reduced ^{99m}Tc-HIDA uptake with bile stasis proximal to obstruction [43]. Complete obstruction, on the other hand, shows marked reduction or no uptake at all in the region affected by the tumor [44]. Involvement of the left hepatic duct, for example, may show no uptake at all over the entire left lobe.

Most patients with cholangiocarcinoma present late, after the onset of jaundice, when hyperbilirubinemia and ductal dilatation are evident. A typical pattern consists of bile pooling in the duct proximal to the site of obstruction, and increased liver to duodenal transit time, often as long as 24 h. Multimodality imaging including ultrasonography, cholescintigraphy, CT, ERCP, and MRCP are complementary imaging modalities [45]. Biopsy is required prior to deciding on a definitive therapeutic strategy.

Stent Patency

Placement of a palliative endoprosthesis to relieve bile duct obstruction due to malignancy is now a standard treatment [46]. The endoprosthesis relieves the obstruction promptly and establishes bile flow immediately. The plastic stents tend to occlude prematurely or move away from the site of obstruction. Gianturco-Rosch self-expanding metal prostheses are preferred, and they function much better and for a longer period of time than the plastic variety [47, 48]. The stent patency is easily documented with ^{99m}Tc-HIDA cholescintigraphy.

Surgery is recommended for the early stages. Some prefer surgery even for tumors located proximally at the bifurcation (Klatskin tumor). Pylorus-preserving partial pancreatoduodenectomy or the Kausch-Whipple resection is the preferred surgical procedure [49, 50]. Insertion of an endoprosthesis is now a popular therapeutic option, especially in the terminal stage. Migration, infection, or occlusion are frequent complications of the endoprosthesis. Recent progress in stent design, and improvements in stent insertion techniques, have contributed towards a longer duration of stent function, for up to 3–4 months. Occluded stents are easily replaced and it is currently not a one-off procedure [51].

References

1. Andren-Sandberg A, Alinder G, Bengmark S. Accidental lesions of the common bile duct at cholecystectomy. Pre- and perioperative factors of importance. Ann Surg 1985;201:328–332
2. A prospective analysis of 1518 laparoscopic cholecystectomies. The southern surgeons club. N Engl J Med 1991;324:1073–1078
3. Terblanche J, Allison HF, Northover JM. An ischemic basis for biliary strictures. Surgery 1983;94:52–57
4. Mueller PR, vanSonnenberg E, Ferrucci JT Jr, et al. Biliary stricture dilatation: multicenter review of clinical management in 73 patients. Radiology 1986;160:17–22
5. Martenson JA Jr, Gunderson LL, Buskirk SJ, et al. Hepatic duct stricture after radical radiation therapy for biliary cancer: recurrence or fibrosis? Mayo Clin Proc 1986;61:530–536
6. Itoh H; Shimono R, Hamamoto K. Evaluation of common bile duct stenosis in chronic pancreatitis using cholescintigraphy. Eur J Nucl Med 1988;14:137–140
7. Ward EM, Kiely MJ, Maus TP, Wiesner RH, Kron RA. Hilar biliary strictures after liver transplantation: cholangiography and percutaneous treatment. Radiology 1990;177:259–263
8. Krishnamurthy GT, Bobba VR, McConnell D, Turner F, Mesgarzadeh M, Kingston E. Quantitative biliary dynamics: introduction of a new non-invasive scintigraphic technique. J Nucl Med 1983;24:217–223
9. Brown PH, Juni JE, Lieberman DA, Krishnamurthy GT. Hepatocyte vs biliary disease: a distinction by deconvolutional analysis of technetium-99m-HIDA time-activity curve. J Nucl Med 1988;29:623–630
10. Honickman SP, Mueller PR, Wittenberg J, et al. Ultrasound in obstructive jaundice: prospective evaluation of site and cause. Radiology 1983;147:511–515
11. Lapis JL, Orlando RC, Mittlesteadt CA, Staab EV. Ultrasonography in the diagnosis of obstructive jaundice. Ann Intern Med 1978;89:61–63
12. Compton RA. Bursting forces within the human body. Radiology 1973;107:77–80
13. Itoh H, Murase K, Hamamoto K. Reflux sign in cholescintigraphy after administration of a gallbladder contracting agent. J Nucl Med 1989;30:1192–1197
14. Brar HS. Scintigraphic cholecystokinin-induced bile reflux named as Krishnamurthy-Bobba sign. J Nucl Med 1990;31:248–249
15. Cooperberg PL, Burhenne HJ. Real-time ultrasonography. Diagnostic technique of choice in calculous gallbladder disease. N Engl J Med 1980;302:1277–1279
16. Laing FC, Jeffrey RB Jr. Choledocholithiasis and cystic duct obstruction: difficult ultrasonographic diagnosis. Radiology 1983;146:475–479
17. Krishnamurthy S, Krishnamurthy GT. Quantitative assessment of hepatobiliary diseases with Tc-99m-HIDA scintigraphy. In: Freeman LM, Weissman HS. eds. Nuclear Medicine Annual 1988. Raven Press, New York, pp 309–330
18. Doo E, Krishnamurthy GT, Eklem MJ, Gilbert S, Brown PH. Quantification of hepatobiliary function as an integral part of imaging with technetium-99m-mebrofenin in health and disease. J Nucl Med 1991;32:48–57
19. Krishnamuthy GT, Lieberman DA, Brar HS. Detection, localization, and quantitation of degree of common bile duct obstruction by scintigraphy. J Nucl Med 1985;26:726–735
20. Krishnamurthy S, Krishnamurthy GT. Biliary dyskinesia: role of the sphincter of Oddi, gallbladder and cholecystokinin. J Nucl Med 1997;38:1824–1830
21. Krishnamurthy S, Krishnamurthy GT. Evolution of nuclear hepatology as a clinical entity. J Nucl Med Technol 1995;23 (suppl)35S–45S
22. Zeman RK, Lee C, Jaffe MH, Burrell MI. Hepatobiliary scintigraphy and sonography in early biliary obstruction. Radiology 1984;153:793–798
23. Darweesh RMR, Dodds WJ, Hogan WJ, et al. Efficacy of quantitative hepatobiliary scintigraphy and fatty meal sonography for evaluating patients with suspected partial common bile duct obstruction. Gastroenterology 1988;94:779–786
24. Lecklitner ML, Austin AR, Benedetto AR, Growcock GW. Positive predictive value of cholescintigraphy in common bile duct obstruction. J Nucl Med 1986;27:1403–1406
25. Juni JE, Reichle R. Measurement of hepatocellular function with deconvolutional analysis: Application in the differential diagnosis of acute jaundice. Radiology 1990;177:171–175

26. Lieberman DA, Krishnamurthy GT. Intrahepatic vs extrahepatic cholestasis. Discrimination with biliary scintigraphy combined with ultrasound. Gastroenterology 1986;90:734–743
27. Lieberman DA, Brown PH, Krishnamurthy GT. Improved scintigraphic assessment of severe cholestasis with the hepatic extraction fraction. Dig Dis Sci 1990;35:1385–1390
28. Lee AW, Ram MD, Shih WJ, Murphy K. Technetium-99m-BIDA biliary scintigraphy in the evaluation of the jaundiced patient. J Nucl Med 1986;27:1407–1412
29. Madacsy L, Velosy B, Lonovics J, Csernay L. Differentiation between organic stenosis and functional dyskinesia of the sphincter of Oddi with amyl nitrite-augmented quantitative hepatobiliary scintigraphy. Eur J Nucl Med 1994;21;203–208
30. Bhatnagar A. Nifedipine interventional cholescintigraphy: a new method for assessing sphincter of Oddi? Indian J Nucl Med 1997;12:93–96
31. Gilbert SA, Brown PH, Krishnamurthy GT. Quantitative nuclear hepatology. J Nucl Med Technol 1987;15:38–43
32. Spackman J, Bartlett ME, Ryals L, et al. Reproducibility of technetium-99m-mebrofenin hepatic functional parameters obtained with semiautomatic soft ware. J Nucl Med Technol 1991;19:228–231
33. Krishnamurthy S, Krishnamurthy GT. Functional imaging in nuclear hepatology. Indian J Nucl Med 1997;12:216–232
34. Tomkins RK, Saunders KD, Roslyn JJ, Longmire WP Jr. Changing patterns in diagnosis and management of bile duct cancer. Ann Surg 1990;211:614–620
35. Klatskin G. Adenocarcinoma of the hepatic duct at its bifurcation within the porta hepatis. An usual tumor with distinctive clinical and pathologic features. Am J Med 1965;38:24
36. Wise L, Pizzimbono C, Dehner LP. Periampullary cancer. A clinicopathologic study of sixty-two patients. Am J Surg 1976;131:141–148
37. Sherlock S, Dooley J. Diseases of the liver and biliary system. 10th edition, Blackwell Science, Malden, MA, 1997, pp 641–649
38. Reiman TH, Balfe DM, Weyman PJ. Suprapancreatic biliary obstruction: CT evaluation. Radiology 1987;163:49–56
39. Bismuth H, Nakache R, Diamond R. Management strategies in resection for hilar cholangiocarcinoma. Ann Surg 1992;215:31–38
40. Courvoisier LG: Kasuistisch-statistiche Beitrage zur Pathologie und Chirurgie der Gallenwege. Leipzig FCV, Vogel, 1890
41. DeGroen PC, Gores GJ, LaRusso NF, Gunderson LL, Nagorney DM. Biliary tract cancers. N Engl J Med 1999;341:1368–1378
42. Burke EC, Jarnagin WR, Hochwald SN, Pisters PWT, Fong Y, Blungart LH. Hilar cholangiocarcinoma. Pattern of spread, the importance of hepatic resection for curative operation, and a pre-surgical staging system. Ann Surg 1998;228:385–394
43. Zeman RK, Gold JA, Gluck L, Caride VJ, Burrell M, Hoffer PB. Tc-99m-HIDA scintigraphy in segmental biliary obstruction. J Nucl Med 1981;22:456–458
44. Gupta S, Owshalimpur D, Cohen G, Margules R, Herrera N. Scintigraphic detection of segmental bile-duct obstruction. J Nucl Med 1982;23:890–891
45. Zeman RK, Lee C, Stahl RS, Cahow CE, Viscomi GN, Neumann RD, Gold JA, Burrell MI. Ultrasonography and hepatobiliary scintigraphy in the assessment of biliary-enteric anastomoses. Radiology 1982;145:109–115
46. Mueller RR, Ferrucci JT Jr, Teplick SK, vanSonnenberg E, Haskin PH, Butch RJ, Papanicolaou N. Biliary stent endoprosthesis: analysis of complications in 113 patients. Radiology 1985;156:637–639
47. Mathieson JR, McLoughlin RE, Cooperberg PL, Prystai CC, Stordy SN, MacFarlane JK, Schmidt N. Malignant obstruction of the common bile duct: long-term results of Gianturco-Rosch metal stents used as initial treatment. Radiology 1994;192:663--667
48. Boguth L, Tatalovic S, Antonucci F, Heer M, Susler H, Zollikofer CL. Malignant biliary obstruction: clinical and histopathologic correlation after treatment with self-expanding metal 9) prostheses. Radiology 1994;192:669–674
49. Beger HG, Treitschke F, Gansauge F, Harada N, Hiki N, Mattfeldt T. Tumor of the ampulla of Vater. Experience with local or radical resection in 171 consecutively treated patients. Arch Surg 1999;134:526–532
50. Launois B, Terblanche J, Lakehal M, Catheline JM, Bardaxoglou E, Landen S, Campion JP, Sutherland F, Meunier B. Proximal bile duct cancer: high resectability rate and 5 year survival. Ann Surg 1999;230:266–275
51. Lee MJ, Mueller PR, Saini S, Morrison MC, Brink JA, Hahn PF. Occlusion of biliary endoprosthesis: presentation and management. Radiology 1990;176:531–534

8.3 Combined Intrahepatic and Extrahepatic Cholestasis (Sclerosing Cholangitis)

By involving both intrahepatic and extrahepatic ducts sequentially, or simultaneously, sclerosing cholangitis is a typical example of a disease that combines features of both intrahepatic and extrahepatic cholestasis. Sclerosing cholangitis (SC) is a slowly progressive disease of unknown etiology characterized by chronic inflammation, fibrosis, and narrowing of both intrahepatic and extrahepatic ducts at multiple levels [1]. Several contributing factors have been identified (Table 8.3.1). Multiple strictures with a normal duct in between gives the characteristic beaded appearance on the contrast cholangiogram. The term "primary" is used when all other possible causes of cholangitis have been excluded. Cholangitis associated with choledocholithiasis, biliary tract surgery, carcinoma, chemotherapy, or acquired immunodeficiency syndrome (AIDS) are called secondary sclerosing cholangitis. Only after exclusion of these secondary causes is the term primary applied.

Table 8.3.1. Cholescintigraphic features of primary sclerosing cholangitis, isolated common bile duct obstruction, and primary biliary cirrhosis

Parameter	Primary sclerosing cholangitis	Isolated common bile duct obstruction	Primary biliary cirrhosis
Level of CBD obstruction	Proximal	Distal	None
Number of obstructions	Multiple	Single	None
Beading of ducts	Common	Rare	None
Bile pooling proximal to obstruction	Uncommon	Very common	Uncommon
Cystic duct obstruction	Common	Rare	Rare
Liver clearance half-time	Marked increase	Moderate increase	Marked increase
Regional variations in clearance half-time	Wide variation from region to region	Uniform increase from all regions	Uniform increase from all regions

Primary Sclerosing Cholangitis

Primary sclerosing cholangitis affects patients usually in their 40s, men more often (75%) than women [2]. An association with inflammatory bowel disease is found in 75% of patients [3,4]. The clinical onset is insidious with fatigue, pruritus, and malaise. Biochemical changes are characterized by moderate elevation of serum alkaline phosphatase, and mild elevation of alanine amino transferase. Elevation of serum bilirubin is a late event. Urinary copper excretion is increased [3]. Unlike primary biliary cirrhosis, there is no specific serological marker for primary sclerosing cholangitis.

Pathophysiology

Histologically four stages are identified. Stage I represents the initial degenerative changes in the duct lining epithelial cells and infiltration by lymphocytes and neutrophils. Stage II is characterized by periportal necrosis, stage III consists of portal to portal fibrous septa and disappearance of bile ducts, and stage IV represents the end stage with cirrhosis and onion skin appearance on biopsy, a characteristic histologic finding. The cholangiogram shows a typical beaded appearance of the extrahepatic ducts. Both intrahepatic and extrahepatic ducts are involved but the contrast cholangiogram is often incapable of detecting the involvement of the intrahepatic ducts [5]. In 100 patients with primary sclerosing cholangitis, 87% had involvement of both intrahepatic and extrahepatic ducts, 11% had involvement of only the intrahepatic ducts, and 2% had involvement of only the extrahepatic ducts [4].

The disease progresses slowly over 10–15 years before reaching the stage of cirrhosis, portal hypertension, liver failure, and death. The median survival is 12 years [5]. The course of the disease is reversible during stage I, and may be reversible in stage II, but irreversible at stage III and IV. The following criteria are required for the diagnosis: (1) increased alkaline phosphatase, more than ×1.5 normal for at least 6 months, and (2) multiple strictures or beading of the ducts on the cholangiogram. Characteristic planar and SPECT images on the ^{99m}Tc-HIDA study may be included as one of the required criteria [6].

Secondary Sclerosing Cholangitis

Secondary sclerosing cholangitis follows an identifiable cause such as surgery on the biliary tract, choledocholithiasis, intraarterial infusions of chemotherapeutic agents [8,], cholangiocarcinoma [9], acquired immunodeficiency syndrome [10], and congenital biliary abnormalities. The diagnosis of primary sclerosing cholangitis is made only after excluding all of the above causes. Inflammatory bowel disease (ulcerative colitis or Crohn's disease) is now considered an accompaniment of primary sclerosing cholangitis and when found either before or in association with cholangitis, the condition is still labeled primary sclerosing cholangitis. The scintigraphic findings of secondary sclerosing cholangitis have not been studied as thoroughly as primary sclerosing cholangitis. The ERCP findings of secondary sclerosing cholangitis are indistinguishable from those of primary sclerosing cholangitis.

Cholescintigraphic Diagnosis

Cholescintigraphic planar images are obtained for 60 min with 3–5 mCi ^{99m}Tc-HIDA. SPECT images are obtained between 60 and 90 min [6, 11]. Early planar images (within 10 min) show a patchy uptake by the liver. Late images show a typical pattern of beading of the right hepatic, left hepatic, common hepatic, or common bile ducts, depending upon the extent of the disease (Fig. 8.3.1). The hepatic extraction fraction remains within the normal range early in the course of the disease and begins to decrease in advanced stages [6, 11]. The excretion half-time increases from the very beginning. Due to multiple duct involvement at various levels, the excretion half-time varies widely from region to region, often with values as high as 6–7 times normal. The gallbladder is often non-visualized due to obstruction of the cystic duct.

SPECT images show characteristic features of varying parenchymal retention among different regions. Liver parenchyma with normal bile ducts shows rapid clearance while the parenchyma drained by obstructed bile ducts shows retention giving the characteristic scintigraphic images (Fig. 8.3.2). The involvement and extent of cholangitis as indicated by cholescintigraphy may be more critical and much larger

Fig. 8.3.1. Sclerosing cholangitis. Planar image shows beading of right hepatic, left hepatic duct, common hepatic, and common bile ducts. Gallbladder is not seen due to obstruction of the cystic duct

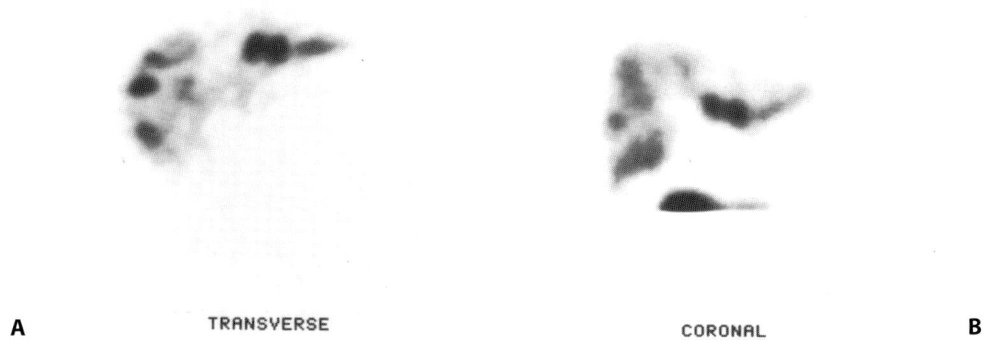

Fig. 8.3.2. SPECT in sclerosing cholangitis. Transaxial (**A**) and coronal (**B**) slices, obtained between 60 and 90 min, show multiple areas of focal parenchymal retention over the involved ducts along with regions of complete clearance from ducts not affected

than the disease shown on the contrast cholangiogram. This underestimation of severity and extent by the cholangiogram is due to the inability of the contrast to enter most of the intrahepatic ducts. Several features characteristic of primary sclerosing cholangitis that help to differentiate it from primary biliary cirrhosis and isolated common bile duct obstruction are shown in Table 8.3.1. Magnetic resonance cholangiopancreatography is an emerging new technique which is capable of demonstrating involvement of both intrahepatic and extrahepatic ducts [12, 13].

Therapy

The medical therapy for primary sclerosing cholangitis includes such drugs as D-penicillamine, cyclosporine, methotrexate, corticosteroids, azathioprine, colchicine, or cholesteramine. Antibiotics are prescribed when there is superimposed infection [5]. Endoscopic stenting is shown to be safe, effective, and works for several years until end stage liver disease sets in [14]. Liver transplantation is recommended for end stage liver disease when medical therapy fails.

References

1. LaRusso NF, Wiesner RH, Ludwig J, MacCarty RL. Current concepts. Primary sclerosing cholangitis. N Eng J Med 1984;310:899–903
2. Wiesner RH, Grambsch PM, Dickson ER, Ludwig J, MacCarty RL, Hunter EB, Fleming TR, Fisher LD, Beaver SJ, LaRusso NF. Primary sclerosing cholangitis: natural history, prognostic factors, and survival analysis. Hepatology 1989;10:430–436
3. Gross JB Jr, Ludwig J, Wiesner RH, McCall JT, LaRusso NF. Abnormalities in tests of copper metabolism in primary sclerosing cholangitis. Gastroenterology 1985;89:272–278
4. Lee YM, Kaplan MM. Primary sclerosing cholangitis. N Eng J Med 1995;332:924–933
5. Wiesner RH. Current concepts in primary sclerosing cholangitis. Mayo Clin Proc 1994;69:969–982
6. Rodman CA, Keeffe EB, Lieberman DA, Krishnamurthy S, Krishnamurthy GT, Gilbert S, Eklem MJ. Diagnosis of sclerosing cholangitis with Technetium 99m-labeled Iminodiacetic acid planar and single photon emission computed tomographic scintigraphy. Gastroenterology 1987;92:777–785
7. Ament AE, Bick RJ, Miraldi FD, Haaga JR, Wiedenmann SD. Sclerosing cholangitis: cholescintigraphy with Tc-99m-labeled DISIDA. Radiology 1984;151:197–201
8. Pien EH, Zeman RK, Benjamin SB, Barth KH, Jaffe MH, Choyke PL, Clark LR, Paushter DM. Iatrogenic sclerosing cholangitis following hepatic arterial chemotherapy infusion. Radiology 1985;156:329–330
9. Shea WJ Jr, Demas BE, Goldberg HI, Hohn DC, Ferrell LD, Kerlan RK. Sclerosing cholangitis associated with hepatic arterial FUDR chemotherapy: radiographic-histologic correlation. AJR Am J Roentgenol 1986;146:717–721
10. MacCarty RL, LaRusso NF, May GR, Bender CE, Wiesner RH, King JE, Coffey RJ. Cholangiocarcinoma complicating primary sclerosing cholangitis: cholangiographic appearances. Radiology 1985;156:43–46
11. Dolmatch BL, Laing FC, Federle MP, Jeffrey RB, CelloJ. AIDS- related cholangitis: radiographic findings in nine patients. Radiology 1987;163:313–316
12. Lee MG, Lee HJ, Kim MH, Kang EM, Kim YH, Lee SG, Kim PN, Ha NK, Auh YH. Extrahepatic biliary diseases: 3D MR cholangiopancreatography compared with endoscopic retrograde cholangiopancreatography. Radiology 1997;202:663–669
13. Asselah T, Ernst O, Sergent G, L'herminé C, Paris J. Caroli's disease: a magnetic resonance cholangiopancreatography diagnosis. Am J Gastroenterol 1998;93:109–110
14. Ponsioen CY, Lam K, van Milligen de Wit AWM, Huibregtse K, Tytgat GNJ. Four years experience with short term stenting in primary sclerosing cholangitis. Am J Gastroenterol 1999;94:2403–2407

8.4 Extrinsic Compression

Extrinsic compression of the bile duct can occur at any point along the course from the small intrahepatic duct to the termination of the common bile duct (Table 8.4.1). Compression due to an enlarged lymph node occurs more frequently at the porta hepatis, where there are many lymph nodes. Lymphosarcoma, reticulum cell sarcoma, and Hodgkin's disease account for the majority of such obstructions [1]. Acute edematous pancreatitis is a frequent cause. Carcinoma of the stomach, pancreas, and gallbladder may invade the bile duct directly, whereas cancer of other distant organs spreads via the hematogenous route [2]. Chronic pancreatitis, which causes obstruction due to thickening of the intraduodenal portion of the duct wall, may also cause obstruction by an extrinsic compression due to fibrosis around the distal common bile duct [3]. Duodenal diverticula are found along the medial duodenal wall, very close to the ampulla of Vater, in about 2% of patients undergoing barium meal examination [4]. On rare occasions, the ampulla of Vater may be found within the diverticulum. Acute cholecystitis and acute pancreatitis often coexist and cause non-visualization of the gallbladder during a ^{99m}Tc-HIDA study [5, 6]. Non-visualization of the gallbladder in a patient with a marked elevation of serum lipase or amylase may indicate acute biliary pancreatitis. Elevation of serum lipase and amylase aids in differentiating pancreatitis from acute cholecystitis. Cancer of the head of the pancreas is a well recognized cause of extrinsic compression (Fig. 8.4.1).

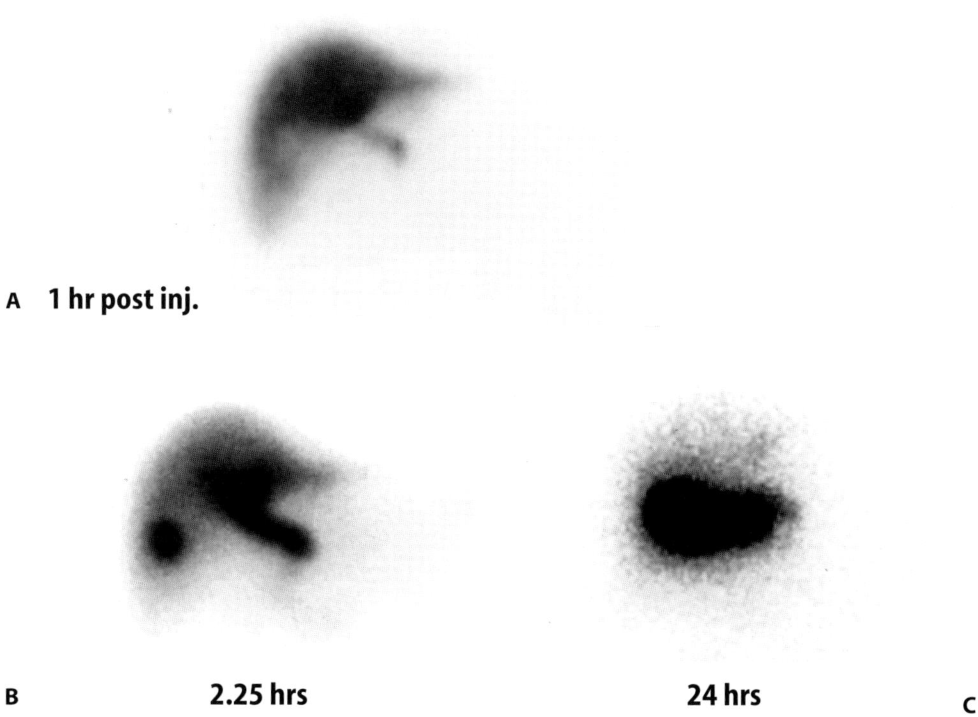

Fig. 8.4.1. Extrinsic compression. Common bile duct obstruction due to extrinsic compression by cancer of the head of pancreas. Distal common bile duct ends abruptly (**A**). Gallbladder is seen late (**B**) and does not empty even at 24 h (**C**)

Table 8.4.1. Causes of bile duct obstruction due to extrinsic compression

1. Periductal lymph node enlargement
2. Carcinoma of head of pancreas
3. Chronic pancreatitis
4. Acute edematous pancreatitis
5. Annular pancreas
6. Duodenal diverticula
7. Pseudocyst of pancreas
8. Mirizzi syndrome

Mirizzi Syndrome

The Mirizzi syndrome is a rare type of common bile duct obstruction due to extrinsic compression from a large gallstone impaction in Hartmann's pouch or at the neck of the gallbladder. Patients with Mirizzi syndrome usually have a long cystic duct that runs parallel to the common hepatic duct before joining it to form the common bile duct [7, 8]. Two types of Mirizzi syndrome are described. Type I Mirizzi syndrome consists of extrinsic compression of the common hepatic duct by the stone in the gallbladder neck or in Hartmann's pouch. In type II Mirizzi syndrome, the stone erodes into the common hepatic duct, forming a cholecystocholedochal fistula. Recent studies have shown a role for non-invasive diagnosis with MR imaging [9]. Laparoscopic cholecystectomy is the preferred initial approach in uncomplicated cases, and open cholecystectomy is recommended when anomalies exist around the Callot triangle [10-12].

References

1. Leuitan R, Diamond HD, Craver LF. Jaundice in Hodgkin's disease. Am J Med 1961;30:99
2. Popp JW Jr, Schapiro RH, Warshaw AL. Extrahepatic biliary obstruction by metastatic breast carcinoma. Ann Intern Med 1979;91:568–571
3. Itoh H, Shimono R, Hamamoto K. Evaluation of common bile duct stenosis in chronic pancreatitis using cholescintigraphy. Eur J Nucl Med 1988;14:137–140
4. McSherry CK, Glenn F. Biliary tract obstruction and duodenal diverticula. Surg Gynecol Obstet 1970;130:829–836
5. Serafini AN, Al-Sheikh W, Barkin JS, Hourani M, Sfakiankis G, Clarke LP, Ashkar FS. Biliary scintigraphy in acute pancreatitis. Radiology 1982;144:591–595
6. Ali A, Turner DA, Fordham EW. Tc-99m-IDA cholescintigraphy in acute pancreatitis: concise communication. J Nucl Med 1982;23:867–869
7. Mirizzi PL. Sindrome del conducto hepatico. J Int Chir 1948;8:731
8. Montefusco P, Spicer N, Geiss AC. Another facet of Mirizzi's syndrome. Arch Surg 1983;118:1221–1223
9. Kim PN, Outwater EK, Mitchel DG. Mirizzi syndrome: evaluation by MR imaging. Am J Gastroenterol 1999;94:2546–2550
10. Sare M, Gürer S, Taskin V, Aladag M, Hilmioglu F, Gürel M. Mirizzi syndrome: choice of surgical procedure in the laparoscopic era. Surg Laparosc Endosc 1998;8:63–67
11. Vezakis A, Davides D, Birbas K, Ammori BJ, Larvin M, McMahon MJ. Laparoscopic treatment of Mirrizzi syndrome. Surg Laparosc Endosc & percut Techn 2000;10:15–18
12. Chowbey PK, Sharma A, Mann V, Knullar R Baijal M, Vashista A. The management of Mirrizzi syndrome in the laparoscopic era. Surg Laparosc Endosc & percut Tech 2000;10:11–14

Diseases of the Gallbladder

Gallbladder disease is one of the most common medical problems in the United States and around the world [1]. There are at least 6.3 million men and 16.6 million women who have some form of gallbladder disease in the United States, and gallstones account for most of them [2]. Women are affected 2–3 times as frequently as men. Race, heredity, gender, age, and obesity are some of the important known risk factors for gallstones (Table 9.1.1). Between the years 60 and 74, the prevalence of gallbladder disease is as high as 25.3% in men and 33.1%% in women (Table 9.1.2), and relatively more common among the Mexican Americans (Table 9.1.3). The highest rate among the Americans is found in Pima Indians in the state of Arizona [3]. By the teenage years, as many as 10–13% of Pima Indian girls develop lithogenic bile, and by the age 35–44 years, about 71% develop gallstones. Almost 90% of Pima Indian women over the age of 65 years develop gallbladder disease, and the prevalence is much higher than in Pima Indian men. Such a high prevalence has also been reported in Mestizo Hispanics of Chile and a high altitude rural population of Peru [4, 5]. The incidence of gallbladder disease varies from country to country; the Italians [6], British [7], Scottish [8], and Swedish [9] people have a much higher rate than people from other parts of Europe. The relative incidence within a country, however, varies depending upon the ethnic, socioeconomic and genetic factors [10].

Table 9.1.1. Risk factors for gallstones

1. Heredity
2. Obesity
3. Gender
4. Diabetes
5. Age
6. Low socioeconomic status
7. Parity
8. Pregnancy
9. Drugs, e.g., somatostatin analogues (octreotide)

Natural History of Gallstones

Most gallstones remain asymptomatic. In a carefully followed prospective study of 24 years, it has been shown that the frequency of biliary pain developing from an asymptomatic gallstone is 10±3% at the end of 5 years, 15±4% at 10 years, and 18.4±4% at 15 years (Fig. 9.1.1). The rate at the end of 20 years remains unchanged from that at 15 years [11]. Generally, the asymptomatic patients with gallstones develop biliary pain (become symptomatic) at an average rate of 2% per year [12, 13]. Both the frequency of

Table 9.1.2. Prevalence of gallstones and gallbladder disease in men and women in the United States [2]

Age (years)	Gallstones		Gallbladder disease	
	Men (%)	Women (%)	Men (%)	Women (%)
20–29	1.3	4.4	1.3	6.5
30–39	1.1	5.2	1.9	10.2
40–49	5.9	8.2	7.3	15.7
50–59	7.3	11.9	11.7	25.0
60–74	17.2	16.4	25.8	33.1
Mean	5.5	8.6	7.9	16.6

Table 9.1.3. Effect of gender and ethnicity on prevalence of gallstones and gallbladder disease in the United States [2]

Gender, ethnicity	Gallstones	Gallbladder disease
Men		
Whites (non-Hispanics)	5.8	8.6
Blacks (non-Hispanics)	3.9	5.3
Mexican Americans	6.1	8.9
Women		
Whites (non-Hispanics)	8.6	16.6
Blacks (non-Hispanics)	7.9	13.9
Mexican Americans	12.8	26.7

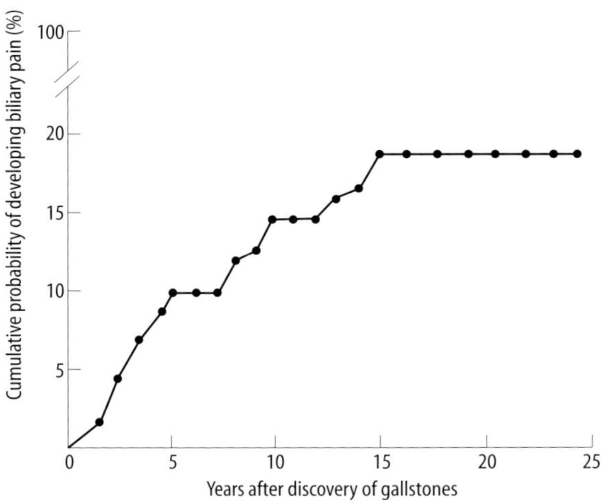

Fig. 9.1.1. Natural history of asymptomatic gallstones. Cumulative probability of onset of biliary pain in patients with asymptomatic gallstones increases with time: 10±3%, 15±4%, 18±4%, and 18±4%, at the end of 5, 10, 15 and 20 years, respectively [11]

gallstones and onset of biliary pain increase during pregnancy to as high as 30%. Stones smaller than 10 mm pass spontaneously after delivery [14]. The higher incidence of gallstones during pregnancy is attributed to elevation of serum estrogen, which induces bile stasis, crystallization, and stone growth within the gallbladder. Gallstones form 7 times more frequently in obese women than in non-obese women of comparable age [10].

Composition of Gallstones

Gallstones are classified into two main types: cholesterol and pigment stones [15, 16]. Cholesterol stones are the most common, soft in consistency, and consist of layers of cholesterol alternating with mucin glycoproteins [17]. Cholesterol is insoluble in water but it is kept in solution in bile by forming micelles formed of cholesterol, bile salts, and phospholipids (lecithin). As the bile cholesterol concentration increases, a large number of multilayered vesicles and crystals are formed which aggregate and grow into large stones [18, 19]. Pigment stones are more common in patients with cirrhosis or chronic hemolytic anemia. They are black or brown in color, hard in consistency, and contain bilirubin or calcium salts [20]. Stones formed within the common bile duct usually belong to the pigment type. The great majority of gallstones (65–70%) seen on a plain abdominal radiograph are pigment stones [21].

9.1 Chronic Calculous Cholecystitis

Clinical Presentation

Patients with chronic calculous cholecystitis usually present with mild to moderate intensity upper abdominal pain without fever or leukocytosis. They ignore pain in the beginning and seek medical aid only when it becomes intolerable. Pain begins 15–30 min after a meal, and this time interval usually corresponds to the time taken for the serum endogenous cholecystokinin level to rise above the threshold to induce gallbladder contraction and emptying. The site of origin and direction of propagation of biliary pain are variable. The most common location is the epigastrium or the right

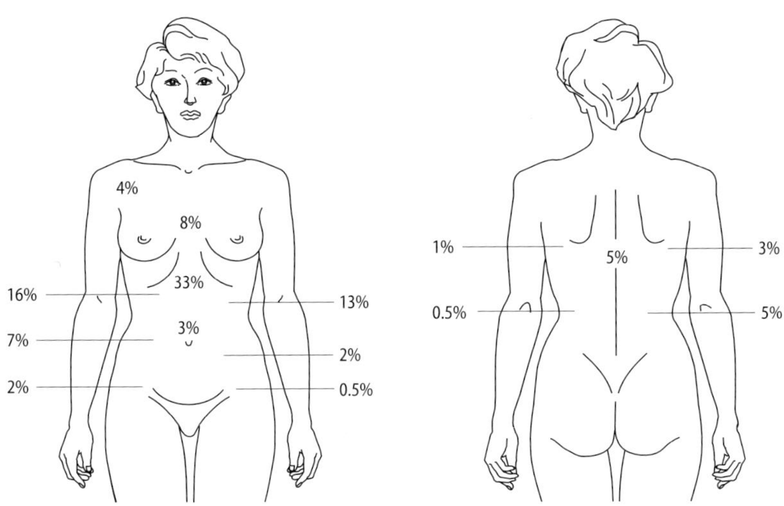

Fig. 9.1.2. Location and propagation of biliary pain. Epigastrium is the most common location, followed by the right hypochondrium. The pain may radiate to the chest and shoulder mimicking an anginal attack, or to the back mimicking pancreatitis. Radiation to the lower quadrants of the abdomen may mimic appendicitis or diverticulitis [22]

hypochondrium (Fig. 9.1.2). The pain beginning in the right lower quadrant may mimic acute appendicitis, or that beginning on the left side of the abdomen may simulate gastritis or diverticulitis. The pain may radiate to the chest and shoulder, mimicking an anginal attack. The pain deep in the abdomen and radiating to the interscapular region in the back may simulate an attack of acute pancreatitis [22]. The pain following dinner usually reaches its peak intensity at midnight [23]. Biliary pain is attributed to distension of the gallbladder or common bile duct when they contract against obstruction to bile flow. Pain intensity correlates directly with the degree of wall distension [24]. Stones lying free within the gallbladder lumen do not cause pain. Pain is intermittent with weeks or months of pain free intervals between attacks. In a given patient, however, the pain frequency, duration, and intensity remain constant despite wide variations among patients [25].

Biliary Pain Pathway

The liver and biliary tract receive both a somatic and an autonomic (sympathetic and parasympathetic) nerve supply. Somatic intercostal nerves from thoracic T8, 9, and 10 spinal segments supply the parietal peritoneum. The phrenic nerve from the cervical third and fourth segments supplies the diaphragm and the underlying parietal peritoneum and the gallbladder. Pain originating from the gallbladder, bile ducts, and peritoneum is also carried centrally through the branches of the right phrenic nerve. The axons from the sympathetic preganglionic neurons located in thoracic T7 to T11 spinal segments travel along the ventral root and the corresponding sympathetic ganglion to reach the celiac ganglion via the greater and lesser splanchnic nerves. Postganglionic sympathetic fibers from the celiac ganglion supply the liver and the biliary tree (Fig. 1.1.7, Chap. 1). Biliary tract pain is carried centrally through these afferent sympathetic fibers. Afferent nerve fibers originating from the corresponding somatotomes and dermatomes join the liver and biliary tract afferent fibers in the spinal cord and serve as a common channel for referred pain. Afferent fibers cross the midline to enter the opposite spinothalamic tract before reaching the thalamus, where pain is processed and sent to higher centers in the cortex.

The parasympathetic nerve supply is via the right and left vagal nerves, which originate in the medulla. After entering the abdomen, vagal fibers pass through the posterior and anterior hepatic plexus before entering the liver, bile ducts, and gallbladder. The parasympathetic branches to the gallbladder and intrahepatic ducts come mainly from the left (anterior) vagus and branches to the extrahepatic bile ducts and the sphincter of Oddi arrive mainly from the right (posterior) vagus. The parasympathetic system supplies the efferent nerve fibers and control motor function of the gallbladder, bile ducts, and sphincter of Oddi. Pain from the gallbladder and common bile duct is referred to the epigastrium, right hypochondrium, right shoulder or anterior chest (Fig. 9.1.2).

Histopathologic Features

The gallbladder of chronic cholecystitis is often small in size and consists of thickening, fibrosis, and microcalcification of the wall. A single large stone or multiple small stones are common. Bile is viscous and contains debris which often settles at the fundus as sludge. The wall shows chronic inflammation and infiltration with lymphocytes, without any hemorrhage or necrosis, which are features of acute cholecystitis. The mucous membrane shows ulceration and scarring. Fibrosis and wall thickening reduce absorption of water through the wall, which accounts for delayed visualization or non-visualization of the gallbladder on an oral cholecystogram. Yet most such non-visualized gallbladders in an oral cholecystogram are usually seen in a ^{99m}Tc-HIDA study, because the entry of even a single drop of high specific activity hepatic bile enables visualization of the gallbladder in a cholescintigram.

Diagnosis of Cholelithiasis

Ultrasonography is the diagnostic procedure of choice for detection of gallstones within the gallbladder. The gallstones are hyperechoic and produce an acoustic shadow beyond the wall (Fig. 9.1.3). A confirmatory diagnosis of cholelithiasis by ultrasound requires demonstration of stone movement with gravity, by taking gallbladder images at several different angles [26]. The stones are readily demonstrated in a fully filled gallbladder but are often missed when the gallbladder is small in size, incompletely filled or filled with stones, or empty of bile. Small stones mixed with sludge settle at the fundus and may fail to produce an acoustic shadow. Bile sludge is a thick, echo-dense fluid, and consists of mucin, protein, calcium bilirubinate granules, and cholesterol monohydrate crystals [27, 28]. Bile sludge produces an irregular echo-dense pattern within the gallbladder and does not produce an acoustic shadow (Fig. 9.1.4). Sludge formation increases after prolonged fasting or parenteral nutrition and it clears after a fatty meal. Sludge formed during pregnancy disappears after delivery [14]. The sludge may collect at the dependent part of the gallbladder in a layered fashion and simulate settlement of the contrast agent (Fig. 9.1.5). About 15% of the gallstones contain enough calcium to be seen on a plain abdominal X-ray film or on a CT scan [29]. Oral contrast cholecystography, once the most popular and common diagnostic test, is rarely used today for the diagnosis of cholelithiasis.

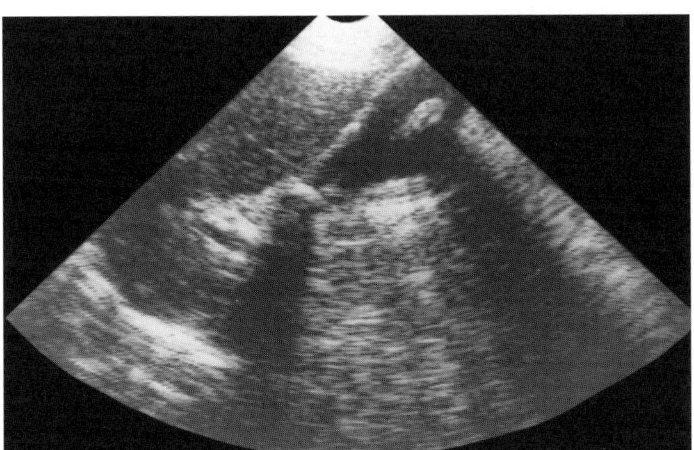

Fig. 9.1.3. Detection of gallstone with the ultrasound. Typically the gallstone appears as hyperechoic mass within the gallbladder and produces an acoustic shadow beyond the wall. Note: one stone in the neck and another in the body of the gallbladder

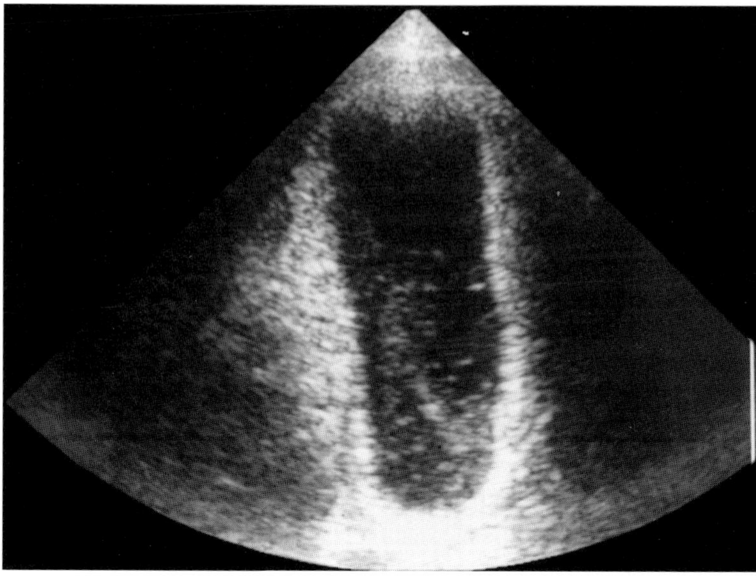

Fig. 9.1.4. Bile sludge. On the ultrasound study the sludge appears as an irregular echo-dense mass without an acoustic shadow. Gallbladder of wall is thickened

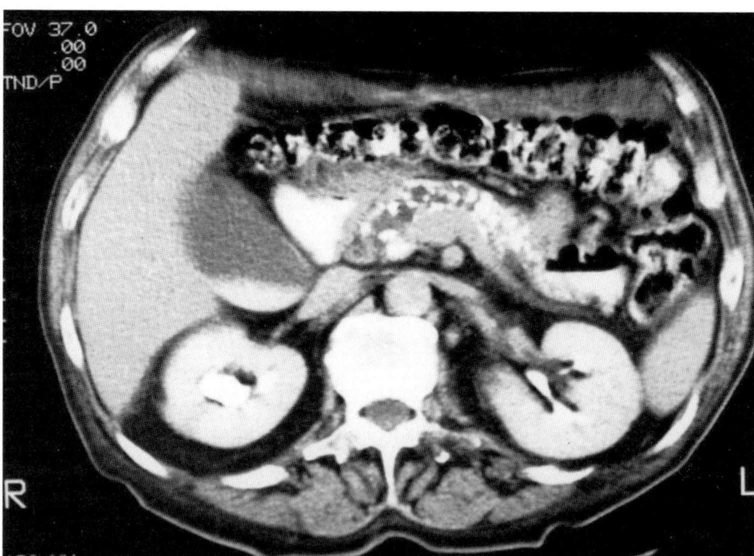

Fig. 9.1.5. Layering of radiocontrast. High density radiocontrast agent settles at the dependent part of the gallbladder and appears as a separate layer from bile

Bile Aspiration

When standard imaging procedures fail, duodenal bile aspiration is performed sometimes to demonstrate cholesterol crystals, the forerunner of gallstones. After positioning the tip of an orally passed tube in the second part of the duodenum, 0.02 µg/kg CCK-8 is infused intravenously to induce contraction and emptying of the gallbladder. The bile emptied from the gallbladder into the duodenum is aspirated through the nasoduodenal tube and examined under the microscope or subjected to biochemical analysis [30]. The test is relatively invasive and expensive and is used mostly for research purposes when all other simple methods fail to demonstrate gallstones.

Quantitative Cholescintigraphy

Cholescintigraphy is used for measuring gallbladder motor function (ejection fraction), and for differentiating symptomatic from asymptomatic gallstones by closely monitoring the temporal relationship between the onset of pain with the phase of gallbladder emptying. A geometric technique for measurement of gallbladder volume was first introduced in 1948 by deSilva by using an oral cholecystogram [31]. A slightly modified method has been adopted for volume measurement with ultrasound [32]. Both oral cholecystogram and ultrasound are geometric methods and require that the gallbladder be of a particular shape (pear) before contraction, and maintain that shape during and after contraction. It is widely recognized that the gallbladder has many different shapes when it is full, and changes its shape to different forms during and after its contraction.

To overcome the theoretical disadvantages of a geometric technique, a count based, non-geometric cholescintigraphic method was introduced in 1981 for measurment of gallbladder emptying [33]. This method does not require that the gallbladder be of a particular shape. Counts originating from the gallbladder accurately represent the bile volume (see Fig. 5.1.6, Chap. 5). Emptying is expressed as an ejection fraction by dividing counts emptied by the total counts before emptying. The technique is highly reproducible either with a fatty meal ingestion or after intravenous administration of cholecystokinin [34, 35]. The short serum half-life (2.5 min) of cholecystokinin enables measurement of serial ejection fractions by administering two to four sequential doses of CCK-8 on a single occasion [36]. Such techniques may enable the study of the effect of various drugs on the gallbladder or on the sphincter of Oddi (Fig. 6.1.7, Chap. 6).

Cholescintigraphy is usually obtained 6–10 h after fasting (minimum 4 h) to ensure a maximum tightness of the sphincter of Oddi and maximum relaxation of the gallbladderwall. In patients with serum bilirubin of less than 2 mg%, a dose of 2–3 mCi (74–111 MBq) HIDA will suffice. Larger doses are required in patients with hyperbilirubinemia. During the first 60 min of data collection (hepatic phase imaging), a relatively larger fraction of the hepatic bile enters the gallbladder in both normal subjects and patients with gallstones. A gallbladder count rate of more than 35,000/min by 30 min, and more than 70,000/min by 45 min, is usual with a 5-mCi dose of ^{99m}Tc-HIDA (Table 9.1.4). A gallbladder which appears early (within 10–15 min) shows a much higher count rate at 60 min (Fig. 9.1.6A) than a gallbladder which visualizes late, between 30 and 60 min (Fig 9.1.6B). In those 5–10% of patients in whom the gallbladder appears late (after 50 min), it is necessary to wait for 90 min or more to

Table 9.1.4. Gallbladder counts following intravenous injection of 5 mCi ^{99m}Tc-HIDA in normal subjects and patients with gallstones [34]

Time (min)	Normal subjects (n=15)	Gallstone patients (n=15)
15	5,100±70	4,200±60
30	40,600±520	38,700±490
45	75,200±680	70,800±630
60	72,000±620	78,100±710

A

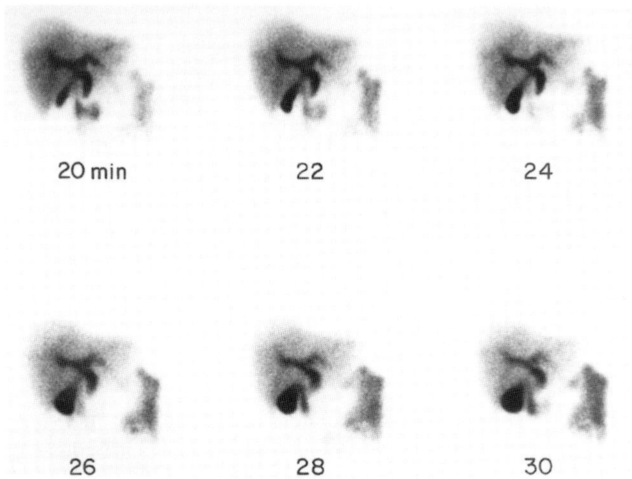

B

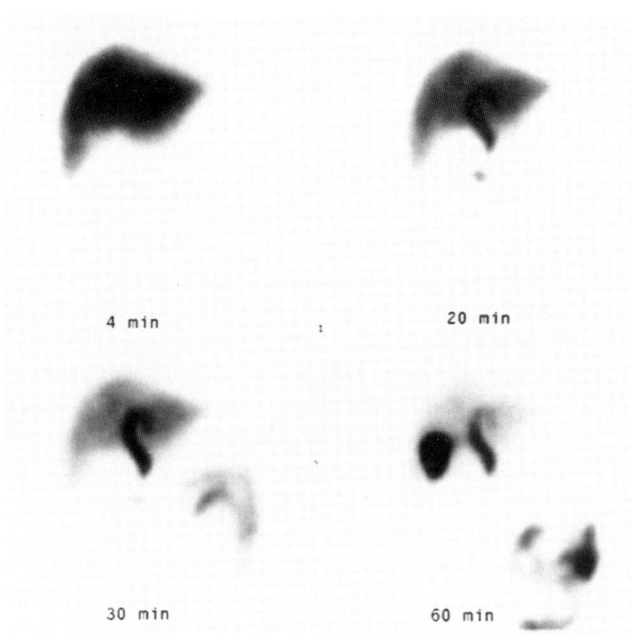

Fig. 9.1.6. Normal cholescintigram: gallbladder, intrahepatic and extrahepatic bile ducts, and duodenum all appear within 30 min in one patient (**A**), whereas the gallbladder appears by 30–60 min in another patient (**B**). Distal common bile duct has a convex left margin. Radioactivity in the first part of the duodenum stays close to the gallbladder in **A** but not in **B**

ensure adequate counts within the gallbladder. Variations in the time of appearance and rate of filling of the gallbladder are common and should be taken into account (Fig. 9.1.6B) before proceeding with quantitative cholescintigraphy [37].

Fatty Meal Stimulation

Gallbladder emptying is under both nervous and hormonal control [38]. Nervous control is exerted via the cholinergic (vagus) and adrenergic nervous system. Gallbladder emptying in response to a sham feeding occurs via the cholinergic nerve stimulation and can be blocked completely with atropine or after vagotomy [39]. Gallbladder emptying after a meal, however, occurs predominantly through release of endogenous cholecystokinin (hormonal control), while the nervous control plays a minor role.

It may take 10–20 min after a meal for serum CCK level to rise above a threshold to induce contraction and emptying of the gallbladder. The mean latent period (time from fatty meal ingestion to the beginning of gallbladder emptying) is 15.5 min. Postprandial serum CCK levels stay above the threshold for 2–3 h postmeal [40, 41] and the gallbladder emptying is maintained as long as the serum CCK levels remain above the threshold for contraction (Fig. 9.1.7).

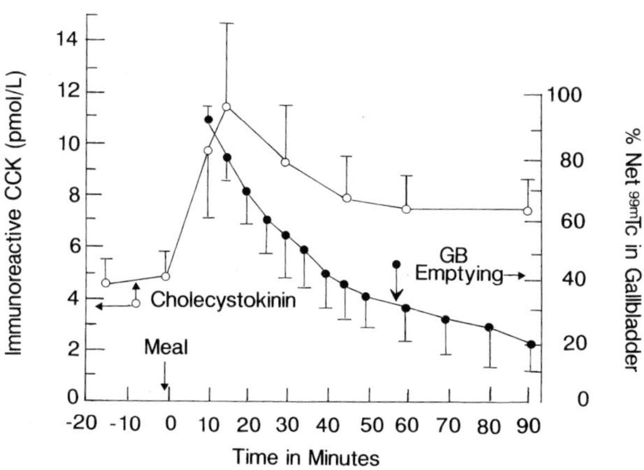

Fig. 9.1.7. Relationship between serum cholecystokinin (CCK) level and gallbladder emptying. Serum CCK level begins to rise soon after a meal, peaks by 10–30 min, and the level is maintained above the threshold for contraction for more than 90 min. Gallbladder maintains its emptying as long as post-prandial serum CCK level remains above the threshold for contraction (modified from [41])

Effect of Nutrients on Gallbladder Emptying

The degree of gallbladder emptying postmeal is dependent upon various factors, including the quality, quantity, total calorie intake, and the proportion of proteins, fats, and carbohydrates in the meal. A mean ejection fraction of 71% has been reported with a liquid meal consisting of 300 ml meritene, with 15 ml lipomul (36 g carbohydrates, 20 g fats, and 10 g proteins), and an ejection fraction of 64% with half and half milk [39, 42]. These results clearly show that one must strictly follow the investigator's protocol while adopting values reported in the literature, or must establish local values if a different type of meal is used.

Causes of Gallbladder Low Ejection Fraction

Many conditions associated with a gallbladder low ejection fraction are listed in Table 9.1.5. A decrease in emptying is attributed to various factors including wall fibrosis, a

Table 9.1.5. Causes of gallbladder low ejection fraction

1. Cystic duct syndrome (chronic acalculous cholecystitis)
2. Diabetes
3. Chronic calculous cholecystitis
4. Obesity
5. Common bile duct obstruction
6. Sphincter of Oddi spasm
7. Opiates
8. Somatostatin analogues (octreotide)
9. Anticholinergic drugs (atropine)
10. Congenital anomalies (septum, bilobed, etc.)

decrease in the total number of CCK receptors in the gallbladder wall, or inactivation of cholecystokinin by anti-cholecystokinin peptides in the serum [43]. The total number of CCK receptors in the gallbladder smooth muscle shows a direct correlation with the degree of emptying; the higher the receptor number, the greater is the ejection fraction, and vice versa [40]. Although a decrease in gallbladder emptying is a common feature of patients with cholelithiasis, a normal or even an exaggerated emptying has been reported in a few selected patients with cholelithiasis [44].

Delay in the appearance of the gallbladder and low ejection fraction in response to CCK stimulation both indicate a functional abnormality [45, 46]. The efficiency with which the wall absorbs water, sodium, and other electrolytes from the lumen is a reflection of the concentration function of the gallbladder and determines the time of appearance of the gallbladder in a ^{99m}Tc-HIDA study. It has been argued in the past whether the abnormal concentration and contraction functions of the gallbladder precede or follow the development of the gallstones. Most of the conditions with a decrease in gallbladder emptying are associated with a higher incidence of gallstones (Table 9.1.5). Patients with colectomy for ulcerative colitis, for example, show a lower gallbladder ejection fraction and a higher incidence of gallstones when compared with a control group [47]. Treatment with octreotide, a somatostatin analogue, which decreases gallbladder emptying, also increases the incidence of cholelithiasis and cholecystitis [48]. Octreotide decreases gallbladder emptying by interfering with the release of both acetylcholine (cholinergic stimulation) and cholecystokinin (hormonal stimulation), and also by directly blocking the effect of cholecystokinin on gallbladder wall [49]. The recent literature, therefore, appears to support the hypothesis that the functional abnormalities precede the development of gallstones by months or years.

Some of the investigators suggest using ultrasound for measurement of both the gallbladder volume and emptying, and claim that it can substitute cholescintigraphy for measurement of emptying [50]. Ultrasound emptying measurements are subject to error due to change of shape, shift of axis, and other technical artifacts introduced during contraction and emptying of the gallbladder. More recent studies have shown a poor correlation between geometric ultrasound and non-geometric cholescintygraphy in the measurement of gallbladder emptying casting doubts on the accuracy of ultrasound [51]. Combining the geometric ultrasound technique for measurement of the resting volume (after making the necessary volume correction) and non-geometric cholescintigraphy for measurement of gallbladder emptying overcomes many of the theoretical limitations of a geometric method. A combination offers the best features of both techniques for evaluation of gallbladder morphology and function [52].

References

1. Ingelfinger FJ. Digestive disease as a national problem. V. Gallstones. Gastroenterology 1968;55:102–104
2. Everhart JE, Khare M, Hill M, Maurer KR. Prevalence and ethnic differences in gallbladder disease in the United States. Gastroenterology 1999;117:632–639
3. Sampliner RE, Bennett PH, Comess LJ, Rose FA, Burch TA. Gallbladder disease in pima indians. Demonstration of high prevalence and early onset by cholecystography. N Engl J Med 1979;283:1358–1364
4. Miquel JF, Covarrubias M, Villaroel L, Mingrone G, Greco AV, Puglielli L, Carvallo P, Marshall G, Del Pino G, Nervi F. Genetic epidemiology of cholesterol cholelithiasis among Chilean Hispanics, Amerindians, and Maoris. Gastroenterology 1998;115:937–946
5. Moro PL, Checkley W, Gilman RH, Lescano G, Bonilla JJ, Silva B, Garcia HH. Gallstone disease in high-altitude Peruvian rural population. Am J Gastroenterol 1999;94:153–158
6. Prevalence of gallstone disease in an Italian adult female population. Rome Group for the Epidemiology and Prevention of Cholelithiasis (GREPO): Am J Epidemiol 1984;119:796–805
7. Godrey PJ, Bates J, Harrison M, King MB, Padley NR. Gallstones and mortality: a study of all gallstone related deaths in a single health district. Gut 1984;25:1029–1033
8. Layde PM, Vessey MP, Yeates D. Risk factors for gall-bladder disease: a cohort study of young women attending family planning clinics. J Epidemiol Community Health 1082;36:274–278
9. Lindstrom CG. Frequency of gallstone disease in a well-defined Swedish population. A prospective necropsy study in Malmo. Scand J Gastroenterol 1977;12:341–346
10. Way LW. Cholelithiasis and chronic cholecystitis. In: Way LW, Pelligrini CA, eds. Surgery of the gallbladder and bile ducts. WB Saunders, Philadelphia 1987, pp 231–250
11. Gracie WA, Ransohoff DF. The natural history of silent gallstones: the innocent gallstone is not a myth. N Engl J Med 1982;307:798–800
12. McSherry CK, Ferstenberg H, Calhoun WF, Lahman E, Virshup M. The natural history of diagnosed gallstone disease in symptomatic and asymptomatic patients. Ann Surg 1985;202:59–63
13. Thistle JL, Cleary PA, Lachin JM, Hersh T. The natural history of cholelithiasis: the National Cooperative Gallstone Study. Ann Intern Med 1984;101;171–175
14. Valdivieso V, Covarrubias C, Siegel F, Cruz F. Pregnancy and cholelithiasis: pathogenesis and natural course of gallstones diagnosed in early puerperium. Hepatology 1993;17:1–4
15. Donovan JM, Carey MC. Physical-chemical basis of gallstone formation. Gastroenterol Clin North Am 1991;20:47–66
16. Holzbach RJ, Busch N. Nucleation and growth of cholesterol crystals. Kinetic determinates in supersaturated native bile. Gastroenterol Clin North Am 1991;20:67–84
17. LaMont JT, Smith BF, Moore JRL. Role of gallbladder mucin in pathophysiology of gallstones. Hepatology 1984;4 (Suppl):51S–56S
18. Admirand WH, Small DM. The physicochemical basis of cholesterol gallstone formation in man. J Clin Invest 1968;47:1043–1052
19. Somjen GJ, Gilat T. Contribution of vesicular and micellar carriers to cholesterol transport in human bile. J Lipid Res 1985;26:699–704
20. Johnston DE, Kaplan MM. Pathogenesis and treatment of gallstones. N Engl J Med 1993;328:412–421
21. Trotman BW, Petrella EJ, Soloway RD, Sanchez HM, Morris TA 3d, Miller WT. Evaluation of radiographic lucency or opaqueness of gallstones as a means of identifying cholesterol or pigment stones. Correlation of lucency or opaqueness with calcium and mineral. Gastroenterology 1975;68:1563–1566
22. Gunn A, Kiddie N. Some clinical observations on patients with gallstones. Lancet 1972;2:239–241
23. Rigas B, Torosis J, McDougall CJ, Vener KT, Spiro HM. The circadian rhythm of biliary colic. J Clin Gastroenterol 1990;12:409–414
24. Sullivan FJ, Eaton SB Jr, Ferrucci JT Jr, Dreyfuss JR, Sloan RW. Cholangiographic manifestations of acute biliary colic. N Engl J Med 1973;288:33–35
25. Doran FS. The sites to which pain is referred from the common bile-duct in man and its implications for the theory of referred pain. Br J Surg 1967;54:599–606

26. Cooperberg PL, Burhenne HJ. Real time ultrasonography. Diagnostic technique of choice in calculous gallbladder disease. N Engl J Med 1980;302:1277–1279
27. Ko CW, Sekijima JH, Lee SP. Biliary sludge. Ann Intern Med 1999;130:301–311
28. Portincasa P, van Erpecum KJ, Jansen A, Renooij W, Gadellaa M, vanBerge-Henegouwen GP. Behavior of various cholesterol crystals in bile from patients with gallstones. Hepatology 1996;23:738–748
29. Berk RN, Ferrucci JT Jr, Fordtran JS, Cooperberg PL, Weissmann HS. The radiological diagnosis of gallbladder disease. An imaging symposium. Radiology 1981;141:49–56
30. Delchier JC, Benfredj P, Preaux AM, Mentreau JM, Dhumeaux D. The usefulness of microscopic bile examination in patients with suspected microlithiasis: a prospective evaluation. Hepatology 1986;6:118–122
31. deSilva GS. A simple method for computing the volume of the human gallbladder. Radiology 1949;52:94–102
32. Everson GT, Braverman DZ, Johnson MA, Kern F Jr. A critical evaluation of real time ultrasonography for the studies of gallbladder volume and contraction. Gastroenterology 1980;69:40–46
33. Krishnamurthy GT, Bobba VR, Kingston E. Radionuclide ejection fraction: a technique for quantitative analysis of motor function of the human gallbladder. Gastroenterology 1981;80:482–490
34. Fisher RS, Stelzer F, Rock E, Malmud LS. Abnormal gallbladder emptying in patients with gallstones. Dig Dis Sci 1982;27:1019–1024
35. Krishnamurthy GT, Bobba VR, Kingston E, Turner F. Measurement of gallbladder emptying sequentially using a single dose of 99mTc-labeled hepatobiliary agent. Gastroenterology 1982;83:773–776
36. Krishnamurthy GT, Bobba VR, Langrell K. The gallbladder emptying response to sequential exogenous and endogenous cholecystokinin. Nucl Med Commun 1984;5:27–33
37. Williams W, Krishnamurthy GT, Brar HS, Bobba VR. Scintigraphic variations of normal biliary physiology. J Nucl Med 1984;25:160–165
38. Hopman WPM, Jansen JBMJ, Rosenbusch G, Lamers CBHW. Cephalic stimulation of gallbladder contraction in humans: role of cholecystokinin and the cholinergic system. Digestion 1987;38:197–203
39. Fisher RS, Rock E, Malmud LS. Cholineric effects on gallbladder emptying in humans. Gastroenterology 1985; 89:716–722
40. Upp JR Jr, Nealon WH, Singh P, Fagan CJ, Jonas AS, Greeley GH Jr, Thompson JC. Correlation of cholecystokinin receptors with gallbladder contractility in patients with gallstones. Ann Surg 1987;205:641–648
41. Vezina WC, McAlister VC, Wall WJ, Engel CJ, Grant DR, Ghent CN, Hutton LC, King ME, Chey WY. Normal fasting volume and postprandial emptying of the denervated gallbladder in liver transplant recipients. Gastroenterology 1994;107:847–853
42. Bobba VR, Krishnamurthy GT, Kingston E, Turner FE, Brown PH, Langrell K. Gallbladder dynamics induced by fatty meal in normal subjects and patients with gallstones: concise communication. J Nucl Med 1984;25:21–24
43. Sarles H, Hags G, Lanier R, Demol P, Bataille D. Present status of the anticholecystokinin hormone. Digestion 1979;19:73–76
44. Northfield TC, Kupfer RM, Maudgal DP, Zenter-Munro PL, Meller ST, Garvie NW, McCready R. Gallbladder sensitivity to cholecystokinin in patients with gallstones. Br Med J 1980;280:143–144
45. Krishnamurthy S, Krishnamurthy GT. Evolution of nuclear hepatology as a clinical subspeciality. J Nucl Med Technol 1995;23:35S–45S
46. Nahrwold DL, Rose RC, Ward SP. Abnormalities in gallbladder morphology and function in patients with cholelithiasis. Ann Surg 1976;184:415–421
47. Damiao AO, Sipahi AM, Vezozzo DP, Goncalves PL, Habr-Gama A, Teixeira MG, Fukushima JT, Laudanna AA. Effects of colectomy on gallbladder motility in patients with ulcerative colitis. Dig Dis Sci 1997;42:259–264
48. Trendle MC, Moertel CG, Kvols LK. Incidence and mortality of cholethiasis in patients receiving chronic octreotide for metastatic carcinoid and malignant islet cell tumors. Cancer 1997;79:830–834
49. Fisher RS, Rock E, Levin G, Malmud L. Effects of somatostatin on gallbladder emptying. Gastroenterology 1987;92:885–890
50. Pallotta N, Corazziari E, Scopinaro F, Bonino R, Schillaci O, Vignoni A, Mangano M, Torsoli AT. Noninvasive estimate of bile flux through the gallbladder in humans. Am J Gastroenterol 1998;93:1877–1885
51. Siegel A, Kuhn C, Crow H, Holtzman S. Gallbladder ejection fraction. Correlation of scintigrahic and ultrasonographic techniques. Clin Nucl Med 2000;25:1–6
52. Krishnamurthy GT, Krishnamurthy S. Hazards of formulating new theories about gallbladder (GB) function based on ultrasound volume data. Am J Gastroenterol 1999;94:1703–1705

9.2 Cystic Duct Syndrome (Chronic Acalculous Cholecystitis)

Cystic duct syndrome, also known as chronic acalculous cholecystitis, is one of two diseases which come under the broad title of "biliary dyskinesia," the other being the spasm of the sphincter of Oddi (Chap. 10). Biliary dyskinesia is a purely functional abnormality without an easily identifiable morphologic abnormality. The term "cystic duct syndrome" merely indicates the major site of functional abnormality. The syndrome was first described by Cozzolino et al. in 1961, but did not receive much clinical recognition until a reliable and easily reproducible diagnostic procedure became available for measurement of gallbladder emptying [1].

Clinical Presentation

Patients with cystic duct syndrome usually present with symptoms very similar to those with chronic calculous cholecystitis (Fig 9.1.2). Intermittent mild to moderate intensity right upper quadrant or epigastric pain is the most common presenting symptom. Pain begins 30–60 min after a meal and is often associated with nausea. Postprandial pain after dinner reaches its peak intensity at midnight. Women in their 30s and 40s are affected 3–4 times more frequently than men of similar age. The physical examination, liver function tests, blood counts, and serum amylase and lipase levels are normal. No gallstones are found within the gallbladder.

Histopathologic Features

Histopathologic abnormalities are confined mostly to the cystic duct. There is kinking and narrowing of the cystic duct lumen due to thickening and fibrosis of the wall [2]. Adhesion and angulation of the infundibulum are common. The connection of the cystic duct with the common hepatic duct normally shows wide variations (Fig. 9.2.1). About 50% of cystic ducts join with the common hepatic duct along its right margin at a 45° angle, 18% pass behind the common hepatic duct before joining it along its left margin, and the remaining 32% show a spiral form before joining the common hepatic duct either in front or behind [3]. Microscopic examination of the cystic duct shows infiltration with chronic inflammatory cells, concentric thickening and fibrosis of the media and adventitia with narrowing of the duct lumen (Fig. 9.2.2).

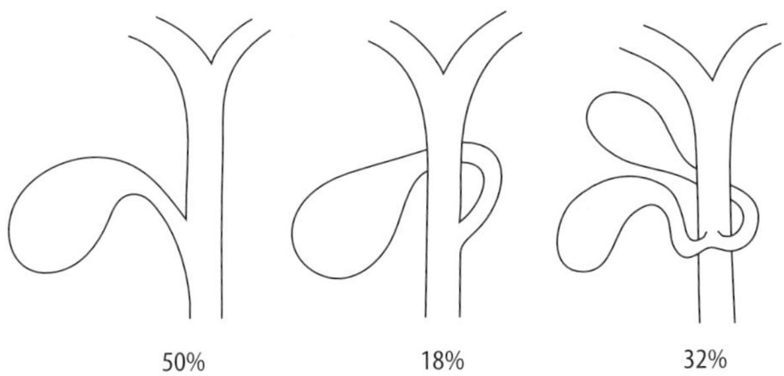

Fig. 9.2.1. Variations in the union of the cystic duct with the common hepatic duct. The cystic duct usually joins the common hepatic duct at a 45° angle along its right margin (50%). It may pass behind the common hepatic duct before joining it on the left side (18%). A spiral cystic duct joins in front in 32% of patients [3]

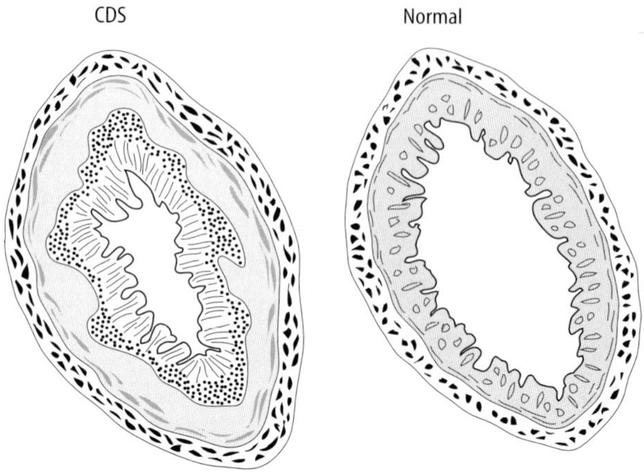

Fig. 9.2.2. Cystic duct histopathology in patients with cystic duct syndrome (*CDS*) and normal subjects. Normal cystic duct wall shows thin mucosal, muscular and adventitial layer. All three layers show inflammation and concentric thickening with narrowing of the lumen in CDS

Functional Abnormality

The major abnormality pertains to concentration and contraction functions of the gallbladder. Bile aspirated from the duodenum in patients with cystic duct syndrome shows a lower concentration of bile salts and phospholipids than in patients without the syndrome [4]. Hepatic bile enters the gallbladder slowly through the narrowed cystic duct. In a ^{99m}Tc-HIDA study, the gallbladder may appear within 40 min (Fig. 9.2.3), but a delayed appearance (after 40 min) is more common (Fig. 9.2.4). Some of the gallbladders may take as long as 2–3 h for their appearance. A late appearance is attributed to delayed and decreased entry of hepatic bile into the gallbladder primarily due to slow absorption of sodium and water through the wall. Gallbladder low ejection

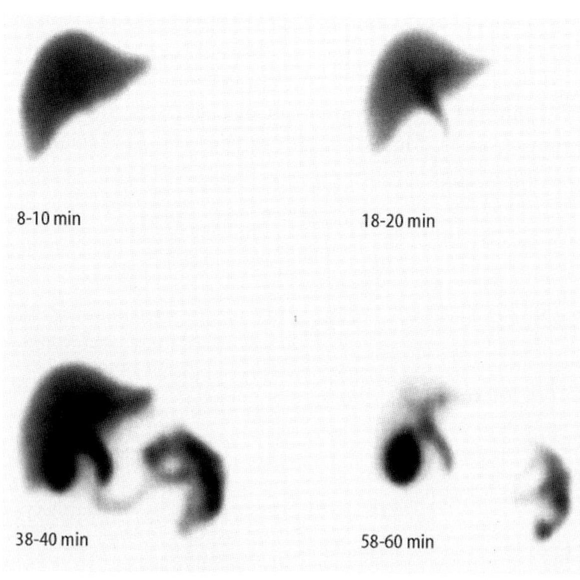

Fig. 9.2.3. Normal bile formation and flow. Bile flow into the gallbladder may remain normal in some of the patients with cystic duct syndrome. The gallbladder, intrahepatic ducts, extrahepatic ducts, and small intestine are seen within 40 min. Radioactivity clears almost completely from the liver and enters the gallbladder and small intestine by 60 min.

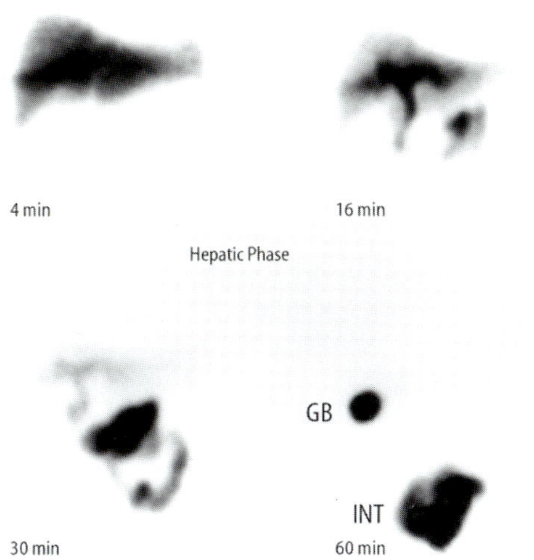

Fig. 9.2.4. A gallbladder (GB) which does not appear by 30 min fills in by 60 min with fewer counts than normal. Intrahepatic and extrahepatic ducts are normal

fraction in response to intravenous cholecystokinin or after fatty meal ingestion is the characteristic feature. Low ejection fraction is attributed to a combination of several factors of which the wall fibrosis, a decrease in the total number of CCK receptors in the gallbladder wall, and/or a decrease in cystic duct threshold for CCK are considered very important (Fig. 9.2.5). The decrease in threshold with paradoxical contraction is attributed to an activation of CCK receptors which induce contraction of the cystic duct [5, 6]. Cystic duct contraction before the contraction of the fundus and body, results in non-emptying of the gallbladder [7]. Unable to empty bile against a contracted cystic duct, the gallbladder contracts and assumes many different shapes,

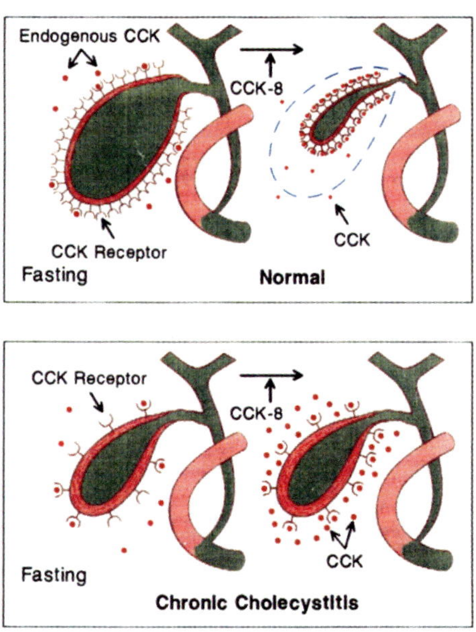

Fig. 9.2.5. Gallbladder cholecystokinin (*CCK*) receptors in health and disease. A normal gallbladder rich with CCK receptors produces almost complete emptying, while the gallbladder with chronic cholecystitis elicits poor emptying due to sparseness of CCK receptors [11]

globular being the most common form. Usually there is no bile reflux into the common hepatic duct or to the right and left hepatic ducts [8].

During fasting, the serum endogenous cholecystokinin reaches its lowest level, which promotes a maximum increase in the tone of the sphincter of Oddi and a maximum relaxation of the gallbladder wall. An increase in sphincter tone raises the sphincter of Oddi mean basal pressure to 15 cmH_2O. The common bile duct and the gallbladder pressure are maintained at 12 cmH_2O and 10 cmH_2O, respectively. The pressure differences at these three levels promote preferential entry of the hepatic bile into the gallbladder, as the bile seeks the path of least resistance. During cholescintigraphy, ^{99m}Tc-HIDA simply follows the path taken by the hepatic bile [8].

After 4–6 h of fasting, a normal gallbladder is filled completely to its maximum capacity of 50 ml, but the liver continues to secrete bile at the rate of 0.4/min, of which about 70% (0.3 ml/min) enters the gallbladder. A completely filled gallbladder is still able to accommodate an additional 0.3 ml hepatic bile per minute simply by absorbing an equal volume of water through the wall. Absorption of water takes place along the lateral intercellular channels situated between the columnar cells of the mucosa (see Fig. 2.1.4, Chap. 2). These lateral intercellular spaces are wide open during fasting when the gallbladder is completely relaxed, and they close tightly when the gallbladder contracts after a meal. These two factors, an increase in sphincter tone and absorption of water through the wall, are the primary mechanisms by which the gallbladder sequesters most bile salts during fasting. The process by which the gallbladder concentrates bile salts during fasting by selective absorption of water and electrolytes through the wall is called the concentration function of the gallbladder [9].

Measurement of Gallbladder Ejection Fraction

Imaging Procedure. Patient preparation and data acquisition and analysis are monitored carefully. The patient fasts for a minimum of 4 h, preferably for 8–10 h. A detailed drug history is taken to ensure that the patient is not currently taking any medications that act either on the gallbladder or on the sphincter of Oddi. Opioids, calcium channel blockers, nitrates, sympathetic and parasympathetic agonists or antagonists, and other drugs that are known to act on the gallbladder or the sphincter of Oddi are withdrawn for a day or two before scheduling the patient for measurement of the gallbladder ejection fraction.

The data are collected with the large field of view gamma camera interfaced to an online computer in two separate phases: the hepatic phase between 0 and 60 min, and the gallbladder phase between 61 and 90 min. The hepatic phase data are collected on a 64×64 matrix at one frame per minute for 60 min, following intravenous injection of 2–3 mCi (74–111 MBq) ^{99m}Tc-HIDA. After ascertaining the adequacy of counts within the gallbladder (Table 9.1.4), the gallbladder phase data are acquired. When the gallbladder appears late and does not contain adequate counts at the end of 60 min, a second dose of ^{99m}Tc-HIDA is given at 60 min, and the gallbladder phase data collection is delayed for an additional 30–60 min. This delay ensures adequate counts within the gallbladder for measurement of the ejection fraction. Images are carefully scrutinized in cine display to check for superimposition of structures over one another, especially the superimposition of the gallbladder and duodenal radioactivity.

In the supine position, the gallbladder fundus lies anteriorly and the neck posteriorly. Small gallstones often gravitate to the dependent posterior part and settle at the neck, blocking bile entry into the gallbladder. Changing the patient position to the right lateral decubitus position or asking the patient to walk for a few minutes usually dislodges the stones from the neck and allows bile entry into the gallbladder. A septum at the neck may allow filling of the proximal segment first and delay entry of radiolabeled bile into the distal segment (Fig. 9.2.6).

Gallbladder Phase Data Acquisition and Analysis. This data collection usually occurs between 61 and 90 min after ^{99m}Tc-HIDA injection, unless there is a delay in filling of the gallbladder [10, 11]. If there is superimposition of structures during the hepatic phase data collection, the gamma camera angle is changed to the position that maximally separates the gallbladder from the common bile duct and the duodenum. When the gallbladder and duodenum are superimposed, drinking a glass of water moves the duodenal radioactivity away from the gallbladder region of interest [12]. The data are collected at one frame per minute for 30 min. Beginning at 5 min, 10 ng/kg CCK-8 is infused over 3 min (3.3 ng/kg/min for 3 min) through an infusion pump [8, 11, 13].

Before the test begins, the patient is instructed to raise a hand when pain is experienced and raise the hand again when pain is relieved. The time of onset and relief of pain are noted on the gallbladder time/activity curve to critically establish the temporal relationship between pain and the phase of gallbladder emptying. Biliary pain typically occurs during the gallbladder ejection period. Pain experienced after the ejection period is considered non-biliary in origin. Saline may be infused as

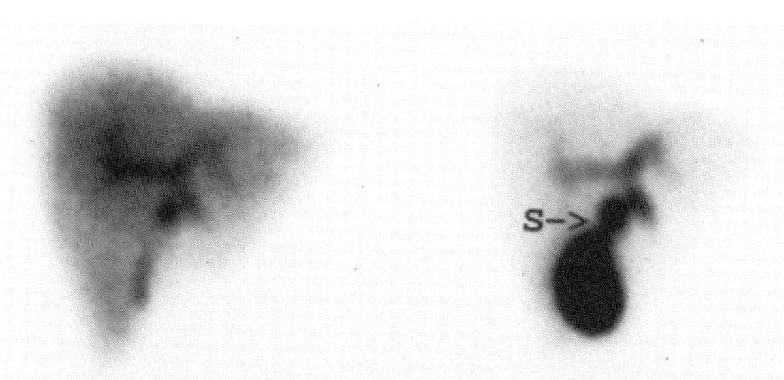

A

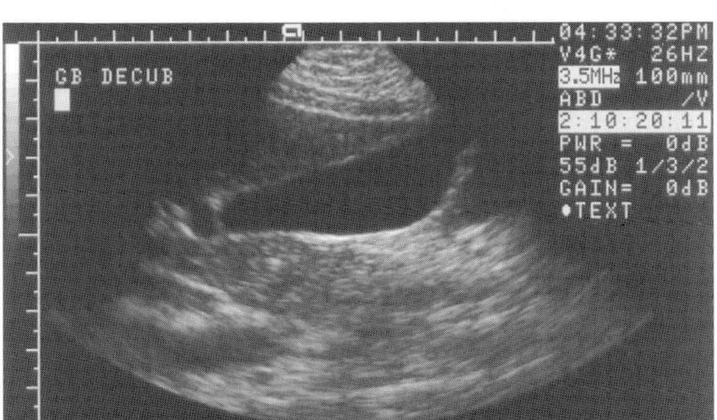

B

Fig. 9.2.6. Septa at t4he neck (*S*): bile enters the small proximal segment at the neck first (*left*) followed by delayed filling of the body and fundus (*right*) forming the distal segment (**A**). Ultrasound shows a septa at the neck (**B**).

placebo prior to CCK-8 infusion. Gallbladder ejection fraction depends upon various factors including the dose, dose rate, and duration of infusion of CCK-8. These variables are controlled strictly to obtain a consistent result. The gallbladder ejection fraction is calculated using the counts before and after emptying [13, 14]. The normal gallbladder ejection fraction is 35% and higher when 10 ng/kg CCK-8 is infused over 3 min. Large bolus doses of CCK-8 produce a non-physiological response and should be avoided.

Contraction and emptying of the gallbladder is initiated when CCK-8 binds to its receptors located in the smooth muscle which distributed is irregularly in the wall (Fig. 9.2.5). The smooth muscle is much thicker in the fundus and neck than in the body and cystic duct. Cholecystokinin receptors located in the smooth muscle of the body, fundus, and cystic duct show varied thresholds for contraction. In the dog, for example, the smooth muscle in the cystic duct shows a much higher threshold (less sensitive) than the smooth muscle in the fundus [5]. The cystic duct, therefore, does not contract when the fundus and body contract in response to a physiologic dose of CCK-8. A dose within a physiologic range causes smooth and coordinated contraction and emptying of the gallbladder.

CCK-8 Dose. A low ejection fraction is often obtained in normal subjects when a large, non-physiologic dose of CCK-8 is given as a rapid bolus. The CCK-8 dose (0.02 μg/kg, given in 30–60 s) recommended in the package insert (Kinevac, Bracco Lab., Princeton, NJ) is for an oral cholecystogram or for stimulation of pancreatic enzyme secretion. This dose is found to be too large for cholescintigraphy and often causes a low ejection fraction in normal subjects and should be avoided [7, 15, 16]. An optimal dose rate for cholescintigraphy is 0.01 μg/kg infused over 3 min (or 3.3 ng/kg/min for 3 min). This dose is much lower (about one-half) than the dose recommended in the package insert. Local normal values should be established when a different CCK-8 dose, dose rate, or duration of infusion are chosen.

Congenital Abnormalities of the Gallbladder. Congenital folds or septa often cause abnormalities in filling and emptying of the gallbladder [17]. An intrahepatic gallbladder may cause a filling defect in the liver in the early images (within 10 min), which fills later with radiolabeled bile, and may not empty normally in response to CCK due to adhesion of its wall to the liver parenchyma. Often a gallbladder is divided into two segments of equal size (Valentine gallbladder) by a fold, and each segment may fill differently and empty at different rates in response to CCK-8 (Fig. 9.2.7). An epithelial fold near the neck creates a pouch-like compartment (Hartmann's pouch) where gallstones may lodge and delay or prevent bile entry into the distal compartment (Fig. 9.2.8). A septum in the middle of the gallbladder may allow normal filling of the proximal segment only during the 1st h, and delay the filling of the distal segment for 2–3 h. In such instances, only the proximal segment may empty bile while the distal segment is prevented from emptying by the septa, which acts as a one-way valve (Fig. 9.2.9). Shorter frame rate imaging enables easy recognition of such morphologic variations. Failure to recognize such abnormalities may provide false information. The distal segment which fills late may not empty bile at all while the proximal segment shows a normal ejection fraction. A non-emptying distal segment may promote formation of gallstones but not the proximal segment with normal emptying [18]. When the shape of the gallbladder in the anterior view mimics the duodenal loop, a right lateral view helps to separate them (Fig. 9.2.10). The gallbladder projects at the middle of the anterior liver border while the duodenum and common bile duct remains posterior in location. Cholescintigra-

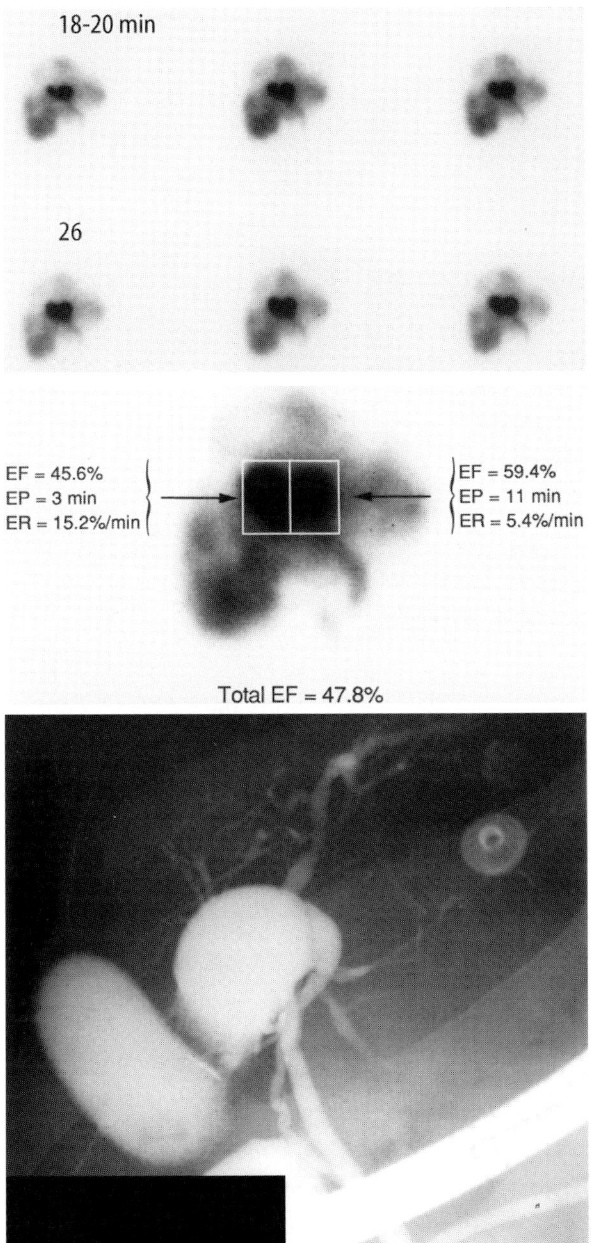

Fig. 9.2.7. Valentine gallbladder. A bilobed gallbladder high in position fills with bile (**A**). Each segment empties at a different rate in response to CCK-8 infusion, with a total ejection fraction of 47.8% (**B**). A cholangiogram (**C**) shows the septa in between two segments [17]

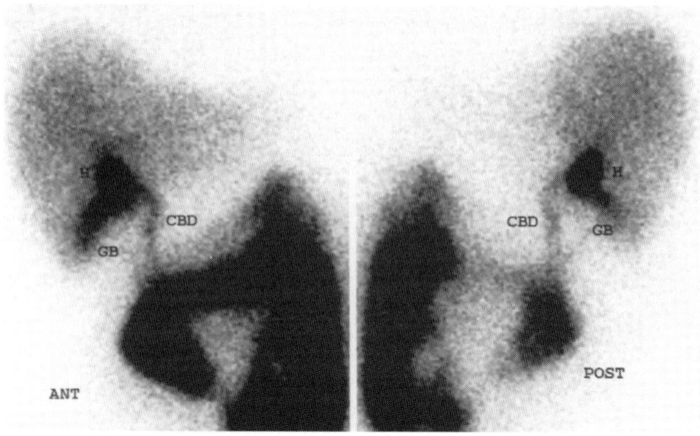

A

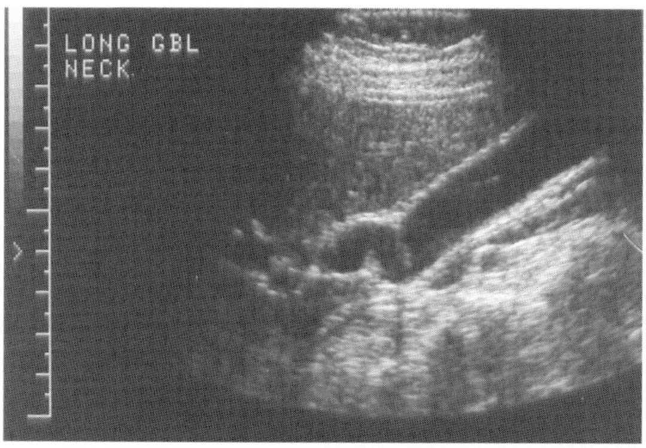

B

Fig. 9.2.8. Hartmann's pouch. Anterior (*Ant*) and posterior (*Post*) view cholescintigram **(A)** show a pouch (*H*) at the neck (Hartmann's pouch) of the gallbladder (*GB*). An ultrasound of the gallbladder **(B)** confirms the pouch at the neck.

phy usually does not show gallstones as a filling defect within the gallbladder due to rapid mixing of ^{99m}Tc-HIDA with gallbladder bile. A large gallstone, however, may occasionally become visible within the gallbladder when most of the bile empties in response to CCK-8 (Fig. 9.2.11).

Irritable Bowel. At the end of the hepatic phase imaging (60 min), most of the bile entering the duodenum moves and collects at the ligament of Treitz, jejunum, and proximal ileum. In a patient with an irritable bowel syndrome, the bile moves much more rapidly through the small and large bowel, resulting in the visualization of the distal ileum and proximal colon. Administration of CCK-8 during the gallbladder phase in such patients increases the intestinal peristalsis and moves the bile much further away, resulting in the delineation of the entire transverse and descending colon. This observation is essential in separating the biliary from bowel pain (Fig. 9.2.12).

Therapeutic Response to Cholecystectomy

Laparoscopic or open cholecystectomy is the most appropriate therapy for cystic duct syndrome (Table 9.2.1). Of a total of 320 patients with cystic duct syndrome who underwent cholecystectomy solely on the basis of a low ejection fraction, 287 patients

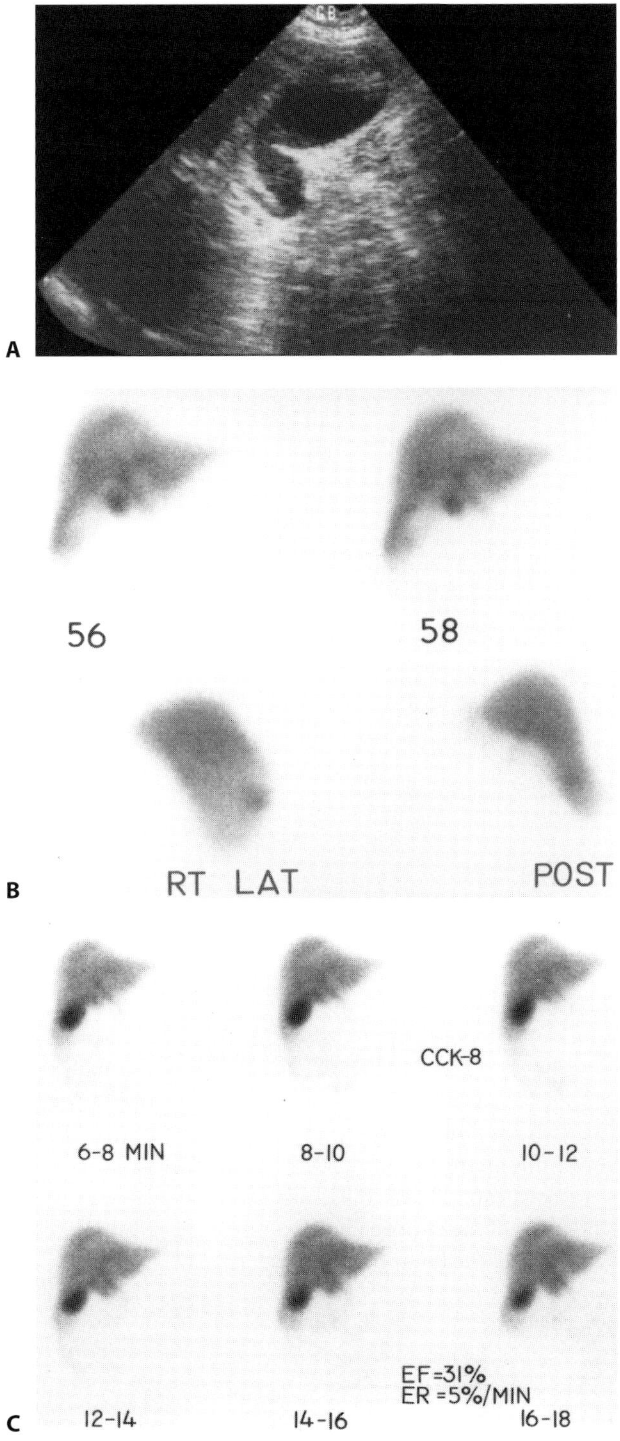

Fig. 9.2.9. Septa in the body of the gallbladder. An ultrasound study shows a prominent septum in the body (**A**). The proximal segment fills in by 58 min (**B**) whereas the distal segment takes 3 h to fill in the cholescintigram Ï(**C**). Mostly the proximal segment empties with CCK-8 with a total ejection fraction of 31%

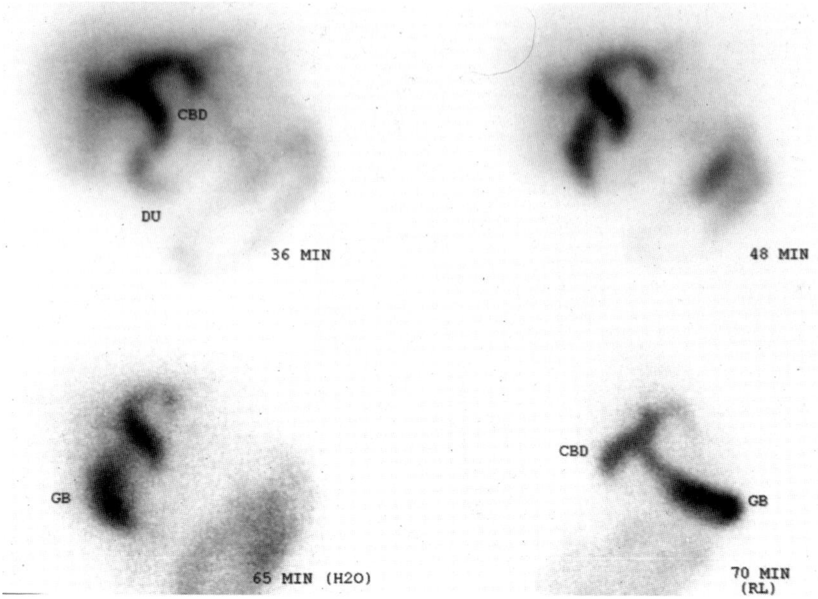

Fig. 9.2.10. A curved gallbladder (*GB*) may mimic first part of the duodenum (*DU*). A right lateral view (*RL*) helps to visualize the long axis of the gallbladder and its relationship with the common bile duct (*CBD*) and duodenum of which are posterior in location.

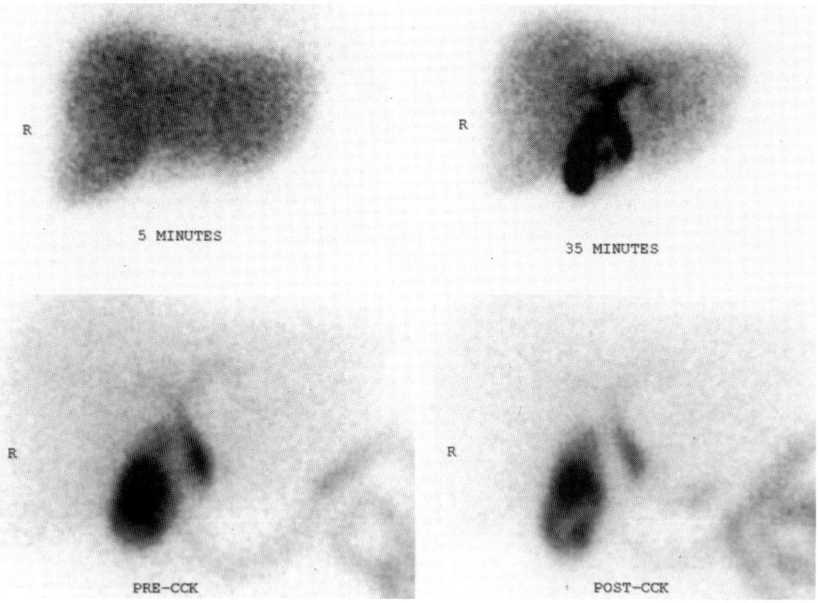

Fig. 9.2.11. Gallstone within the gallbladder. Radiolabeled hepatic bile enters the gallbladder (35 min), surrounds the gallstone, and obscures it (pre-CCK). The stone becomes obvious as a filling defect only after CCK-8 induced gallbladder emptying

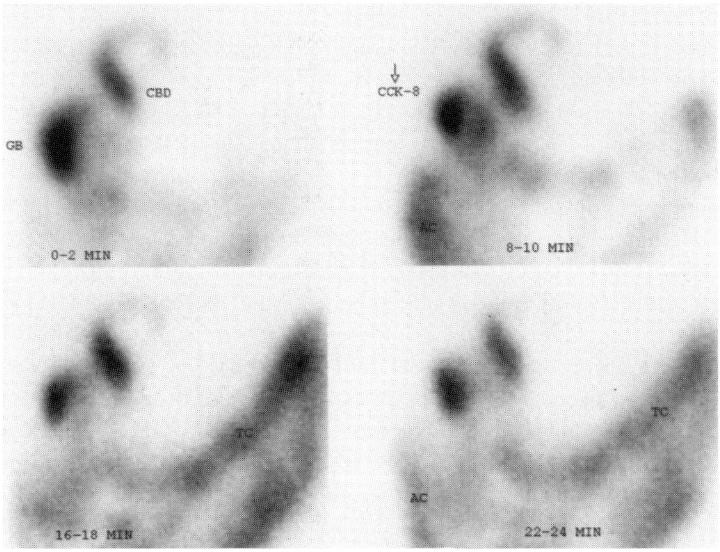

Fig. 9.2.12. Irritable bowel. Bile transit is hastened by CCK-8 infusion. The bile emptied from the gallbladder mixes with rest of the intestinal bile and moves rapidly through the ascending (*AC*), transverse (*TC*), and descending colon.

(90%) had relief of pain [19–25]. Histopathological examination showed evidence of gallbladder or cystic duct disease in 285 patients (89%). A high therapeutic success rate, however, is not universal. One report showed pain relief in only 69% of patients with the cystic duct syndrome [26]. Recent studies have identified *Helicobacter* DNA in both bile and the gallbladder wall of patients with chronic cholecystitis, raising the possibility of an infection as a forerunner of chronic cholecystitis and that antibiotics may have a role in the treatment [27, 28]. These therapeutic options may add new dimensions to the role of quantitative functional imaging in the diagnosis and management of patients with various types of gallbladder disease [29].

Table 9.2.1. Cholescintigraphic, histopathologic, and postcholecystectomy results in patients with cystic duct syndrome (chronic acalculous cholecystitis)

Authors [ref.]	No. patients with pain and low EF (cholecystectomy)	No. patients with abnormal histopathology of gallbladder	No. patients with postcholecystectomy relief of pain
Pickelman et al. [19]	19	11	18
Fink-Bennet et al. [20]	124	115	105
Zack et al. [21]	59	54	56
Misra et al. [22]	67	60	58
Halverson et al. [23]	12	10	10
Sorenson et al. [24]	11	11	11
Kleiger et al. [25]	28	26	27
Total	320	287 (90%)	285 (89%)

Standardization of Technique

In the literature, many different values have been reported for post CCK-8 gallbladder ejection fraction. This wide variation is primarily due to differences in methodology. Variations in the dose, dose rate, and duration of infusion of CCK-8 influence the gallbladder ejection fraction. Unlike the left ventricular ejection fraction, which is controlled solely by the ventricle, the gallbladder ejection fraction can be controlled to any desired level simply by controlling the dose, dose rate, and duration of infusion of CCK-8. The widely reported normal gallbladder ejection fraction value of 35% or higher was obtained with 10 ng/kg CCK-8, infused over 3 min (3.3 ng/kg/min).

The gallbladder contracts and empties bile as long as the serum CCK-8 level is maintained above the threshold level. After cessation of CCK-8 infusion, the gallbladder emptying continues for an additional 8–12 min and then stops. The emptying resumes upon CCK-8 reinfusion. One can obtain as many as two to four sequential gallbladder ejection fractions following a single dose of ^{99m}Tc-HIDA [14]. The CCK-8 receptors in the cystic duct usually do not respond when the hormonal dose is within the physiologic limit. Large, non-physiologic doses, however, induce cystic duct contraction with subsequent non-emptying of a normal gallbladder [16]. The physiologic dose rate ranges from 1 to 4 ng/kg/min. A steady state serum CCK level can be achieved for 1–2 h by continuously infusing doses as low as 0.3 ng/kg/min. A basal serum CCK level of less than 1 pmol/l, raises to above 4 pmol/l by 10 min, reaches a peak level of 6.5 pmol/l by 30 min, and a steady state level between 5 and 6 pmol/l, which can be maintained for as long as 70 min by constant infusion [15]. Infusion of a smaller dose over a longer period of time simulates postprandial CCK release, and is much more effective than an infusion of a larger dose as a bolus [7, 16, 30].

References

1. Cozzolino HJ, Goldstein F, Greening RR, Wirts CW. The cystic duct syndrome. JAMA 1963;185:920–924
2. Goldstein F, Grunt R, Margulies M. Cholecystokinin cholecystography in the differential diagnosis of acalculous gallbladder disease. Am J Dig Dis 1974;19:835–849
3. Shaw MJ, Dorsher PJ, Vennes JA. Cystic duct anatomy : an endoscopic perspective. Am J Gastroenterology. 1993;88:2102–2106
4. Venkataramani A, Strong RM, Anderson DS, Gilmore IT, Stokes K, Hoffman AF. Abnormal duodenal bile composition in patients with acalculous chronic cholecystitis. Am J Gastroenterol 1998;93:434–441
5. Upp JR Jr, Nealon WH, Singh P, Fagan CJ, Jonas AS, Greeley GH Jr, Thompson JC. Correlation of cholecystokinin receptors with gallbladder contractility in patients with gallstones. Ann Surg 1987;205:641–648
6. Courtney DF, Clanachan AS, Scott GW. Cholecystokinin constricts the canine cystic duct. Gastroenterology 1983;85:1154–1159
7. Krishnamurthy GT, Bobba VR, Kingston E. Optimization of octapeptide of cholecystokinin (OP-CCK) dose for gallbladder emptying. In: Raynaud C. ed, Preceding of the third world congress of nuclear medicine and biology. Paris, Pergamon Press 1982 pp 2244–2247
8. Krishnamurthy S, Krishnamurthy GT. Biliary dyskinesia: role of the sphincter of Oddi, gallbladder, and cholecystokinin. J Nucl Med 1997;38:1824–1830
9. Wheeler HO. Concentrating function of the gallbladder. Am J Med 1971;51:588–595
10. Balon HR, Fink-Bennett DM, Brill DR, Fig LM, Freitas JE, Krishnamurthy GT, Klingensmith WC 3rd, Royal HD. Procedure guideline for hepatobiliary scintigraphy. J Nucl Med 1997;38:1654–1657
11. Krishnamurthy S, Krishnamurthy GT. Evolution of nuclear hepatology as a clinical subspeciality. J Nucl Med Technology 1995;24:35S-45 S (supplement)

12. Keller IA, Weissman HS, Kaplun LL, freeman LM. The use of water ingestion to distinguish the gallbladder and duodenum on cholescintigraphy. Radiology 1984;152:811–813
13. Krishnamurthy GT, Bobba VR, Kingston E. Radionuclide ejection fraction: a technique for quantitative analysis of motor function of the human gallbladder. Gastroenterology 1981;80:482–490
14. Krishnamurthy GT, Bobba VR, Kingston E, Turner F. Measurement of gallbladder emptying sequentially using a single dose of Tc-99m-labeled hepatobiliary agent. Gastroenterology 1982;83:773–776
15. Toftdahl DB, Hojgaard L, Winkler K. Dynamic cholescintigraphy: induction and description of gallbladder emptying. J Nucl Med 1996;37:261–266
16. Krishnamurthy S, Krishnamurthy GT. Gallbladder ejection fraction: a decade of progress and future promise (editorial). J Nucl Med 1992;33:542–543
17. Gad MA, Krishnamurthy GT, Glowniak JV. Identification and differentiation of congenital gallbladder abnormality by quantitative Tc-99 m HIDA cholescintigraphy. J Nucl Med 1992;33:431–434
18. Kramer EL, Rumancik WM, Harkavy L, Tiu S, Banner HJ, Sanger JJ. Hepatobiliary scintigraphy of the compartmentalized gallbladder. Am J Roentgenol (AJR) 1985;145:1205–1206
19. Pickelman J, Peiss RL, Henkin R, Salo B, Nagel P. The role of sincalide cholescintigraphy in the evaluation of patients with acalculous gallbladder disease. Arch Surg 1985;120:693–697
20. Fink-Bennett D, DeRidder P, Kolozsi WZ, Gordon R, Jaros R. Cholecystokinin cholescintigraphy: detection of abnormal gallbladder motor function in patients with chronic acalculous gallbladder disease. J Nucl Med 1991;32:1695–1699
21. Zech ER, Simmons LB, Kendrick RR, Soballe PW, Olcese JA, Goff WB 2d, Lawrence DPl, DeWeese RA. Cholecystokinin enhanced hepatobiliary scanning with ejection fraction calculation as an indicator of disease of the gallbladder. Surg Gynecol Obstet 1991;172:21–24
22. Misra DC Jr, Blossom GB, Fink-Bennett D, Glover JL. Results of surgical therapy for biliary dyskinesia. Arch Surg 1991;126:957–960
23. Halverson JD, Garner BA, Siegel BA, Alexander R, Edmundowicz SA, Campbell W, Miller JE. The use of hepatobiliary scintigraphy in patients with acalculous biliary disease. Arch Intern Med 1992;152:1305–1307
24. Sorenson MK, Francher S, Lang NP, Eidt JF, Broadwater JR. Abnormal gallbladder nuclear ejection fraction predicts success of cholecystectomy in patients with biliary dyskinesia. Am J Surg 1993;166:672–675
25. Klieger PS, O'Mara RE. The clinical utility of quantitative cholescintigraphy: the significance of gallbladder dysfunction. Clin Nucl Med 1998;23:278–282
26. Westlake PJ, Hershfield NB, Kelly JK, Kloiber R, Liu R, Sutherland LR, Shaffer EA. Chronic right upper quadrant pain without gallstones: does HIDA scan predict outcome after cholecystectomy ? Am J Gastroenterol 1990;85:986–990
27. Fox JG, Dewhirst FE, Shen Z, Feng Y, Taylor NS, Paster BJ, Ericson RL, Lau CN, Correa P, Araya JC, Roa I. Hepatic Helicobacter species identified in bile and gallbladder tissue from Chileans with chronic cholecystitis. Gastroenterology 1998;114:755–763
28. Blaser MJ. Helicobacters and biliary tract disease. Gastroenterology 1998;114:840–841
29. Krishnamurthy S, Krishnamurthy GT. Functional imaging in nuclear hepatology. Indian J Nucl Med 1997;12:216–232
30. Ziessmann HA. Cholecystokinin Cholescintigraphy: Victim of its own success? J Nucl Med 1999;40:2038–2042

9.3 Acute Cholecystitis

Acute cholecystitis is one of the common abdominal emergencies that requires immediate diagnosis and therapy. It usually presents with right upper quadrant pain, fever, and leukocytosis. Since gallstones are found in nearly 10% of all Americans, a mere association between gallstone and abdominal pain with fever cannot be equated with a diagnosis of acute cholecystitis [1, 2]. The great majority of gallstones remain silent and only about 15–20% ever become symptomatic [3]. About 85–90% of cases of acute cholecystitis associated with gallstones are called acute calculous cholecystitis and the remaining 10–15% without gallstones are called acute acalculous cholecystitis [4].

Clinical Presentation

Acute cholecystitis clinically presents as right upper quadrant or epigastric pain and fever, mimicking other abdominal and lower thoracic acute emergencies (Table 9.3.1). Pain may radiate to the right shoulder, mediastinum, or lower anterior chest, mimicking an acute myocardial infarction [5]. The pain radiation to the right lower quadrant may mimic an acute appendicitis, or that radiating to the left lower quadrant may mimic an acute diverticulitis. Pain is due to distension of the inflamed gallbladder wall. On deep inspiration when the liver moves downwards, the fundus of the gallbladder extends below the right costal margin and is felt as a soft mass during deep palpation. When the palpating finger touches the inflamed gallbladder wall, the patient experiences pain and abruptly stops breathing. This is called "Murphy's" sign.

Acute cholecystitis is 3–4 times more common in women than men, and the incidence increases with age. The clinical presentation of a calculous or an acalculous acute cholecystitis is very similar. A combination of fever with chills, right upper quadrant abdominal tenderness, and clinical jaundice is called the "Charcot triad." The triad is found more frequently when acute cholecystitis occurs in association with obstruction of the common bile duct. The place of maximum tenderness over the gallbladder fundus corresponds to the point where a line drawn between the left superior iliac spine and umbilicus meets the right costal margin, when the line is extended upwards (Fig. 9.3.1). This point also corresponds to the intersection of the

Table 9.3.1. Differential diagnosis of acute cholecystitis

1. Acute pancreatitis
2. Acute hepatitis
3. Gastritis
4. Acute appendicitis
5. Acute cholangitis
6. Acute nephritis
7. Angina or acute myocardial infarction
8. Pleurisy
9. Right lower lobe pneumonia
10. Acute diverticuliti

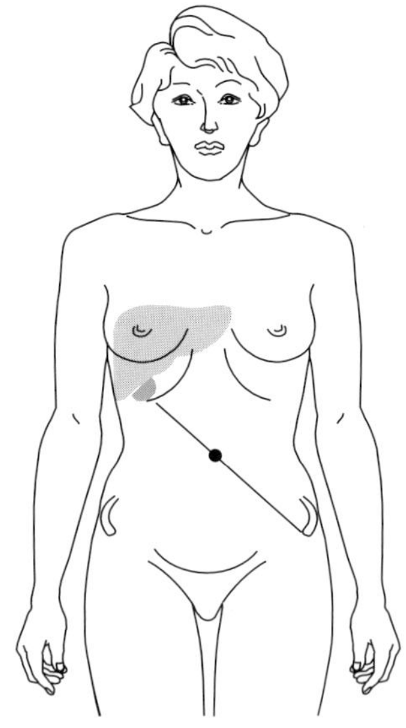

Fig. 9.3.1. Clinical location of the gallbladder fundus and Murphy's sign. A straight line drawn between the left anterior superior iliac spine and the umbilicus points to the fundus of the gallbladder when extended upwards to meet the right costal margin. This is also the point of Murphy's sign

lateral border of the right rectus abdominis muscle with the right ninth costal cartilage. Murphy's sign is readily elicited by beep palpation at this point. Clinical presentation of acute cholecystitis is variable, and mimics varieties of other abdominal diseases, and hence clinical diagnosis alone is not reliable to plan for a definitive therapy. The accuracy of clinical diagnosis alone ranges from 45% to 77% [6].

Acute cholecystitis is usually accompanied by leukocytosis; about 75% of patients have greater than 10,000 white cells/dl. Liver function tests usually remain normal, especially when patients present early in the course of the disease. A few patients who present late may show a mild elevation of serum alkaline phosphatase and transaminase. An elevation of serum bilirubin indicates a complicated acute cholecystitis, such as acute cholangitis or obstruction of the common bile duct.

Pathophysiology

The macroscopic appearance of the gallbladder wall as seen directly by the surgeon just prior to cholecystectomy may reflect the true pathology much more accurately than the histopathological changes seen under the microscope after laparoscopic cholecystectomy. The microscopic findings after laparoscopic cholecystectomy may show changes secondary to tissue damage sustained during surgical manipulation and not necessarily the changes due to acute cholecystitis.

The histopathologic changes are divided into six evolving stages: (1) edema, (2) congestion, (3) focal necrosis, (4) suppuration, (5) gangrene, and (6) perforation. Edema is the earliest change initiated by infection or a gallstone impaction in the cystic duct or in Hartmann's pouch. Edema leads to obstruction of the cystic duct and distension of the gallbladder [7]. When the gallbladder distends, the stone may become dislodged and fall back into the lumen and the pathologic changes initiated by the stone may then subside completely with spontaneous recovery. When inflammation and edema of the cystic duct continue, on the other hand, a full blown picture of acute cholecystitis sets in and edema extends to involve the rest of the gallbladder wall. Either wall edema or stone or a combination of both is the most common cause of obstruction of the cystic duct which prevents entry of hepatic bile into the gallbladder, resulting in its non-visualization in a ^{99m}Tc-HIDA study [8]. Acute inflammation increases the vascularity of the gallbladder wall and infiltration with inflammatory cells: neutrophils and monocytes during the acute phase, and lymphocytes as it enters the subacute phase. Edema and infiltration with inflammatory cells produces thickening of the gallbladder wall which is seen often on the ultrasonogram [9].

As the focal necrosis progresses and becomes more diffuse, it may lead onto developing suppuration and abscess formation. Inflammation from the superior gallbladder wall, which lies in direct contact with the liver, often spreads to the adjoining liver tissue and causes edema and pericholecystic fluid collection along the gallbladder fossa, manifesting a "rim sign" of acute cholecystitis on cholescintigraphy [10]. When the necrosis becomes diffuse, the pain receptors often lose their sensation and produce a negative Murphy's sign. A negative Murphy's sign, therefore, is an ominous feature and calls for immediate action. Necrosis leads to ulceration and occasional perforation and bile leak. Due to its faraway location from the entrance of the cystic artery, the fundus is more vulnerable to ischemic necrosis, rupture, and bile leak than the body and neck. When the diagnosis and treatment of acute cholecystitis are delayed, the incidence of perforation and bile peritonitis increases to as high as 12% [11].

Cholescintigraphic Approach

The patient should fast for a minimum of 4 h, preferably for 8–10 h, but not more than 24 h. Serum endogenous cholecystokinin reaches its lowest level during fasting, which promotes a maximum increase in the tone of the sphincter of Oddi and a maximum relaxation of the gallbladder wall. A wide basal pressure difference between these two structures during fasting promotes preferential bile entry into the gallbladder when the cystic duct is patent, and ^{99m}Tc-HIDA simply follows the path taken by the hepatic bile [12, 13].

Hepatic Phase Imaging. With the patient in the supine position, a large field of view gamma camera fitted with a low energy all purpose collimator is positioned anteriorly over the upper abdomen to cover the entire liver. In patients with a normal bilirubin level, a dose of 2–3 mCi (74–111 MBq) ^{99m}Tc-HIDA is injected intravenously and the data are acquired at 1 frame/min for 60 min. Hypervascularity of the acutely inflamed gallbladder wall can be demonstrated by obtaining a radionuclide perfusion study by collecting the 1st min data at 1 frame/2 s [14]. A higher dose (3–6 mCi or 111–222 MBq) is needed when a perfusion study is desired. After completion of 60-min data collection, the images are viewed in cine mode display and reformatted at two frames/image and recorded on X-ray film for interpretation.

Delayed Imaging vs Morphine Administration. Two options are available when the gallbladder is not seen by 60 min (during hepatic phase imaging) in a patient with clinically suspected acute cholecystitis. One option is to choose a delayed imaging protocol by obtaining images at 3–4 h after injection of ^{99m}Tc-HIDA, sometimes even at 24 h. The other option is to administer morphine (0.04 mg/kg) intravenously at 60 min and take images immediately for an additional 30 min (total imaging time 90 min). In both cases, a second dose of ^{99m}Tc-HIDA (1–3 mCi) is administered if the radiotracer from the first dose clears almost completely from the liver by 60 min.

The diagnostic sensitivity, specificity, and accuracy of cholescintigraphy using the delayed imaging protocol varies from 92% to 100% [15–20]. A mean sensitivity of 97%, a specificity of 96%, and an accuracy of 97% have been reported from a total of 1426

Table 9.3.2. Sensitivity, specificity, and accuracy of ^{99m}Tc-HIDA cholescintigraphy in the diagnosis of acute cholecystitis by using a delayed imaging protocol (without using morphine)

Authors [ref.]	No. of patients	Sensitivity (%)	Specificity (%)	Accuracy (%)
Fonseca et al. [15]	113	100	100	100
Freitas et al. [16]	186	97	87	94
Matolo et al. [17]	619	92	97	95
Mauro et al. [18]	95	100	94	96
Szlabick et al. [19]	117	100	98	99
Weissmann et al. [20]	296	95	99	98
Total	1426	97%	96%	97%

Table 9.3.3. Sensitivity and specificity of ^{99m}Tc-HIDA cholescintigraphy in the diagnosis of acute cholecystitis with morphine augmentation

Authors [ref.]	Sensitivity	Specificity
Choy et al. [22]	23/24 (96%)	35/35 (100%)
Kim et al. [23]	11/11 (100%)	18/18 (100%)
Keslar et al. [24]	19/19 (100%)	12/12 (100%)
Mehta et al. [25]	18/18 (100%)	13/13 (100%)
Vasquez et al. [26]	10/10 (100%)	22/26 (85%)
Fig et al. [27]	12/12 (100%)	14/17 (96%)
Kistler et al. [28]	13/14 (93%)	14/18 (78%)
Fink-Bennett et al. [29]	35/36 (97%)	115/117 (98%)
Kim et al. [30]	24/28 (86%)	15/17 (88%)
Total	165/172 (96%)	258/273 (94%)

patients from six reports (Table 9.3.2). The major disadvantage of the delayed imaging protocol is that it simply delays the diagnosis and hence the therapy.

Morphine administration and Dose. Currently, the most popular imaging protocol for suspected acute cholecystitis is to administer morphine intravenously at 60 min if the gallbladder is not seen by then. Morphine acts immediately on the sphincter of Oddi and raises the sphincter pressure by increasing the frequency and amplitude (Fig 6.2.2 of Chapter 6)of phasic waves [21]. The usual dose of morphine is 0.04 mg/kg, infused intravenously over 1 min. A standard 70-kg-weight patient would require a minimum total dose of 2.8 mg. Since morphine sulfate is packaged in a 2-mg unit dose for intravenous use, it is convenient to dispense a 4-, 6-, or 8-mg dose for adults. Morphine increases the sphincter of Oddi pressure and forces the hepatic bile entry into the gallbladder when the cystic duct is patent [22–30]. Hepatic bile does not enter the gallbladder, despite morphine, if the cystic duct is not patent, as is the case in patients with acute cholecystitis. A sensitivity of 96% and a specificity of 94% have been shown with the morphine protocol (Table 9.3.3).The major advantage of intravenous morphine is that it enables an early diagnosis, usually within 90 min, allowing the referring physician to plan for an appropriate therapy immediately. The disadvantage of intravenous morphine is its central sedation. Caution is exercised while giving morphine to outpatients and the patient is instructed not to drive for at least 8–10 h after receiving morphine.

Scintigraphic Features of Acute Cholecystitis

Obstruction of the cystic duct is the salient pathophysiologic feature of acute cholecystitis (Fig. 9.3.2A). The most common cause of cystic duct obstruction is edema of the wall [7, 8]. Gallstones which may initiate inflammation often fall back into the lumen when the gallbladder distends, but the edema continues. A diagnostic test that establishes the status of the cystic duct (patency or obstruction), therefore, carries a much higher sensitivity and specificity than other imaging modalities that may show gallstones, wall thickening, or pericholecystic fluid collection as indicators of acute cholecystitis (Fig. 9.3.2B). Documentation of the cystic obstruction in an appropriate clini-

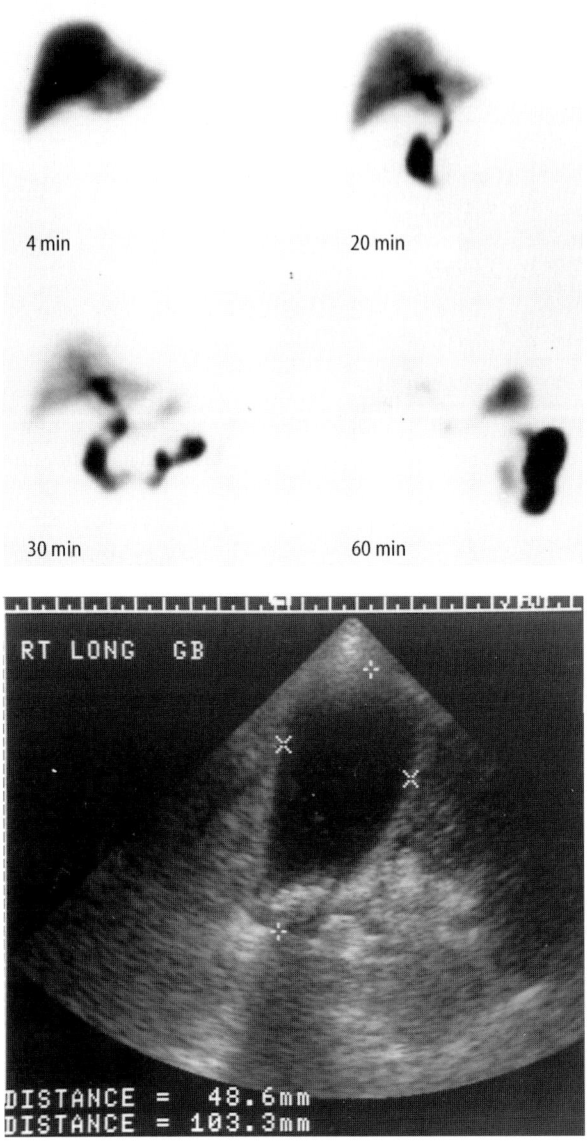

A B

Fig. 9.3.2. Acute cholecystitis. Cholescintigraphic non-visualization of the gallbladder due to obstruction of the cystic duct is the most characteristic feature. Liver shows normal uptake excretion and the bile enters the duodenum (**A**). Ultrasound shows gallstones in the neck and thickening of the gallbladder wall (**B**)

cal setting confirms the diagnosis of acute cholecystitis with a high degree of certainty [31]. Hypervascularity of an acutely inflamed gallbladder wall is seen in 72% of patients with acute cholecystitis, and can be shown by including a ^{99m}Tc-HIDA perfusion study as a part of the imaging protocol. Hypervascularity of the wall correlates with severity of acute cholecystitis [14, 32].

Pericholecystic Hepatic Retention of ^{99m}Tc-HIDA or "Rim Sign". An acute inflammation along the superior gallbladder wall often spreads to the adjoining liver parenchyma causing focal hepatitis when pericholecystitic hepatocytes show a normal pattern of uptake but a delayed excretion of ^{99m}Tc-HIDA relative to the hepatocytes far away from the gallbladder, manifesting a thin strip of increased radioactivity along the gallbladder fossa in the late images (Fig. 9.3.3A). This is called a "rim sign" [33]. The spread of infection from the gallbladder wall into the adjacent liver tissue takes place via a special set of bile ducts called the "aberrant ducts of Luschka" [34]. These aberrant ducts connect the pericholecystic hepatocytes with the adventitia of the gallbladder wall, where they end blindly (Fig. 9.3.3B). An increase in intraluminal pressure due to inflammation produces pseudodiverticulum in the gallbladder wall. Microorganisms from the superior gallbladder wall travel along these aberrant channels and pseudodiverticulum and infect the hepatocytes and Kupffer cells of liver parenchyma.

On histopathological examination, the liver tissue from the rim sign region shows edema, sinusoidal congestion, hyperplasia of Kupffer cells, and obliteration of the canalicular lumen, impeding bile flow from the rim sign region [35]. The rim sign is

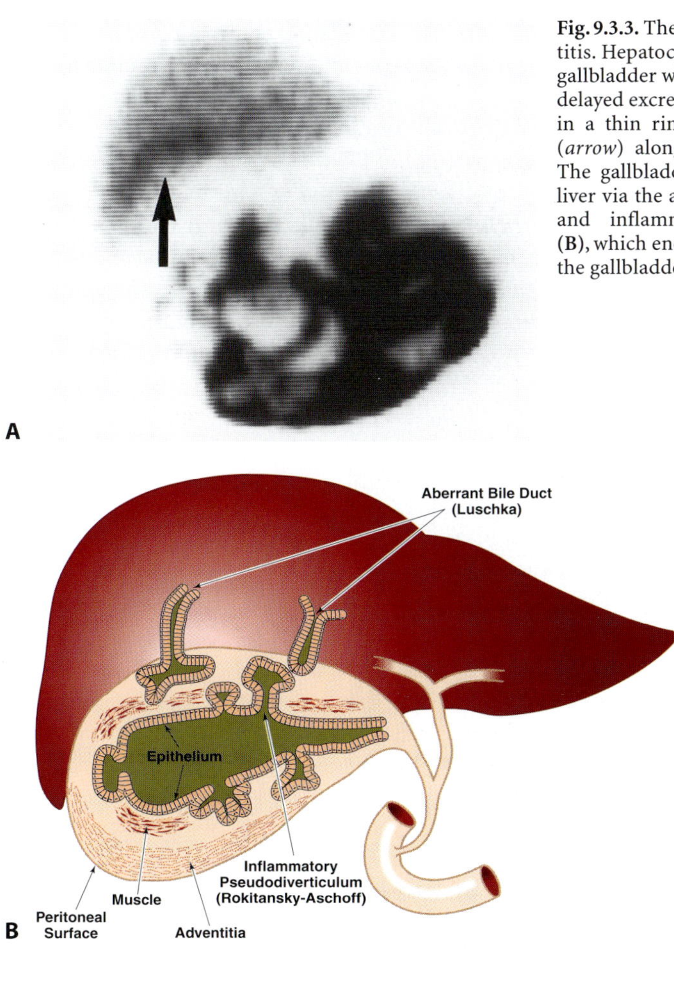

Fig. 9.3.3. The "rim sign" of acute cholecystitis. Hepatocytes adjacent to the superior gallbladder wall show normal uptake but a delayed excretion of ^{99m}Tc-HIDA, resulting in a thin rim of increased radioactivity (*arrow*) along the gallbladder fossa (**A**). The gallbladder infection spreads to the liver via the aberrant bile ducts (Luschka) and inflammatory pseudodiverticulum (**B**), which ends blindly in the adventitia of the gallbladder wall

found in 34–60% of patients with acute cholecystitis. Despite a strong positive predictive value, the rim sign alone does not carry a high enough specificity for acute cholecystitis to terminate cholescintigraphy at 60 min, when the gallbladder is not seen. Morphine augmentation is necessary to increase the sensitivity, specificity, and overall diagnostic certainty (Table 9.3.3) before planning for a definitive therapeutic strategy [36]. Gangrene, abscess, and perforation of the gallbladder wall with bile leak are some of the complications of acute cholecystitis [37, 38]. Among patients with a definite rim sign, the frequency of complications is often as high as 45%. A gangrenous acute cholecystitis on the ultrasound study shows an edematous wall with thick sludge or pus within the gallbladder (Fig. 9.3.4).

Gallbladder Preemptying with CCK

Some authors advocate intravenous cholecystokinin with the notion that preemptying, prior to cholescintigraphy, facilitates rapid gallbladder filling, when the cystic duct is patent. Administration of cholecystokinin prior to cholescintigraphy is counterproductive as it creates the physiological conditions that are just the opposite of what is required for diversion of hepatic bile into the gallbladder. By stimulating contraction of the gallbladder and relaxation of the sphincter of Oddi, cholecystokinin promotes free bile flow directly into the duodenum (Chap. 6). Comparison of studies with and without CCK-8 preemptying show a much lower specificity for studies using CCK-8 preemptying protocol. The specificity of cholescintigraphy without CCK-8 preemptying is 94%, and only 81% with the CCK-8 preemptying protocol. Preemptying with CCK-8, however, does not alter the sensitivity (94%) of cholescintigraphy [39]. In a study of 86 patients using the CCK-8 preemptying protocol, the gallbladder did not visualize by 60 min in 43 patients. In 18 of these 43 patients, the gallbladder filled in only after the use of intravenous morphine, indicating the necessity of maximizing the tonus of the sphincter of Oddi just prior to cholescintigraphy [40]. Preemptying is appropriate in patients on hyperalimentation or those who have fasted for longer than 24 h (Fig. 9.3.5).

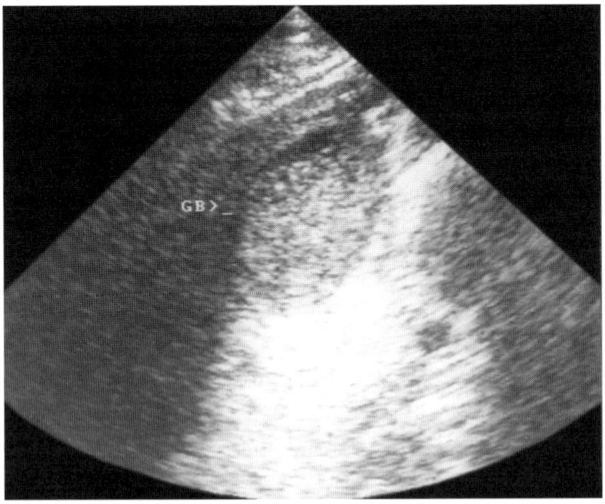

Fig. 9.3.4. Gangrenous acute cholecystitis. Ultrasound shows an edematous gallbladder wall (GB) and the lumen contains hyperechoic pus or bile sludge

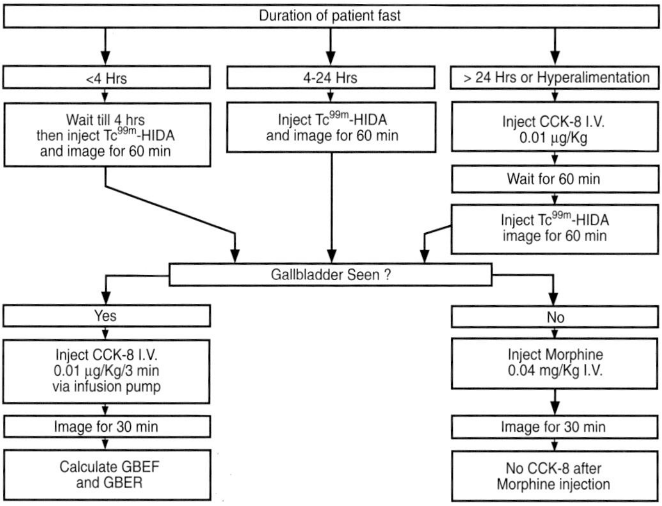

Fig. 9.3.5. Protocol for ^{99m}Tc-HIDA study. Four-hour fasting is the minimum, 8–10 h is ideal, and more than 24-h fasting should be avoided. Morphine or CCK-8 use depends upon the clinical situation at hand [42]

The decision as to when to use morphine vs cholecystokinin is dependent upon the clinical challenge at hand. Administration of morphine is appropriate in a clinical setting of acute cholecystitis and its use is inappropriate in a clinical setting of biliary dyskinesia. Administration of cholecystokinin, on the other hand, is appropriate in a clinical setting of biliary dyskinesia but not in patients with acute cholecystitis [39]. Rarely is there a need to use both agents sequentially in a given patient [41, 42].

Cholangitis

The superior gallbladder wall not covered by the peritoneum lies directly against the inferior surface of the liver (the bare area). The aberrant ducts of Luschka and inflammatory pseudodiverticulum serve as the shortest and direct route for the spread of infection from the gallbladder wall to the biliary canaliculi and hepatocytes (Fig. 9.3.3B). The microorganisms responsible for acute cholecystitis travel along these aberrant ducts and cause acute cholangitis. Clinically acute cholangitis is suggested by the onset of the "Charcot triad," which consists of fever and chills accompanied by gallbladder tenderness and jaundice, in the absence of obstruction of the common bile duct. Characteristic features of a combined acute cholecystitis and acute cholangitis on cholescintigraphy include non-visualization of the gallbladder (despite morphine), delayed clearance of ^{99m}Tc-HIDA from the entire liver (intrahepatic cholestasis), leukocytosis, right upper quadrant pain, fever, and jaundice (Fig. 9.3.6). The rim sign is typically absent due to diffuse retention of ^{99m}Tc-HIDA by the liver, not just by the pericholecystic hepatocytes.

Differential Diagnosis of Acute Cholecystitis

Many diseases are to be considered in the differential diagnosis in any patient who presents clinically with abdominal pain, fever, and leukocytosis (Table 9.3.1). Pain due to a right renal stone is colicky in nature and very severe in intensity when compared with pain due to acute cholecystitis, which tends to be of moderate intensity. A renal

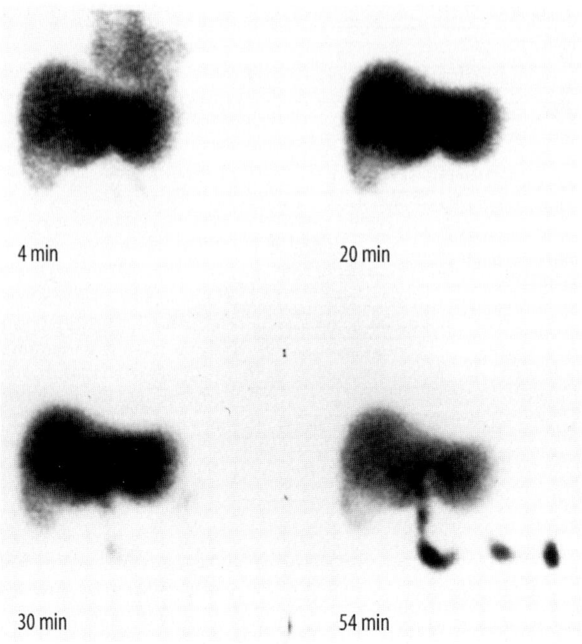

Fig. 9.3.6. Acute cholecystitis and acute cholangitis. The gallbladder is non-visualized and there is diffuse retention of ^{99m}Tc-HIDA by the liver parenchyma. The rim sign is absent and bile enters the duodenum

stone often causes hematuria as it passes through the ureter. The pain due to viral hepatitis is accompanied by abnormal liver function tests and a hepatitis profile confirms the diagnosis. Acute pancreatitis and acute cholecystitis often coexist. Non-visualization of the gallbladder in association with a rise in serum amylase or lipase indicates the coexistence of acute cholecystitis and acute pancreatitis [43,44]. A peptic ulcer may cause epigastric pain mimicking cholecystitis. Infection with *Helicobacter pylori* is now the most common cause of peptic ulcer. These bacteria produce the enzyme urease, which splits ^{14}C-labeled urea in the stomach and liberates ^{14}C-labeled carbon dioxide, which is eliminated in the expired breath. A positive ^{14}C-urea breath test confirms active *H. pylori* infection. Radiation of gallbladder pain upwards into the chest and shoulder may mimic anginal pain. An electrocardiogram, measurement of cardiac enzymes, or ^{99m}Tc-pyrophosphate myocardial imaging help confirm the cardiac origin of acute pain. A thorough clinical evaluation along with measurement of the appropriate biochemical profile, aids the primary care physician in requesting the most appropriate imaging test to either confirm or rule out each diagnostic possibility.

Comparison of Cholescintigraphy and Ultrasound

Immediately after the introduction of ^{99m}Tc-HIDA agents in 1976 and up until 1984, most cholescintigraphic studies were carried out with the first generation agents using a delayed imaging protocol, which often delayed diagnosis, sometimes for up to 24 h. The diagnostic time interval using the current generation ^{99m}Tc-HIDA agents is now reduced to less than 90 min by administering morphine intravenously at 60 min, when the gallbladder is not seen in a patient with suspected acute cholecystitis. A meta analysis of 2466 patients from 30 reports revealed cholescintigraphy as the test of choice for acute cholecystitis and ultrasound for cholelithiasis [45]. For acute cholecystitis, the cholescintigraphic sensitivity is 97% (95% confidence interval, 0.96–0.98) and specificity 90% (95% confidence interval, 0.86–0.95). Morphine administration shortens the diagnostic time interval but does not alter the sensitivity or specificity when compared with delayed imaging protocol (Tables 9.3.2, 9.3.3). Adjusted sensitivity of ultrasound for acute cholecystitis is 88% (95% confidence interval, 0.74–1.0) and specificity 80% (95% confidence interval, 0.62–0.98). Adjusted sensitivity for detection of cholelithiasis with the ultrasound is 84% (95% confidence limit, 0.76–0.92) and adjusted specificity is 99% (95% confidence interval, 0.97–1.0). Since the salient pathophysiology of acute cholecystitis is cystic duct obstruction, cholescintigraphy which establishes the status of the cystic duct (patency or obstruction) is much more reliable than ultrasound or CT, both of which depend upon wall thickness as an indicator of acute cholecystitis.

Application of Bayes' Analysis

Clinical diagnosis is often a probability estimate based on the frequency of the disease in the study population. Because it is impossible to study the entire population, the estimates are made from studies comprising a limited number of samples from the population at risk. After the clinical examination, a clinician makes a rough estimate of the disease probability (pre-test probably) based on the frequency of that disease in that particular population. Imaging tests are requested either to confirm the clinical diagnosis or rule out the disease from consideration with a high degree of certainty. The clinicians feel more comfortable proceeding with a definitive therapeutic strategy after confirmation of acute cholecystitis by an imaging procedure. When the clinical diagnosis is not confirmed by the imaging test, then the clinicians have the option of accepting the results of the imaging test as final or ignoring it completely and obtaining additional diagnostic tests.

Most imaging procedures are interpreted subjectively, and they provide a dichotomous result in the form of either the disease is present or absent. The probability of a disease being present or absent after an imaging test (post-test probability) depends upon various factors including the sensitivity, specificity, false-positive, and false-negative ratio of the test, and the prevalence of the disease in the study population. Probabilities are assessed by applying Bayesian analysis [46, 47]. After conducting a thorough clinical evaluation and obtaining a basic biochemical profile, the clinician arrives at a tentative clinical diagnosis and then chooses one of the diagnostic imaging tests for confirmation. In the case of acute cholecystitis, ^{99m}Tc-HIDA cholescintigraphy and ultrasound are two of the most common imaging options and the clinician may decide to choose either one or both. The previously popular oral cholecystography is no longer used today. Sensitivity and specificity of an imaging test are calculated by using the following format:

	Target disease	
Test result	Present	Absent
Positive	a	b
Negative	c	d

$$\text{Sensitivity} = \frac{a}{a+c} \qquad \text{specificity} = \frac{d}{b+d}$$

The probability of acute cholecystitis when the imaging test is positive or negative is given by the following formulas:

$$\text{Probability of acute cholecystitis when the test is positive (abnormal)} = \frac{\left[\text{Sensitivity} \times \text{Prevalence of acute cholecystitis in the study population}\right]}{\left[\text{Sensitivity} \times \text{Prevalence of acute cholecystitis in the study population}\right] + \left[\text{False positive fraction} \times \text{Prevalence of no acute cholecystitis in the study population}\right]}$$

$$\text{Probability of acute cholecystitis when the test is negative (normal)} = \frac{\left[\text{False-negative fraction} \times \text{Prevalence of acute cholecystitis in the study population}\right]}{\left[\text{False-negative fraction} \times \text{prevalence of acute cholecystitis in the study population}\right] + \left[\text{Specificity} \times \text{Prevalence of no acute cholecystitis in the study population}\right]}$$

Pre-test probability (prevalence): The proportion of patients who have the target disease, as determined before the test is carried out $= \dfrac{a+c}{a+b+c+d}$

Post-test probability: The proportion of patients with the target disease with a positive test.

Likelihood ratio (LR): This is the ratio of the probability of a test result among the patients with the target disease to the probability of the same test result among patients who do not have the target disease.

$$\text{The likelihood ratio for a positive test} = \frac{\text{sensitivity}}{1\text{–specificity}}$$

$$\text{The likelihood ratio for a negative test} = \frac{1\text{–specificity}}{\text{sensitivity}}$$

After knowing the pre-test (clinical evaluation) and post-test (after an imaging procedure) probability, the clinicians can calculate the Bayes factor or likelihood ratio of the target disease, prior to subjecting the patient to a definitive therapy. The Bayes factor is considered to be more objective and can substitute for the "*P*" value of a null hypothesis [48, 49]. By referring to the nomogram (Fig. 9.3.7), the post-test likelihood ratio is obtained directly without the need for an actual calculation [50, 51]. The likelihood ratio corresponds to the point where a straight line drawn between the pre-test probability and the post-test probability intersects the likelihood ratio line in the middle. Let us assume that in a patient with right upper quadrant pain and fever, the pre-test probability of acute cholecystitis (after the clinical examination) is 20%. If the gallbladder is not visualized in a ^{99m}Tc-HIDA study (97% sensitivity), the likelihood ratio of acute cholecystitis is approximately 200. The cost-effectiveness of a positive (GB not seen) ^{99m}Tc-HIDA test is greater when the pre-test probably is lower, and the cost-effectiveness decreases as the pre-test probably increases to a very high level.

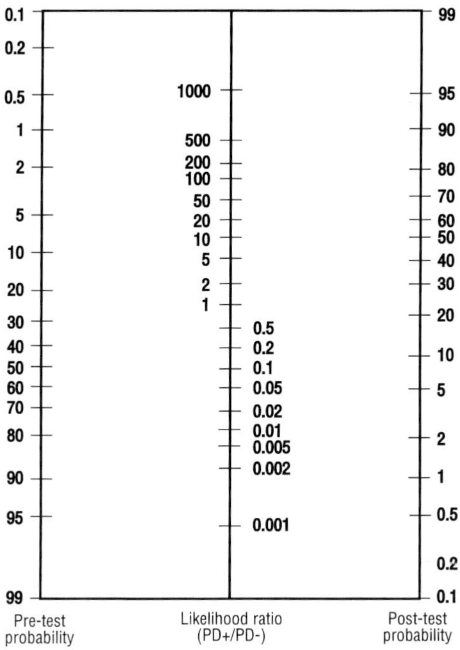

Fig. 9.3.7. Nomogram for likelihood ratio. A line drawn between the pre-test (clinical diagnosis) and post-test (after imaging test) probability intersects the line in the middle and indicates the likelihood ratio [51]

The discriminating power of a test is the difference in post-test probability between a positive (gallbladder not seen) and a negative test (gallbladder seen) for acute cholecystitis [31]. The wider the difference between positive and negative tests, the greater is the discriminating power (Fig. 9.3.8). Cholescintigraphy and oral cholecystography, both of which establish the patency or obstruction of the cystic duct (the basic pathology of acute cholecystitis), carry a much better discriminating power than ultrasound. Ultrasound, which detects gallstones and thickness of the gallbladder wall but does not establish the status of the cystic duct, therefore, carries a much lower discriminating power for acute cholecystitis (Fig. 9.3.9). The discriminating power of a test works at its best when the prevalence of disease in the study population is around 50%. The discriminating power decreases precipitously when the prevalence is below 15% or above 85% [31].

Application of Bayesian analysis requires the establishment of true sensitivity and specificity of an imaging test. The ultimate diagnosis of acute cholecystitis, however, is based upon the histopathological criteria chosen by the pathologist. Some pathologists are satisfied with the mere presence of transmural inflammation of the gallbladder wall, while others insist upon the presence of hemorrhage and necrosis before assigning the definitive diagnosis of acute cholecystitis. The best combination of sensitivity and specificity for cholescintigraphy is obtained when the presence of any one of the above two histological criteria is chosen as the basis for the diagnosis of acute cholecystitis [52]. Under an appropriate clinical setting, most clinicians are satisfied with the cholescintigraphic documentation of cystic duct obstruction as sufficient evidence for the diagnosis of acute cholecystitis in planning for a definitive therapy.

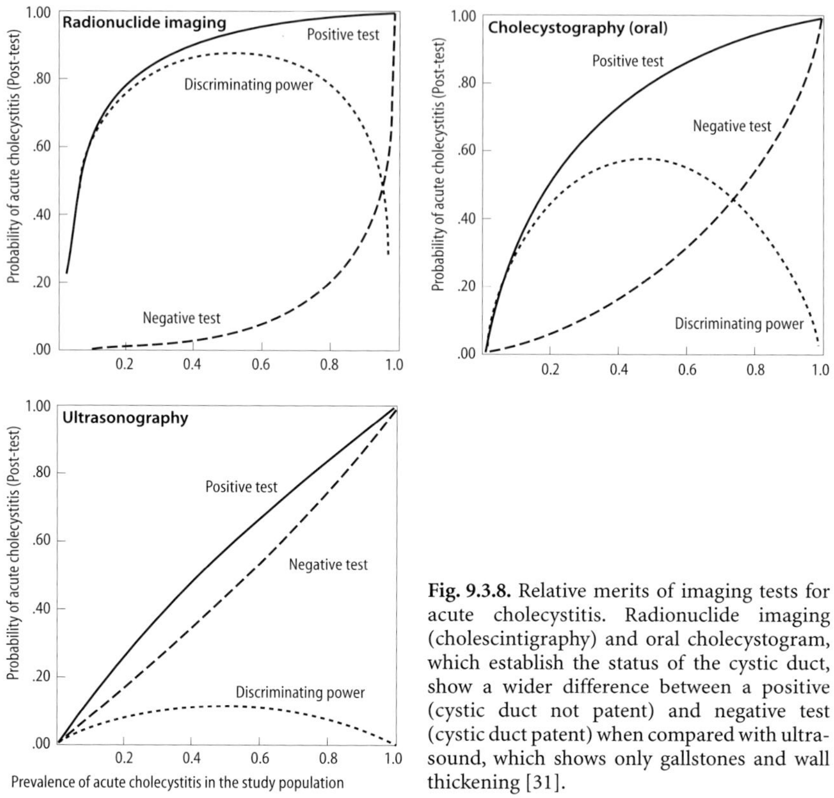

Fig. 9.3.8. Relative merits of imaging tests for acute cholecystitis. Radionuclide imaging (cholescintigraphy) and oral cholecystogram, which establish the status of the cystic duct, show a wider difference between a positive (cystic duct not patent) and negative test (cystic duct patent) when compared with ultrasound, which shows only gallstones and wall thickening [31].

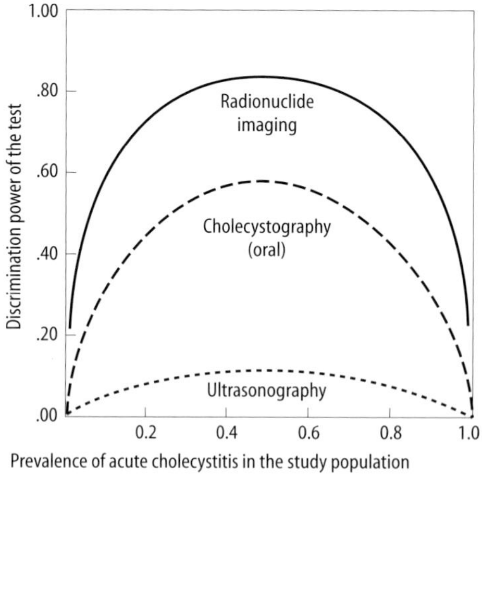

Fig. 9.3.9. Discriminating power. The difference between a positive (gallbladder not seen) and a negative test (gallbladder seen) probability is the discriminating power of the diagnostic test. Positive cholescintigraphy and oral cholecystography in an appropriate clinical setting confirm acute cholecystitis. A negative test (gallbladder seen) rules out acute cholecystitis. Ultrasound shows the least discriminating power for acute cholecystitis [31].

Acute Acalculous Cholecystitis

Clinically acute acalculous cholecystitis presents very similar to that of acute calculous cholecystitis, but has a few unique clinical features of its own. Patients are usually much older, and have additional risk factors such as recent surgery, crush injury, burns, sepsis, or hyperalimentation. About 10–15% of all acute cholecystitis cases belong to the acalculous variety. The incidence of acute acalculous cholecystitis appears to be increasing recently, which may be attributed to increased clinical awareness and sensitivity of the diagnostic tests [53]. The morbidity and mortality of acute acalculous cholecystitis are much higher than those of acute calculous cholecystitis. As obstruction of the cystic duct is common for both conditions, the diagnostic sensitivity of cholescintigraphy is similar for both calculous and acalculous acute cholecystitis [54, 55]. Edema (and not the stone) as the primary cause of cystic duct obstruction is easy to appreciate in the case of acute acalculous cholecystitis, as there are no gallstones associated with it.

References

1. Ingelfinger FJ. Digestive diseases as a national problem. V Gallstones. Gastroenterology 1968;55:102–104
2. Friedman GD, Kannel WB, Dawber TR. The epidemiology of gallbladder disease: observations in the Framingham Study. J Chronic Dis 1966;19:273–292
3. Gracie WA, Ransohoff DF. The natural history of silent gallstones: the innocent gallstone is not a myth. N Engl J Med 1982;307:798–800
4. Pelligrini CA, Way LW. Acute cholecystitis. In: Way LW, Pelligrini CA. Eds. Surgery of the gallbladder and bile ducts. WB Saunders, Philadelphia 1987, pp 251–264
5. Ryan ET, Pak PH, DeSanctis RW. Myocardial infarction mimicked by acute cholecystitis. Ann Intern Med 1992;116:218–220
6. Freitas JE, Fink-Bennet DM, Thrall JH, Resinger WW, Calderon HC, Mirkes SH, Shah PK. Efficacy of hepatobiliary imaging of acute abdominal pain: concise communication. J Nucl Med 1980;21:919–924
7. Schein CJ. Acute cholecystitis. Harper and Row, New York, 1972
8. Eikman EA, Cameron JL, Colman M, Natarajan TK, Dugal P, Wagner HN, Jr. A test for patency of the cystic duct in acute cholecystitis. Ann Intern Med 1975;82:318–322
9. Handler SJ. Ultrasound of gallbladder wall thickening and its relation to cholecystitis. Am J Roentgenol 1979; 132:581–585
10. Brachman MB, Tanasescu DE, Ramanna L, Waxman AD. Acute gangrenous cholecystitis: radionuclide diagnosis. Radiology 1984;151:209–211
11. Ranson JHC. Perforation of the gallbladder. In: Way LW, Pelligrini CA. Eds. Surgery of the gallbladder and bile ducts. WB Saunders, Philadelphia 1987, pp 265–273
12. Krishnamurthy S, Krishnamurthy GT. Evolution of nuclear hepatology as a clinical subspeciality. J Nucl Med Technol 1995;23:35S–45S (Supplement)
13. Wheeler HO. Concentrating function of the gallbladder. Am J Med 1971;51:588–595
14. Colletti PM, Ralls PW, Siegel ME, Halls JM. Acute cholecystitis: diagnosis with radionuclide angiography. Radiology 1987;163:615–618
15. Fonseca C, Greenberg D, Rosenthall L, Arzoumanian A. Assessment of the utility of gallbladder imaging with 99m-Tc-IDA. Clin Nucl Med 1978,3:437–441
16. Freitas JE, Gulati MD. Rapid evaluation of acute abdominal pain by hepatobiliary scanning. JAMA 1980;244:1585–1587
17. Matolo NM, Stadalnik RC, Dixon SM. Value and limitations of scanning of the biliary tract. Surg Gynecol Obstet 1980;150:521–524
18. Mauro MA, McCartney WH, Melmud JR. Hepatobiliary scanning with 99m-Tc-PIPIDA in acute cholecystitis. Radiology 1982;142:193–197
19. Szlabick RE, Catto JA, Fink-Bennett D, Ventura V. Hepatobiliary scanning in the diagnosis of acute cholecystitis. Arch Surg 1980;115:540–544

20. Weissmann HS, Badia J, Sugarman LA, Kluger L, Rosenblatt R, Freeman LM. Spectrum of 99m-Tc-IDA cholescintigraphic patterns in acute cholecystitis. Radiology 1981;138:167–175
21. Helm JF, Venu RP, Geenen JE, Hogan WJ, Dodd WJ, Toouli J, Arndorfer RC. Effects of morphine on the human sphincter of Oddi. Gut 1988;29:1402–1407
22. Choy D, Shi EC, McLean RG, Hoschl R, Murray IP, Ham JM. Cholescintigraphy in acute cholecystitis: use of intravenous morphine. Radiology 1984;151:203–207
23. Kim EE, Pjura G, Lowry P, Nguyen M, Pollack M. Morphine-augmented cholescintigraphy in the diagnosis of acute cholecystitis. Am J Roentgenol 1986;147:1177–1179
24. Keslar PJ, Turbiner EH. Hepatobiliary imaging and the use of intravenous morphine. Clin Nucl Med 1987;12:592–596
25. Mehta A, Alazraki N. The effectiveness of morphine in expediting the radionuclide diagnosis of acute cholecystitis. J Nucl Med 1987;28:596 (abstract)
26. Vasquez TE, Greenspan G, Evans DG, Halpern SE, Ashburn WL. Clinical efficacy of intravenous morphine administration in hepatobiliary imaging for acute cholecystitis. Clin Nucl Med 1988;13:4–6
27. Fig LM, Stewart RE, Wahl RL, Shapiro B. Potential pitfalls in the use of morphine hepatobiliary scintigraphy. J Nucl Med 1989;30:850 (abstract)
28. Fink-Bennett D, Balon H, Robbins T, Tsai D. Morphine-augmented cholescintigraphy: its efficacy in detecting acute cholecystitis. J Nucl Med 1989;30:850 (abstract)
29. Kistler AM, Ziessman HA, Gooch D, Bitterman P. Morphine-augmented cholescintigraphy in acute cholecystitis. A satisfactory alternative to delayed imaging. Clin Nucl Med 1991;16:404–406
30. Kim CK, Tse KK, Juweid M, Mozley PD, Woda A, Alavi A. Cholescintigraphy in the diagnosis of acute cholecystitis: morphine augmentation is superior to delayed imaging. J Nucl Med 1993;34:1866–1870
31. Krishnamurthy GT. Acute cholecystitis: the diagnostic role for current imaging tests. West J Med 1982;137:87–94
32. Moncada R, Cordoso M, Danley R, Rodriguez J, et al. Acute cholecystitis: 137 patients studied by infusion tomography of the gallbladder. Am J Roentgenol 1977;129:583–585
33. Bushnell DL, Perlman SB, Wilson MA, Polcyn RE. The rim sign: association with acute cholecystitis. J Nucl Med 1986;27:353–356
34. Netter FH. The CIBA collection of medical illustration: Volume 3. Digestive system, part 111. Liver, biliary tract and pancreas. CIBA Pharmaceutical Co. Summit, NJ. 1964. pp 1–31
35. Meekin GK, Ziessman HA, Klappenbach RS. Prognostic value and pathophysiologic significance of the rim sign in cholescintigraphy. J Nucl Med 1987;28:1679–1682
36. Oates E, Selland DG, Chin CT, Achong DM. Gallbladder nonvisualization with pericholecystic rim sign: morphine-augmentation optimizes diagnosis of acute cholecystitis. J Nucl Med 1996;37:267–269
37. Smith R, Rosen JM, Gallow LN, Anderson PO. Pericholecystic hepatic activity in cholescintigraphy. Radiology 1985;156:797–800
38. Swayne LC, Ginsberg HN. Diagnosis of acute cholecystitis by cholescintigraphy: significance of pericholecystic hepatic uptake. Am J Roentgenol 1989;152:1211–1213
39. Krishnamurthy S, Krishnamurthy GT. Cholecystokinin and morphine pharmacological intervention during 99m-Tc-HIDA cholescintigraphy: a rational approach. Semin Nucl Med 1996;26:16–24
40. Chen CC, Holder LE, Maunoury C, Drachenberg CI. Morphine augmentation increases gallbladder visualization in patients pretreated with cholecystokinin. J Nucl Med 1997;38:644–647
41. Kim CK. Pharmacological intervention for the diagnosis of acute cholecystitis: cholecystokinin pretreatment or morphine, or both? J Nucl Med 1997;38:647–649
42. Krishnamurthy S, Krishnamurthy GT. Evolution of nuclear hepatology as a clinical subspeciality. J Nucl Med Technology 1995;24:35S–45S (supplement)
43. Serafini AN, Al-Sheikh W, Barkin JS, Hourani M, Sfakiankis G, Clarke LP, Ashkar FS. Biliary scintigraphy in acute pancreatitis. Radiology 1982;144:591–595
44. Ali A, Turner DA, Fordham EW. Tc-99m-IDA cholescintigraphy in acute pancreatitis: concise communication. J Nucl Med 1982;23:867–869
45. Shea JA, Berlin JA, Escarce JJ, Clarke JR, Kinosian BP, Cabana MD, Tsai WW, Horangic N, Malet PF, Schwartz S, Williams SV. Revised estimates of diagnostic test sensitivity and specificity in suspected biliary tract disease. Arch Intern Med 1994;154:2573–2581
46. Hamilton GW, Trobaugh GB, Ritchie JL, et al. Myocardial imaging with thallium-201: an analysis of clinical usefulness based on Bayes' theorem. Semin Nucl Med 1976;17:439–448
47. McNeil BJ, Adelstein SJ. Determining the value of diagnostic and screening tests. J Nucl Med 1976;17:439–448
48. Goodman SN. Toward evidence-based medical statistics. 1: the *P* value fallacy. Ann Intern Med 1999;130:995–1004

49. Goodman SN. Toward evidence-based medical statistics. 2: the Bayes factor. Ann Intern Med 1999;130:1005–1013
50. Fagan TJ. Nomogram for Bayes's theorem. N Engl J Med 1975;293:257
51. Glossary. Terms used in therapeutics. ACP Journal Club 1998;129:A21
52. Freitas JE, Coleman RE, Nagle CE, Bree RL, Krewer KD, Gross MD. Influence of scan and pathologic criteria on the specificity of cholescintigraphy: concise communication. J Nucl Med 1983;24:876–879
53. Frazee RC, Nagorney DM, Mucha P, Jr. Acute acalculous cholecystitis. Mayo Clin Proc 1989;64:163–167
54. Swayne LC. Acute acalculous cholecystitis: sensitivity in detection using technetium-99m iminodiacetic acid cholescintigraphy. Radiology 1986;160:33–38
55. Weissmann HS, Burkowitz D, Fox MS, Gliedman ML, Rosenblatt R, Sugarman LA, Freeman LM. The role of technetium 99m iminodiacetic (IDA) cholescintigraphy in acute acalculous cholecystitis. Radiology 1983;146:177–180

9.4 Management of Gallbladder Disease

Cholecystectomy is the treatment of choice for most diseases of the gallbladder. The very first cholecystectomy was performed in 1882 by a German surgeon, Langenbach [1]. Today as many as 700,000 cholecystectomies are performed annually in the United States with either laparoscopic or open cholecystectomy. Open cholecystectomy carries a mortality rate ranging from 0% to 2.4% and a morbidity ranging from 4.1% to 14.7%. The incidence of bile duct injury varies from 0.06% to 0.45% [2]. Laparoscopic cholecystectomy, which has now almost replaced open cholecystectomy, carries a similar rate of mortality but a slightly lower morbidity (1.6–12%) than open cholecystectomy [3]. Laparoscopic cholecystectomy in the beginning was restricted mostly to symptomatic cholelithiasis, but now it is performed for varieties of gallbladder diseases, including acute cholecystitis, gangrenous cholecystitis, hydrops, and empyema [4]. Young as well as old patients tolerate the laparoscopic cholecystectomy procedure well, and the hospital stay is much shorter than with open cholecystectomy [5]. Administration of prophylactic antibiotics does not seem to affect the rate of wound infection in the case of elective laparoscopic cholecystectomy [6].

Complications

Complications of acute cholecystitis can occur either before or after treatment. The complications of delayed or untreated acute cholecystitis include acute cholangitis, gallbladder perforation, and bile leak. Postoperative complications include bile leak, cholangitis, infection, and stricture formation. Bile fistula occurs as a chronic complication.

Perforation of the Gallbladder

Perforation of the gallbladder is rare and occurs usually in association with gangrenous acute cholecystitis. Perforation is found in 10% of patients undergoing open cholecystectomy for acute gangrenous cholecystitis [7]. After perforation, the bile may leak into a small closed space or leak freely into the peritoneum, causing bile peritonitis. Localized leaking is the most common type and accounts for 50% of all perforations (Fig. 9.4.1). Free perforation into the peritoneal cavity with peritonitis occurs in 30% and the remaining 20% form fistulas connected with the subhepatic space, duodenum, stomach, or colon. Most of the localized leaks and those that form fistula remain

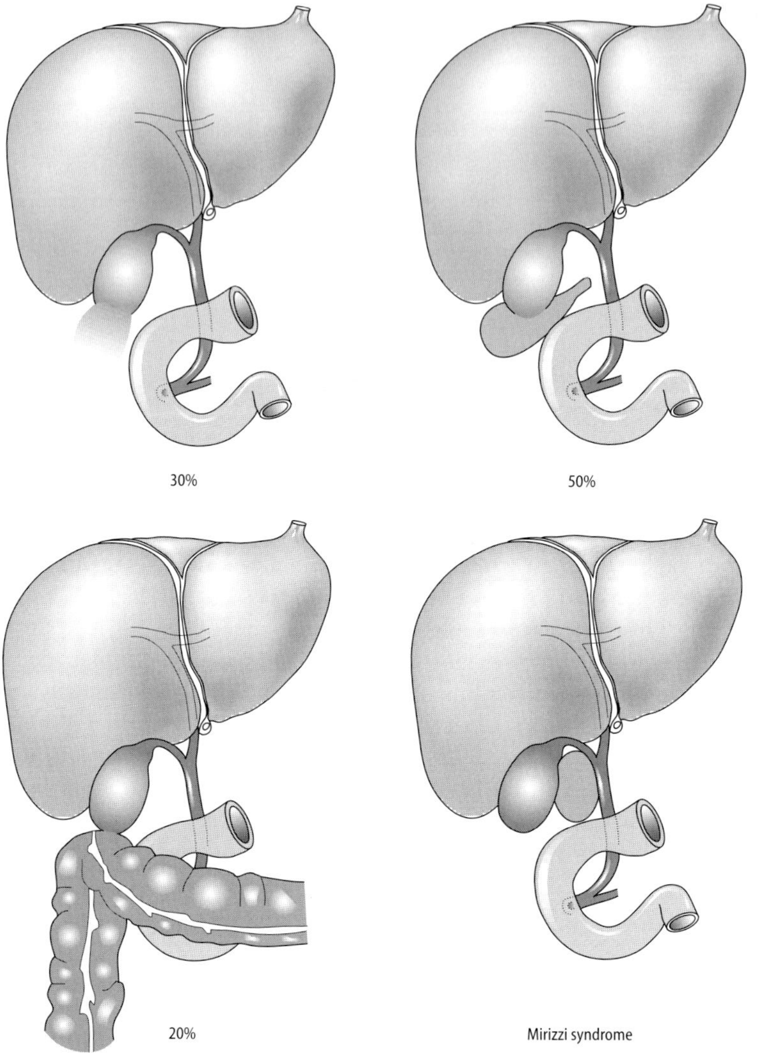

Fig. 9.4.1. Types of gallbladder perforation. The subhepatic bed is the most common site, followed by leak into the free peritoneum and colon. Perforation near the neck and Hartmann's pouch may form a biloma and compress the common bile duct extrinsically, manifesting the Mirizzi syndrome [7]

undiagnosed as they usually do not producc symptoms. Free perforation with bile peritonitis presents with the most disabling symptoms and is responsible for many deaths if not treated immediately. Most perforations into the subhepatic space are walled off and manifest very few symptoms. Perforation into the stomach and hepatic flexure of the colon causes few symptoms. Perforation near the neck or Hartmann's pouch may form a biloma and compress the common bile duct, externally manifesting a Mirizzi syndrome.

Bile Leak

The most common complication of laparoscopic cholecystectomy is bile leak through an unligated cystic duct or from an injury to the bile duct (Fig. 9.4.2). Leak is best defined as bile collection in an unanticipated location or in an anticipated location at an unanticipated time. The exact point of leaking corresponds to the place of its first appearance. Data acquisition at short intervals (one frame/min) and display in cine mode are critical for exact localization of the leak. The common hepatic duct, which lies directly in front of the tip of the laparoscopic instrument, sustains injury more frequently than other bile ducts. The incidence of bile duct injury from laparoscopic cholecystectomy is twice as frequent as from open cholecystectomy. The consequence of bile leak depends upon its volume and location. A small volume subhepatic bile leak (Fig. 9.4.2A) or a large volume bile leak into the stomach (Fig. 9.4.2B) causes a few of the symptoms. A large volume hepatic subcapsular leak (Fig. 9.4.2C) or a leak into the peritoneal cavity (Fig. 9.4.2D) requires treatment. Since the leak offers the path of least resistance, major bile ducts often are not visualized (Fig. 9.4.2A, C, D).

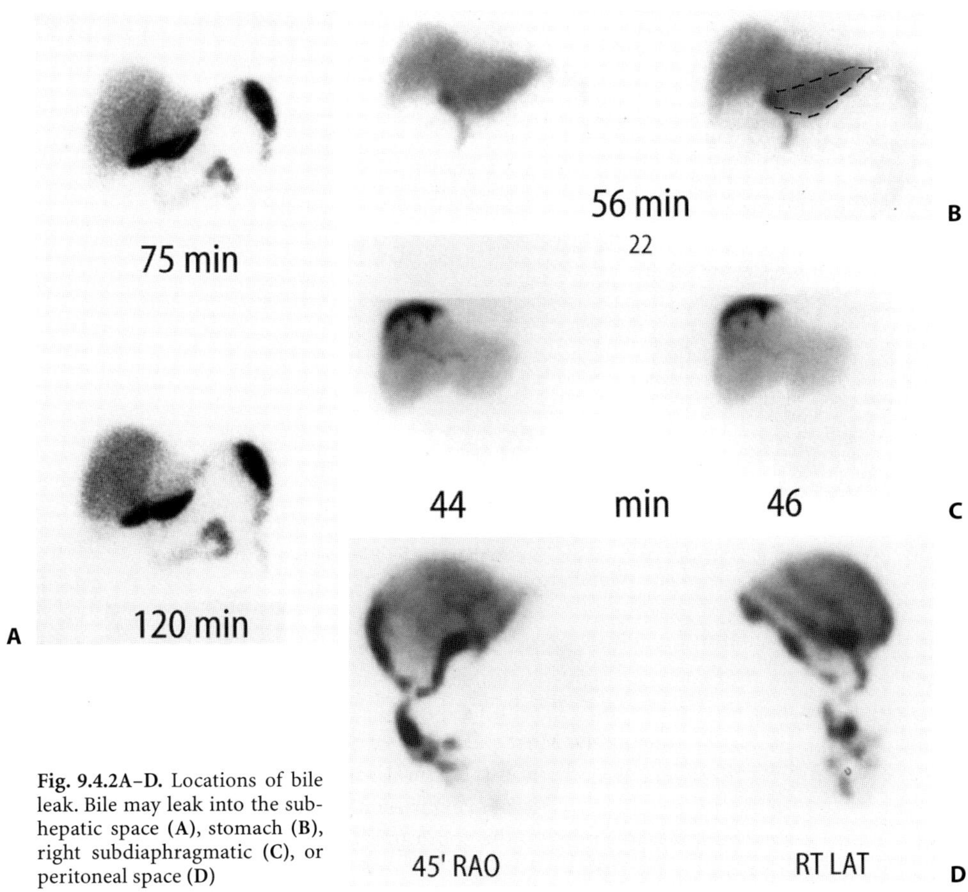

Fig. 9.4.2A–D. Locations of bile leak. Bile may leak into the subhepatic space (**A**), stomach (**B**), right subdiaphragmatic (**C**), or peritoneal space (**D**)

Treatment of Bile Leak

Small volume bile leaks close spontaneously if the tonus of the sphincter of Oddi is maintained at its minimum by treating patients with antispasmodics (Fig. 9.4.3). Use of opioids is avoided. Bile leak can be quantified by choosing one region of interest over the leak and another to include the stomach, small intestine, and colon. Large volume bile leaks may require sphincterotomy for healing. Sphincterotomy creates the path of least resistance for hepatic bile and promotes closure of the leak (Fig. 9.4.4A,B). Few patients may require reopening and ligation of the open cystic duct. Bile leak from the common hepatic or common bile duct may require stents or surgical repair. Postsurgical strictures at the site of bile duct injury may require stents or dilatation through the endoscopic or transhepatic route. Malignant strictures usually require stents [8].

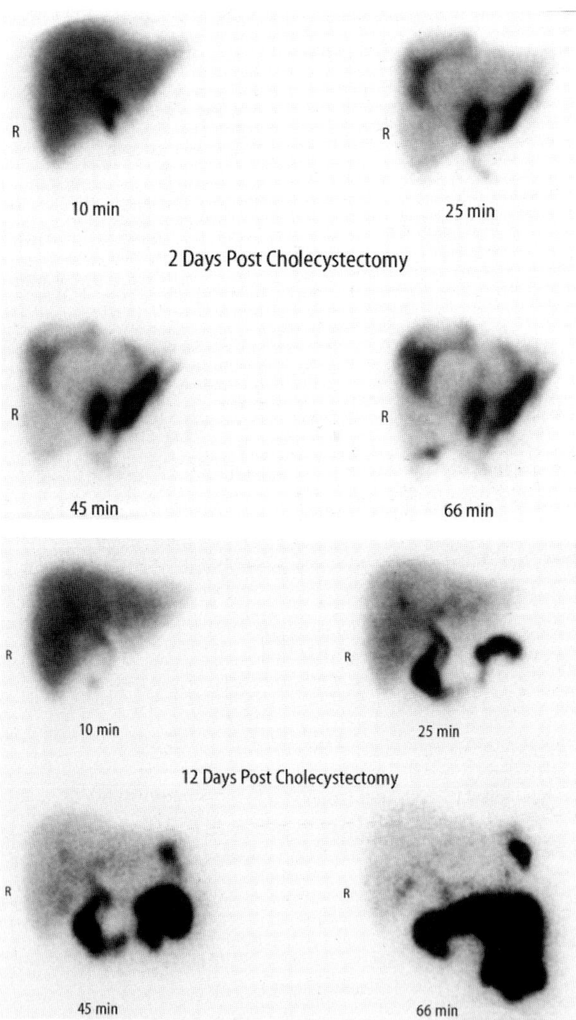

A

B

Fig. 9.4.3. Spontaneous closure of bile leak. Bile leak into the lateral aspect of the right lobe 2 days after cholecystectomy **(A)** stops spontaneously after 12 days **(B)**. Narcotics which constrict the sphincter of Oddi were discontinued during this time period

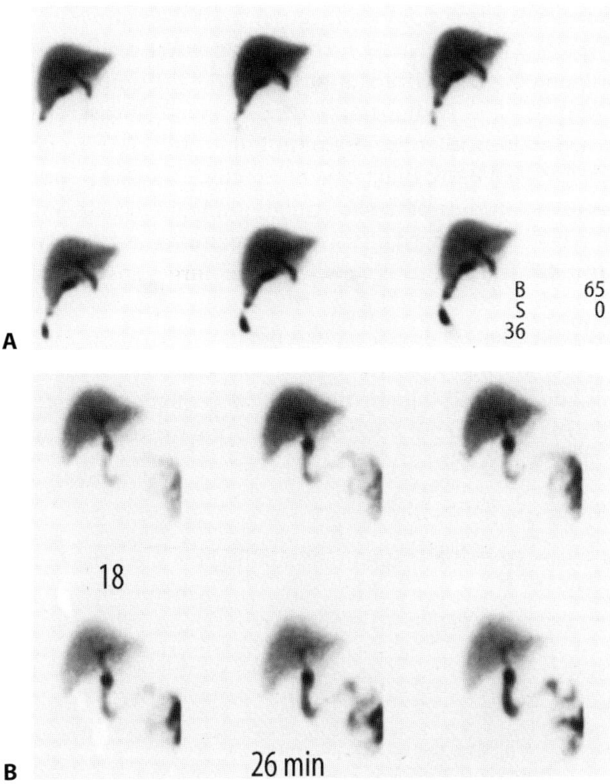

Fig. 9.4.4. Closure of bile leak after sphincterotomy. A large volume bile leak through an unligated cystic duct (**A**) required sphincterotomy for its stoppage (**B**)

Bile Duct Stricture

Stricture is a late complication of cholecystectomy. The frequency of postoperative bile duct stricture is much higher after laparoscopic than after open cholecystectomy (Table 9.4.1). Most postoperative strictures occur in the proximal one-half of the common hepatic duct, often involving its bifurcation into right and left hepatic ducts. Strictures near the bifurcation are treated with Hepp-Couinaud hepaticojejunostomy using the left hepatic duct [9]. Recently, the design of laparoscopic instruments has improved and it is now possible to perform cholecystectomy safely with needles as small as 3 mm in diameter [10]. Postoperative strictures commonly occur at the site of ductal injury

Table 9.4.1. Complications of open vs laparoscopic cholecystectomy [3]

Complication	Open cholecystectomy (%)	Laparoscopic cholecystectomy (%)
CBD injury	0.1	0.2
Bile leak	0.8	5.6
Pancreatitis	1.0	1.1
Jaundice	1.2	1.0
Atelectasis	10.0	5.4
Ileus	12.0	5.3
Urinary retention	17.4	6.5

and are classified into four grades depending upon its location from the bifurcation into the left hepatic with right hepatic duct [11]. Grade I strictures are more than 2 cm, grade II less than 2 cm, from the union, grade III are at or just below the union, and grade IV occur at the site of union.

In the past, controversy existed as to the appropriate time for cholecystectomy (immediate vs late cholecystectomy), once the diagnosis of acute cholecystitis was established. Well designed prospective studies have shown that immediate cholecystectomy is much more cost-effective than delayed elective cholecystectomy [12, 13]. Early laparoscopic cholecystectomy (within 72 h) is now preferred for its cost-effectiveness [14, 15].

Postoperative subhepatic fluid collection is common and is noted in as many as 25% of patients following open cholecystectomy [16]. However, only about 30–45% of these subhepatic fluid cases are due to bile leak [17]. Bile fistulae as a consequence of acute and chronic complications occur in the subhepatic space, duodenum, or stomach, or into the hepatic flexure of the colon (Fig. 9.4.5).

Prophylactic Cholecystectomy

Patients with asymptomatic gallstones or diabetes mellitus usually show a decrease in gallbladder emptying but generally do not require cholecystectomy, when either dis-

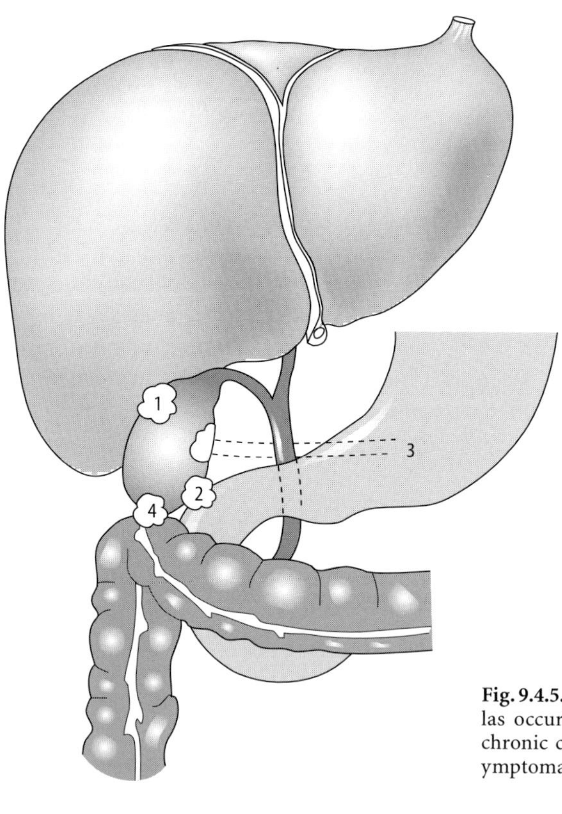

Fig. 9.4.5. Common sites of biliary fistula. Fistulas occur as a complication of either acute or chronic cholecystitis. Most of them remain asymptomatic

ease exists alone [18,19]. However, patients with a combination of asymptomatic gallstones and diabetes mellitus develop acute cholecystitis and its complications 2.2 times more frequently than with either disease alone. Based upon such findings, prophylactic cholecystectomy is recommended for asymptomatic gallstone patients with diabetes mellitus [20]. Prophylactic cholecystectomy is also recommended for patients undergoing cardiac transplantation but not for those undergoing renal transplantation [21, 22]. Newer therapy in the form of oral dissolution, contact dissolution, and extracorporeal biliary lithotripsy are still in the experimental stage, and are being used less and less frequently in recent years [23]. Some of the preventive measures are known to reduce the incidence of gallstones and accompanying complications. A 30-min exercise 5 times a week reduces symptomatic gallstones by 34% in men [24] and recreational physical activity (jogging, running, bicycling) reduces the incidence of symptomatic gallstones and cholecystectomy significantly in women [25].

References

1. Langenbuch CJA: Ein Fall von Extirpation der Gallenblase wegen chronischer Cholelithiasis. Heilung Berl Klin Wochenscher 1882:19;725–727
2. Deziel DJ. Complications of cholecystectomy. Incidence, clinical manifestations, and diagnosis. Surg Clin North Am 1994;74:809–823
3. Shea JA, Berlin JA, Bachwich DR, Staroscik RN, Malet PF, McGuckin M, Schwartz JS, Escarce JJ. Indications for and outcomes of cholecystectomy: a comparison of the pre and postlaparoscopic eras. Ann Surg 1998;227:343–350
4. Eldar S, Sabo E, Nash E, Abrahamson J, Matter I. Laparoscopic cholecystectomy for the various types of gallbladder inflammation. A prospective trial. Surgical Laparoscopy Endoscopy 1998;8:200–207
5. Lujan JA, Sanchez-Bueno F, Parrilla P, Robles R, Torralba JA, Gonzales-Costea R. Laparoscopic vs open cholecystectomy in patients aged 65 and older. Surgical Laparoscopy Endoscopy 1998;8:208–210
6. Higgins A, London J, Charland S, Ratzer E, Clark J, Haun W, Maher P. Prophylactic antibiotics for elective laparoscopic cholecystectomy. Arch Surg 1999;134:611–614
7. Ranson JHC. Perforation of the gallbladder. In: Way LW, Pelligrini CA. eds. Surgery of the gallbladder and bile ducts. WB Saunders, Philadelphia, 1987, pp 265–273
8. Way LW, Biliary stricture. In: Way LW, Pelligrini CA, eds. Surgery of the gallbladder and bile ducts. WB Saunders, Philadelphia, 1987, pp 419–429
9. Murr MM, Gigot J, Nagorney DM, Harmsen WS, Ilstrup DM, Farnell MB. Long-term results of biliary reconstruction after laparoscopic bile duct injuries. Arch Surg 1999;134:604–610
10. Cheah WK, Goh P, Gagner M, So J. Needlescopic retrograde cholecystectomy. Surgical Laparoscopy Endoscopy 1998;8:237–238
11. Martin RF, Rossi RL. Bile duct injuries. Spectrum, mechanisms of injury, and their prevention Surg Clin North Am 1994;74:781–803
12. MacArthur P, Cuschieri A, Sell RA, Shields R. Controlled clinical trial comparing early with interval cholecystectomy for acute cholecystitis. Br J Surg 1975;62:850–852
13. Fowkes FG, Gunn AA. The management of acute cholecystitis and its hospital cost. Br J Surg 1980;67:613–617
14. Lo CM, Liu CL, Fan ST, Lai EC, Wong J. Prospective randomized study of early versus delayed laparoscopic cholecystectomy for acute cholecystitis. Ann Surg 1998;227:461–467
15. Hunter JG. Acute cholecystitis revisited: get it while it's hot. Ann Surg 1998,227:468–469
16. Elboim CM, Goldman L, Hann L. Significance of post-cholecystectomy subhepatic fluid collection. Ann Surg 1983;198:137–141
17. Gilsdorf TR, Phillips M, McLeod MK, Gregg RO. Radionuclide evaluation of bile leakage and the use of subhepatic drains after cholecystectomy. Am J Surg 1986;156:259–262
18. Shreiner DP, Sarva RP, Van Thiel D, Yingvorapant N. Gallbladder function in diabetic patients. J Nucl Med 1986;27:357–360
19. Fisher RS, Stelzer F, Rock E, Malmud LS. Abnormal gallbladder emptying in patients with gallstones. Dig Dis Sci 1982;27:1019–1024

20. Ransohoff DF, Miller GL, Forsythe SB, Hermann RE. Outcome of acute cholecystitis in patients with diabetes mellitus. Ann Intern Med 1987;106:829–832
21. Menegaux F, Dorent R, Tabbi D, Pavie A, Chigot J, Gandjbakhch I. Biliary surgery after heart transplantation. Am J Surg 1998;175:320–321
22. Melvin WS, Meier DJ, Elkhammas EA, Bumgardner GL, Davies EA, Henry ML, Pelletier R, Ferguson RM. Prophylactic cholecystectomy is not indicated following renal transplantation. Am J Surg 1998;175:317–319
23. Johnston DE, Kaplan MM. Pathogenesis and treatment of gallstones. N Engl J Med 1993;328:412–421
24. Leitzmann MF, Giovannucci EL, Rimm EB, Stampfer MJ, Spiegelman D, Wing AL, Willett WC. The relation of physical activity to risk for symptomatic gallstone disease in men. Ann Intern Med 1998;128:417–425
25. Leitzmann MF, Rimm EB, Willet WC, Spiegelman D, Grodstein F, Stampfer MJ, Colditz GA, Giovannucci E. Recreational physical activity and the risk of cholecystectomy in women. N Engl J Med 1999;341:777–784

Biliary Dyskinesia

Biliary dyskinesia consists primarily of two disease entities, sphincter of Oddi spasm (SOS) and cystic duct syndrome (CDS). These two entities are anatomically separate but physiologically related by an abnormal functional response to cholecystokinin. Sphincter of Oddi spasm is located within the sphincter at the distal end of the common bile duct, and cystic duct syndrome is confined mostly to the cystic duct of the gallbladder [1, 2]. In the literature, sphincter of Oddi spasm is also known by such names as papillary stenosis or bile duct dyskinesia, and cystic duct syndrome as chronic acalculous cholecystitis. Both the sphincter of Oddi and gallbladder contain receptors for cholecystokinin which is released endogenously into circulation from the intestinal mucosa upon entry of food into the duodenum [3, 4]. By binding to CCK-A type receptors, cholecystokinin normally stimulates the contraction of the gallbladder with simultaneous relaxation of the sphincter of Oddi. The cystic duct, which also contains CCK receptors, normally does not respond, because its serum threshold for contraction is set at a much higher level than the threshold for contraction of the fundus and body of the gallbladder [5]. Controversy over the existence of the entity of biliary dyskinesia prevailed for many years [6]. The availability of manometric studies has helped to understand the basic sphincter mechanism and the action of cholecystokinin on it in both health (Chap. 6) and disease, especially in patients with SOS (Table 10.1.1). A clear understanding of the bile secretion and flow mechanisms and the pathophysiologic changes associated with biliary dyskinesia are now complete due to the availability of quantitative cholescintigraphy and biliary manometry [7–9].

Pathophysiology

A normal sphincter of Oddi exhibits an average of 6–7 contractions/min with a wave amplitude of 113 mmHg. The mean pressure in the sphincter of Oddi is about 14.9 mmHg, and 8.6 mmHg in the common bile duct. About 54% of the contraction waves progress antegrade, 18% retrograde, and 28% occur simultaneously in the proximal, middle, and caudal segment of the sphincter (Table 10.1.1). Administration of cholecystokinin abolishes the contraction waves and relaxes the sphincter of Oddi immediately, promoting smooth passage of bile emptied from the gallbladder into the duodenum (Fig. 10.1.1). Sphincter of Oddi spasm is characterized manometrically by an increase in basal pressure of the sphincter to 37 mmHg, and that in the common bile duct to 17 mmHg. The total number of basal contractions increase to 17/min and the number of retrograde contractions increases to 41% (Fig. 10.1.2A). Usually dormant contractile receptors in the sphincter become activated. These activated (otherwise

Table 10.1.1. Biliary pressure profile in asymptomatic control subjects and patients with sphincter of Oddi spasm

Structure	Control subjects (n=9)	SOS patients (n=10)	P value
CBD pressure (mmHg)	8.6±1.02 (6–13)	17.0±1.25 (12–22)	0.001
Sphincter of Oddi pressure (mmHg)	14.9±0.99 (11–21)	36.9±5.44 (20–70)	0.005
Phasic contractions			
Amplitude (mmHg)	113.0±8.6 (95–125)	109.5±9.3 (85–160)	0.37
Frequency (/min)	6.89±0.20	7.56±0.41	0.46
Direction of propagation			
Antegrade	54%±6%	29%±7%	0.04
Simultaneous	28%±4%	30%±3%	0.34
Retrograde	18%±6%	41%±9%	0.01

Values are means ± SE, ranges in parentheses (adopted from Meshkinpour et al. [9])

dormant) receptors paradoxically induce contraction of the sphincter in response to cholecystokinin [10, 11]. Cholecystokinin administration increases both the number of waves and the number of retrograde waves per minute (Fig. 10.1.2B). Because of this paradoxical response (contraction) of the sphincter, the bile either fails empty from the gallbladder, or the emptied bile refluxes into the common hepatic duct and right and left hepatic ducts, and reenters the gallbladder soon after cessation of CCK-8 infusion [12].

Cystic duct syndrome is characterized by kinking, fibrosis, and thickening of the wall with narrowing of the cystic duct lumen [13]. Hepatic bile enters the gallbladder slowly but cannot get out readily in response to cholecystokinin (Chap. 9.2). Due to a decrease in the total number of CCK receptors, there is poor contraction and emptying of the gallbladder, postmeal [14, 15]. The threshold of the cystic duct for contraction is presumably lowered, which results in its contraction when cholecystokinin is released. The duodenal bile in patients with cystic duct syndrome is more dilute and contains fewer bile acids than in normal subjects [16].

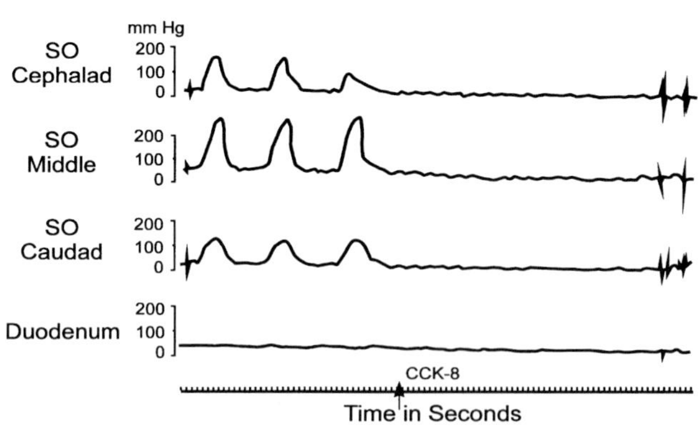

Fig. 10.1.1. Action of CCK-8 on normal sphincter of Oddi. Normal contraction waves are abolished immediately after CCK-8 administration, which facilitates dilatation of the sphincter for smooth passage of bile through it [11]

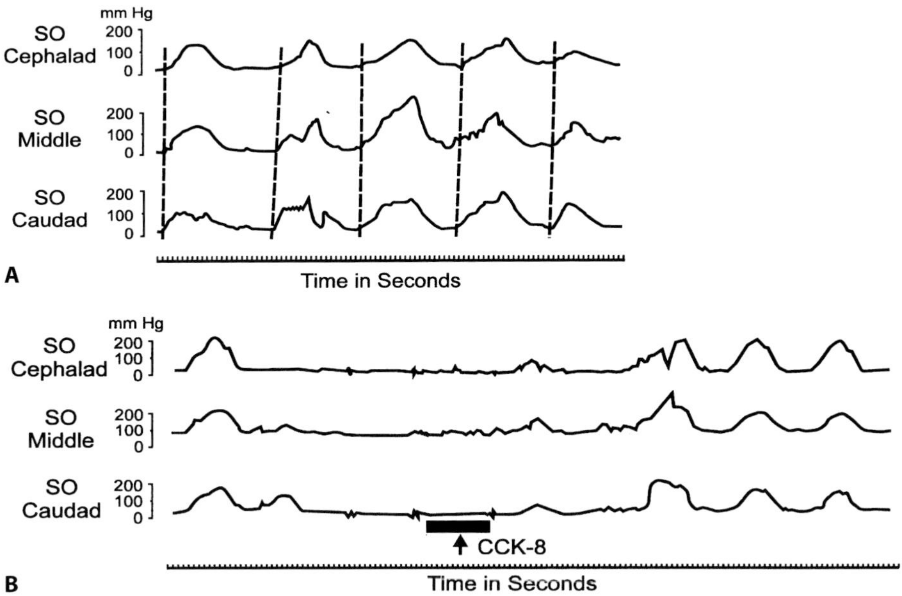

Fig. 10.1.2A,B. Propagation of contraction waves and effect of CCK-8 on the sphincter in SOS. Contraction begins first at the caudal end and travels retrograde towards the middle and cephalic end of the sphincter (A). Administration of CCK-8 paradoxically increases the number of retrograde contractions (B) resulting in closure of the sphincter [11]

Clinical Presentation

Biliary dyskinesia patients are mostly women in their 3rd or 4th decade of life. They present with postprandial right upper quadrant or epigastric pain. Pain usually begins 30 min after a meal and reaches its peak intensity 2–3 h later. Liver function tests and blood counts remain within the normal range. The gallbladder and intrahepatic and extrahepatic bile ducts are morphologically normal and gallstones are absent. On the ultrasound examination, the size of the common hepatic duct and common bile duct remains within the normal range early in the course of the disease. Because of these normal biochemical and morphologic findings, the diagnosis of biliary dyskinesia is frequently delayed for months or years and patients often go from physician to physician seeking relief of postprandial abdominal pain.

Cholescintigraphic Diagnosis

Biliary manometry is considered the gold standard. It is invasive, expensive, and not readily available in most community hospitals. Cholescintigraphy provides a non-invasive alternative. Imaging and quantitative analysis are carried out by acquiring data in two separate phases: hepatic phase and gallbladder phase. Patients are studied after 8–10 h of fasting, for a minimum of 4 h. A detailed clinical and drug history is taken to exclude the intake of opioids, smooth muscle relaxants, calcium channel blockers or other drugs which act either on the sphincter of Oddi or gallbladder. In hypertensive patients, calcium channel blockers are discontinued for 2–3 days prior to the test. With the patient in the supine position, a large field of view gamma camera fitted with a low energy, all purpose, parallel hole collimator is positioned anteriorly and 3–5 mCi (111-185 MBq) ^{99m}Tc-HIDA is injected intravenously. The data are acquired on the computer at one frame/min for 60 min [17–19]. Hepatic phase images usually appear normal (Fig. 10.1.3A) unless the disease is far advanced, when there may be bile stasis in extrahepatic ducts and delay in entry of bile into the duodenum. If

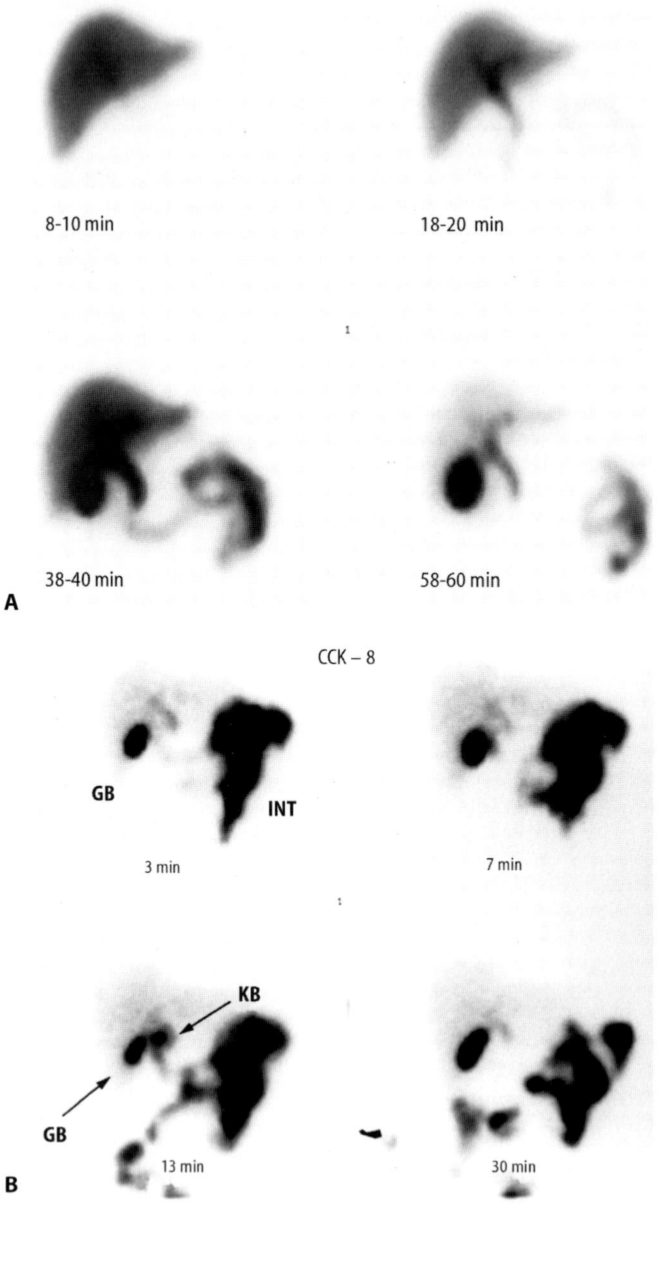

Fig. 10.1.3. Cholescintigraphy in SOS. The uptake and excretion of ^{99m}Tc-HIDA are normal with delineation of the gallbladder and entire biliary tree. Bile enters the small intestine normally **(A)**. After CCK-8 infusion, the gallbladder contracts and empties bile which refluxes into the common hepatic duct (*KB*). Refluxed bile reenters the gallbladder immediately after cessation of CCK-8 infusion **(B)**

the gallbladder is not seen by 60 min, delayed images are obtained at 3–4 h after injection of a second dose of ^{99m}Tc-HIDA. Injection of opioids to induce contraction of the sphincter of Oddi to fill the gallbladder early is avoided.

Gallbladder Phase Imaging

The data are acquired with the gamma camera. Hepatic phase images are carefully scrutinized for superimposition of duodenal or common bile duct radioactivity over the gallbladder. If there is any superimposition, the gamma camera angle is altered to separate the gallbladder from other structures. Often this may require changing the gamma camera angle by 10°–15° to the left or right anterior oblique position. The data are collected at one frame/min for 30 min, between 61 and 90 min after injection of ^{99m}Tc-HIDA (when the gallbladder fills within 60 min). Cholecystokinin at a dose of 10 ng/kg (0.01 μg/kg) is infused intravenously over 3 min (3.3 ng/kg/min for 3 min), beginning at 65 min after HIDA injection (Fig. 10.1.3B). The patient's symptoms (nausea, abdominal cramps, and/or pain) are monitored carefully and their time of onset and relief are noted on the gallbladder time/activity curve (Fig. 10.1.4). Gallbladder

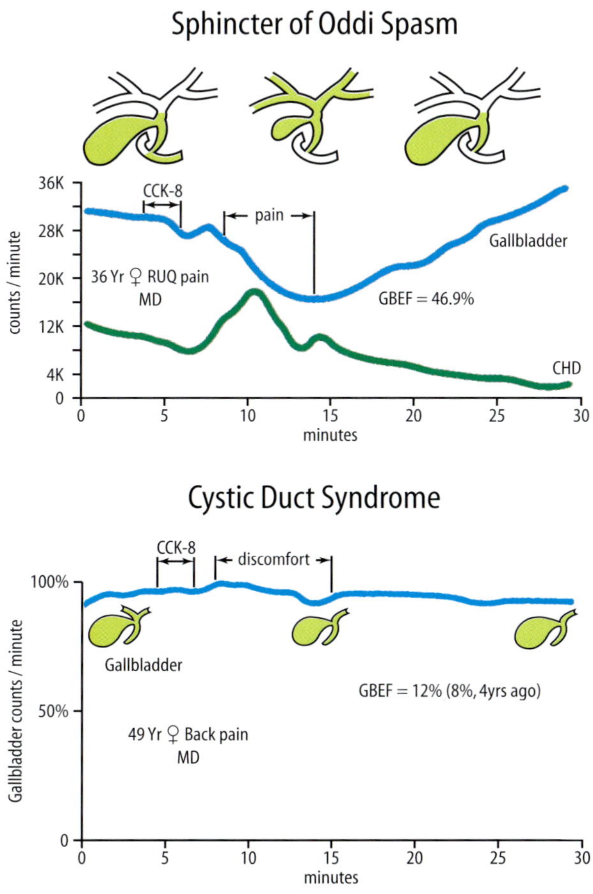

Fig. 10.1.4. Biliary dynamics in biliary dyskinesia. In the case of sphincter of Oddi spasm, the gallbladder contracts and empties bile which refluxes into the common hepatic and intrahepatic ducts. Most of the refluxed bile reenters the gallbladder (*top*). In patients with cystic duct syndrome, the gallbladder empties poorly and no refilling occurs (*bottom*). Pain or discomfort occurs mostly during the gallbladder ejection period [12]

ejection fraction, ejection period, and ejection rate are calculated by drawing an ROI'S over the gallbladder, common hepatic duct including right hepatic and left hepatic ducts, common bile duct, duodenum, and background over the liver [17–19]. The gallbladder, common hepatic duct (including right and left hepatic ducts), common bile duct, and duodenum and their corresponding curves are scrutinized carefully. Sphincter of Oddi spasm is differentiated from cystic duct syndrome by careful analysis of both the image pattern and quantitative functional parameters [12].

Sphincter of Oddi Spasm

Cholescintigraphic findings vary depending upon the presence or absence of the native gallbladder. There is usually no bile pooling within the intrahepatic ducts, a feature distinctly different from those with stricture of the common bile duct [17]. Several types of functional abnormalities have been shown by different authors depending upon the method of data collection and analysis [20, 21]. Shaffer et al. measured hepatobiliary peak uptake time and calculated percentage excretion at 45, 60, and 90 min. Cholecystokinin at a dose of 0.02 units/kg/min was infused slowly between 60 and 90 min. The region of interest included both the liver and bile ducts. In 22 subjects with previous cholecystectomy with no current symptoms (control), hepatobiliary mean peak time was 9.8±0.7 min. Percentage excretion at 45, 60, and 90 min was 50.6±3.6, 66.3±2.8, and 84.7±1.3, respectively. Emptying rates in 0–60 min and 60–90 min (after CCK) were 1.46±0.07/min, and 0.73±0.6/min, respectively. In nine patients with postcholecystectomy SOS, mean peak time was increased to 23 min, and percentage excretions at 45 and 60 min decreased to 20 and 39, respectively. Emptying rate between 0 and 60 min was 1.05±0.13/min and increased to 1.12±0.19/min after CCK infusion between 60 and 90 min [21]. Most of the functional parameters improved after papillotomy (Fig. 10.1.5). Others have shown prolongation of hepatic hilum to duodenal transit time [22, 23].

The hepatic phase images appear normal in most patients with early SOS with an intact gallbladder (Fig. 10.1.3A). The gallbladder shows a normal or a slightly reduced ejection fraction with CCK-8. Cholescintigraphy in SOS is characterized by reflux of gallbladder bile into the common hepatic and right and left hepatic ducts with reentry of refluxed bile into the gallbladder immediately after cessation of CCK-8 infusion (Fig. 10.1.4). The curve shows rapid refilling of the gallbladder almost to its original volume, often even exceeding the original volume due to stimulation and expulsion of hepatic bile by cholecystokinin. Intrahepatic and extrahepatic bile ducts can accommodate almost all of 40–50 ml bile emptied from the gallbladder, without being dilated. Common hepatic duct bile reflux also occurs in patients with stenosis of the common bile duct and is referred to as the Krishnamurthy-Bobba sign, after the original authors [24]. When patients complain of pain during the gallbladder dynamic phase, the pain duration usually corresponds to the gallbladder ejection period. Not every patient with biliary dyskinesia, however, complains of pain at the time of the study. The extrahepatic ducts may appear early and persist for a longer duration, resulting in a marked delay in peak hepatic uptake in advanced cases [22, 25].

Sphincter of Oddi spasm is differentiated from anatomic stricture of the common bile duct by assessing both the image pattern and quantitative curve analysis after a pharmacologic intervention. Amyl nitrite, nitric oxide, or nifedipine relieve the spasm

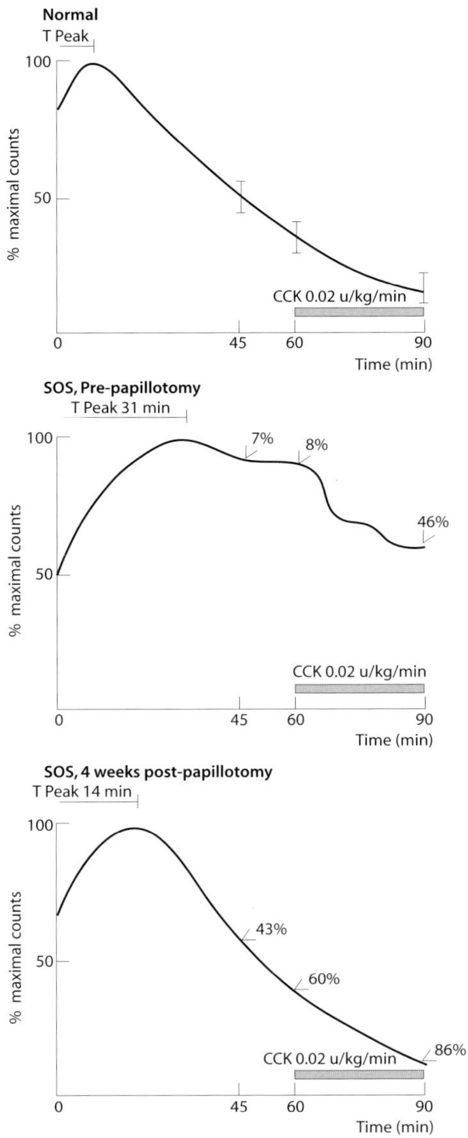

Fig. 10.1.5. Hepatic bile clearance in SOS. Normally, peak uptake of ^{99m}Tc-HIDA occurs within 10 min and 66% is excreted within 60 min. CCK enhances excretion. In patients with SOS, the peak is delayed and 60-min excretion is decreased. CCK administration has only a partial effect before papillotomy. Both uptake and excretion improve after papillotomy [21]

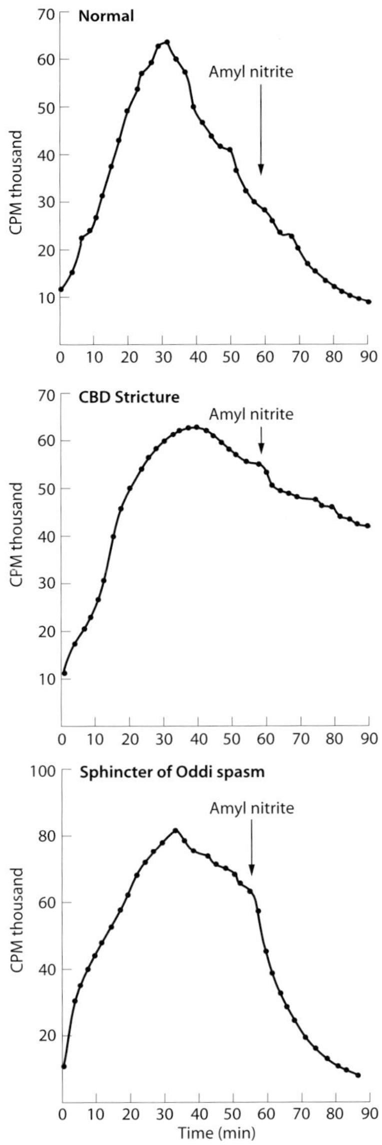

Fig. 10.1.6. Cholescintigraphic differentiation of SOS from CBD stricture. The normal common bile duct time/activity curve shows an early peak with rapid decline before and after amyl nitrite (*top*). The peak is delayed in both stricture and SOS. Following amyl nitrite, there is a rapid decline in patients with SOS (*bottom*), but not with stricture (*middle*) [26]

and dilate the sphincter, promoting rapid bile flow through it in the case of SOS, but not in patients with an anatomic stricture (Fig. 10.1.6) of the common bile duct [26–28]. The sensitivity of cholescintigraphy in SOS varies from 70% to 90% [29].

Cystic Duct Syndrome

Cystic duct syndrome is characterized often by a slow filling of the gallbladder during the hepatic phase with a poor emptying response to cholecystokinin in the gallbladder phase (See also Chapter 9.2). Although most of the gallbladders appear within 60 min after injection of ^{99m}Tc-HIDA, some are delayed for 3–4 h. A reduction in gallbladder ejection fraction below 35% with 10 ng/kg/3 min CCK-8 dose is the salient feature. Many patients, but not all, experience mild to moderate intensity abdominal pain during the gallbladder ejection period. The gallbladder curve appears flat in patients with ejection fractions below 15%, and it is often difficult to note the exact time of onset and end of gallbladder emptying (Fig. 10.1.4). There is usually no bile reflux into the intrahepatic or extrahepatic ducts, and the gallbladder curve does not show refilling after cessation of CCK-8 infusion [12, 18]. The direction of the latter half of the curve is assessed carefully to make sure that there is no refilling of the gallbladder, which will suggest SOS. A large, non-physiological CCK-8 dose when given as a rapid intravenous bolus often produces low ejection fraction and abdominal pain in many of the normal subjects, mimicking cystic duct syndrome. This effect is attributed to exceeding the cystic duct threshold for contraction and should be avoided.

Differentiation of SOS from CDS

The differentiation is critical for appropriate patient management because cholecystectomy is the preferred treatment for CDS and antispasmodics or sphincterotomy for SOS. Cholecystectomy for SOS is inappropriate and may make the patient condition worse by taking away its low pressure reservoir function [30]. Both conditions are relatively more common in women than men. Proper attention is given during patient preparation, data collection, and analysis. The hepatic phase imaging data appear similar in both conditions and there is bile entry into the duodenum in early cases. Only during the gallbladder phase is a difference seen between SOS and CDS. Cholecystokinin induced bile reflux into common hepatic duct (Krishnamurthy-Bobba sign) and paradoxical refilling of the gallbladder are typical for SOS. In the authors' experience, the other condition that may cause such a paradoxical filling is hyperacute (within 48 h) critical obstruction of the common bile duct (Chap. 8). Cholecystokinin stimulates bile secretion by cholangiocytes lining intrahepatic bile ducts and expels bile from the liver by inducing contraction of the bile ducts. The hepatic bile is forced to enter the gallbladder in the presence of critical obstruction of the common bile duct. Other features of hyperacute obstruction include its acute clinical presentation, abnormal liver function tests, and no bile entry into the duodenum during the hepatic phase. On rare occasions, superimposition of jejunal or ileal loops over the gallbladder region of interest may cause false elevation of the gallbladder curve, which is readily recognized with the cine display of the gallbladder phase data. Patients with CDS do not exhibit paradoxical filling of the gallbladder and there is no bile reflux into intrahepatic ducts (Fig. 10.1.7).

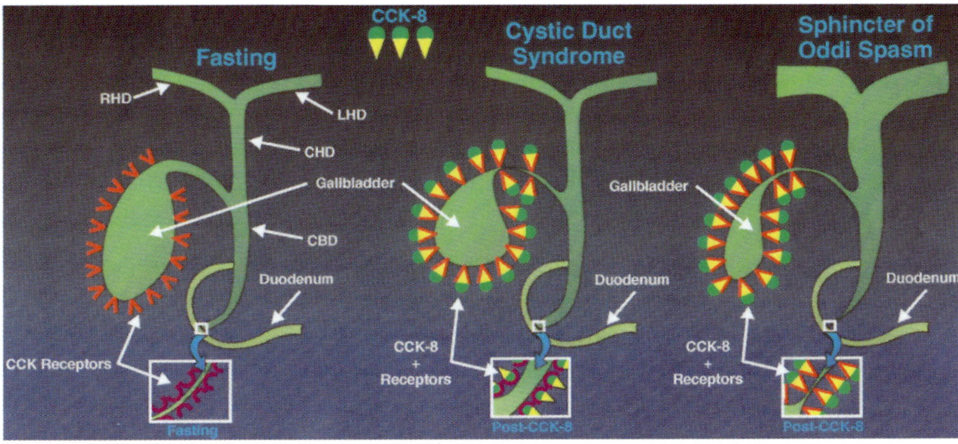

Fig. 10.1.7. Differentiation of CDS from SOS. Cholecystokin (CCK) receptors on the gallbladder smooth mucle remain free in the fasting state (left). In cystic duct syndrome (middle), the gallbladder empties poorly in response to CCK-8 infusion due to a decrease in the total number of CCK receptors in the gallbladder body and fundus and activation of contractile receptors in the cystic duct. In the case of the sphincter of Oddi spasm (right), the sphincter contracts due to activation of the contractile receptors, and the bile emptied from the gallbladder refluxes into the common hepatic and intrahepatic ducts, later reentering the gallbladder (CCK induced paradoxical filling of the gallbladder) after cessation of CCK-8 infusion [12]

Treatment

Treatment for SOS is different from that of CDS. A normal sphincter of Oddi function is modulated by local generation of nitric oxide [27]. Medical treatment with nitrites, nitrates, calcium channel blockers (nifedipine), or other smooth muscle relaxants has been shown to relieve the spasm and dilate the sphincter in patients with SOS [28]. Endoscopic sphincterotomy is reserved for those patients who fail to respond to medical therapy. Sphincterotomy is invasive, expensive, and carries a high rate of procedural complications. An overall endoscopic sphincterotomy complication rate in 2347 patients from 17 institutions in a multicenter study in the United States has been reported to be 9.8%. The complication rate is much higher (21.7%) in patients with sphincter of Oddi dysfunction [31]. Acute pancreatitis (5.4%) and hemorrhage (2.0%) account for the great majority of complications. Special training, a large number of patients, and more frequent sphincterotomy reduce the complication rate [32]. Sphincteroplasty through endoscopic balloon dilatation is shown to be effective in patients with bile duct stones [33]. However, its role in sphincter of Oddi spasm has not been studied. Cholecystectomy is a relative contraindication in SOS. An intact gallbladder acts as a reservoir and accommodates bile that fails to pass through the sphincter in patients with SOS. Cholecystectomy takes away this reservoir function and the symptoms persist or may even become worse, manifesting a postcholecystectomy syndrome [30, 34]. The patient with SOS shown in Fig 10.1.4 responded to antispasmodies and the patient with CDS got relief of abdominal pain after laparoscopic cholecystectomy.

Cholecystectomy

Cholecystectomy is the treatment of choice for CDS. Due to its low morbidity and low mortality, laparoscopic cholecystectomy has become more popular and has replaced open cholecystectomy as the preferred therapy [35]. Of a total of 320 patients with CDS who underwent cholecystectomy solely on the basis of a gallbladder low ejection fraction, 90% had relief of abdominal pain [36–42]. Histopathological examinations showed microscopic changes of disease in the gallbladder wall or cystic duct in 90% of patients (Table 9.2.1 of Chap. 9). Abdominal pain is known to persist in about 20% of patients undergoing cholecystectomy for various reasons [43]. Recent studies seem to suggest that the majority of these patients belong to SOS. Clinically SOS is divided into three types. Only type I responds to endoscopic sphincterotomy and type II and III have a varied response. Type III is considered a duodenal visceral hyperalgesia and the pain may not originate from the biliary tree at all [44].

Postcholecystectomy Syndrome

Postcholecystectomy syndrome can now be considered an iatrogenic disease exaggerated by an inappropriate therapy (cholecystectomy) for patients with SOS. Removal of the gallbladder, which serves as a low pressure reservoir by accommodating hepatic bile, exaggerates the symptoms in patients with SOS. This syndrome can now be studied non-invasively by combining magnetic resonance cholangiopancreatography (MRCP) with quantitative cholescintigraphy. Rubini and Dimonte reported five patients with postcholecystectomy syndrome and showed dilatation of the common hepatic and common bile ducts in four, and the cystic duct remnant in three (two remnants with gallstones) on MRCP. Cholescintigraphy showed bile pooling in both intrahepatic and extrahepatic ducts with no bile entry into the duodenum at 60 min in all five patients. Bile did not enter the duodenum for another 60 min after a high fat meal. Both peak hepatic uptake time and excretion half-time were increased. Hepatic extraction fraction stayed above 80%, suggesting primarily a biliary disease. All four patients who underwent endoscopic sphincterotomy responded well with relief of symptoms [45].

Pitfalls

Cholescintigraphy plays an important role in the evaluation of patients with biliary dyskinesia. A clear understanding of the mechanism of bile secretion and flow and factors that alter bile flow is important in arriving at a proper diagnosis. Functional imaging and measurement of parameters quantitatively require appropriate patient preparation and attention to technical details during data acquisition and analysis. Unlike the left ventricle, the gallbladder ejection fraction can be controlled to any desired level simply by controlling the dose, dose rate, and duration of infusion of cholecystokinin. Cholecystokinin is available in two different molecular forms: an intact molecule with 33 amino acids (CCK-33) and a fragment with 8 amino acids (CCK-8). The dose recommended in the package insert of CCK-8 (Kinevac) kit is found to be too large and often elicits a non-physiologic response during cholescintigraphy [46–48]. The dose should be reduced for cholescintigraphy (Chap. 6). When cholecystokinin is not available, the test is standardized using a fatty meal stimulation, where the total calorie, fat, carbohydrate, and protein contents are controlled strictly for the chosen meal. Use of

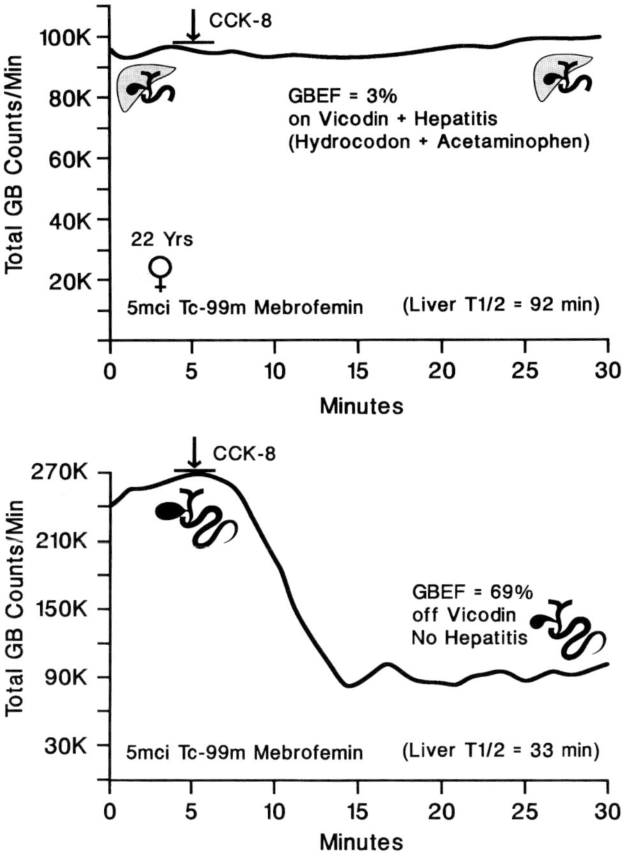

Fig. 10.1.8. Effect of opioids on gallbladder ejection fraction. A patient on vicodin for pain during viral hepatitis A shows slow clearance of the radiotracer from the liver ($T_{1/2}$ = 92 min) and an ejection fraction of only 3% (*top*). Both the clearance and ejection fraction return to normal after discontinuation of vicodin and recovery from hepatics (*bottom*)

opioids for pain is common in both inpatients and outpatients and their use reduces the gallbladder ejection fraction, which returns to normal after discontinuation (Fig. 10.1.8). A commitment to high technical quality control and direct interaction with the patient before, during, and after the procedure results in the best clinical outcome [49].

References

1. Oddi R. D'une disposition a sphincter specille del'ouverture du canal cholidoque. Arch Ital Biol 1887;8:317–322
2. Cozzolino HJ, Goldstein F, Greening RR. The cystic duct syndrome. JAMA 1963;185:920–924
3. Ivy AC, Oldberg E. A hormone mechanism of gallbladder contraction and evacuation. Am J Physiology 1928;86:599–613
4. Sjolund K, Sanden G, Hakanson R, Sundler F: Endocrine cells in human intestine: An immunocytochemical study. Gastroenterology 1983;85:1120–1130
5. Courtney DF, Clanachan AS, Scott GW: Cholecystokinin constricts the canine cystic duct. Gastroenterology 1983;85:1154–1159

6. Steinberg WM. Sphincter of Oddi dysfunction: A clinical controversy. Gastroenterology 1988;95:1409–1415
7. Geenen JE, Hogan WJ, Dodds WJ, Stewart ET, Arndorfer RC. Intraluminal pressure recording from the human sphincter of Oddi. Gastroenterology 1980;78:317–324
8. Thune A, Scicchitano J, Thompson IR, Toouli J: Reproducibility of endoscopic sphincter of Oddi manometry. Dig Dis Sci 1991;36:1401–1405
9. Meshkinpour H, Mollot M, Eckerling GB, Bookman. Bile duct dyskinesia. Clinical and manometric study. Gastroenterology 1984;87:759–762
10. Hogan WJ, Geenen JE: Biliary dyskinesia: Endoscopy 1988;20:179–183
11. Toouli J, Roberts-Thompson IC, Dent J, Lee J. Manometric disorders in patients with suspected sphincter of Oddi dysfunction. Gastroenterology 1985;88 :1243–1250
12. Krishnamurthy S, Krishnamuthy GT. Biliary dyskinesia: role of the sphincter of Oddi, gallbladder, and cholecystokinin. J Nucl Med 1997;38:1824–1830
13. Goldstein F, Grunt R, Margulies M. Cholecystokinin cholescintigraphy in the differential diagnosis of acalculous gallbladder disease. Digestive Diseases 1974;19:835–849
14. Upp JR, Nealon WH, Singh P, Fagan CJ, Jonas AS, Greeley GH, Thompson JC: Correlation of cholecystokinin receptor with gallbladder contractility in patients with gallstones. Ann Surg 1987;205:641–648
15. Steigerwalt RW, Goldfine ID, Williams JA: Characterization of cholecystokinin receptors on bovine gallbladder membranes. Am J Physiol 1984;247:G709–G714
16. Venkataramani A, Strong RM, Anderson DS, Gilmore IT, Stokes K, Hoffman AF. Abnormal duodenal bile composition in patients with acalculous chronic cholecystitis. Am J Gastroenterol 1998;93:434–441
17. Krishnamurthy GT, Bobba VR, McConnell D, et al: Quantitative biliary dynamics: Introduction of a new noninvasive scintigraphic technique. J Nucl Med 1983;24:217–223
18. Krishnamurthy S, Krishnamurthy GT. Evolution of nuclear hepatology as a clinical subspeciality. J Nucl Med Technol 1995;23:35S–45S
19. Krishnamurthy S, Krishnamurthy GT. Technetium-99m-iminodiacetic acid organic anions: Review of biokinetics and clinical application in hepatology. Hepatology 1989;9:139–153
20. Cicala M, Scopinaro F, Corzziari E, Viscardi A, Habib FI, Torsoli A. Quantitative cholescintigraphy in the assessment of choledochoduodenal bile flow. Gastroenterology 1991;100:1106–1113
21. Shaffer EA, Hershfield NB, Logan K, Kloiber R: Cholescintigraphic detection of functional obstruction of the sphincter of Oddi. Effect of papillotomy. Gastroenterology 1986;90:728–733
22. Fullarton GM, Hilditch T, Campbell A, Murray WR: Clinical and scintigraphic assessment of the role of endoscopic sphincterotomy in the treatment of sphincter of Oddi dysfunction. Gut 1990;31:231–235
23. Drane WE, Johnson DA. Sincalide-augmented quantitative hepatobiliary scintigraphy (QHBS): Definition of normal parameters and preliminary relation between QHBS and sphincter of Oddi (SO) manometry in patients suspected of having SO dysfunction. J Nucl Med 1990;31:1462–1468
24. Brar HS. Scintigraphic cholecystokinin-induced bile reflux named as Krishnamurthy-Bobba sign. J Nucl Med 1990;31:248
25. Sostre S, Kalloo AN, Spiegler EJ, Camargo EE, Wagner HN Jr. A noninvasive test of sphincter of Oddi dysfunction in post-cholecystectomy patients: The scintigraphic score. J Nucl Med 1992;33:1216–1222
26. Madacsy L, Velosy B, Lonovics J, Csernay L. Differentiation between organic and functional dyskinesia of the sphincter of Oddi with amyl nitrite-augmented quantitative hepatobiliary scintigraphy, Eur J Nucl Med 1994;21:203–208
27. Mourelle M, Guarner F, Moncada S, Malagelada JR. The arginine/nitric oxide pathway modulates sphincter of Oddi motor activity in guinea pigs and rabbits. Gastroenterology 1993;105:1299–1305
28. Bhatnagar A. Nifedifine interventional cholescintigraphy: a new method for assessing sphincter of Oddi? Indian J Nucl Med 1997;12:93–96
29. Dodds WJ, Thakur S, Collier RD. Quantitative hepatobiliary scintigraphy (editorial). J Nucl Med 1990;31:1468–1469
30. Tanaka M, Ikeda S, Nakayama F. Change in bile duct pressure response after cholecystectomy: loss of gallbladder as a pressure reservoir. Gastroenterology 1984.87:1154–1159
31. Freeman ML, Nelson DB. Sherman S, Haber GB, Herman ME, Dorsher PJ, Moore JP, Fennerty B, Ryan ME, Shaw MJ, Lande JD, Pheley AM. Complications of endoscopic biliary sphincterotomy. N Engl J Med 1996;335:909–918
32. Huibregtse K. Complications of endoscopic sphincterotomy and their prevention. N Engl J Med 1996;335:961–962

33. Mathuna PM, White P, Clarke E, Merriman R, Lennon JR, Crowe J. Endoscopic balloon sphinctero-plasty (papillary dilatation) for bile duct stones: efficacy, safety, and follow-up in 100 patients. Gastrointest Endosc 1995;42:468–474
34. Gregg JA, Clark G, Barr C, McCartney A, Milano A, Volcjak C. Postcholecystectomy syndrome and its association with ampullary stenosis. Am J Surg 1980;139:374–378
35. Frassinelli P, Werner M, Reed III JF, Scagliotti C. Laparoscopic cholecystectomy alleviates pain in patients with acalculous biliary diseases. Surgical Laparoscopy Endoscopy 1998;8:30–34
36. Pickelman J, Peiss RL, Henkin R, Salo B, Nagel P. The role of sincalide cholescintigraphy in the evaluation of patients with acalculous gallbladder disease. Arch Surg 1985;120:693–697
37. Fink-Bennet D, DeRidder P, Kolozsi WZ, Gordon R, Jaros R. Cholecystokinin cholescintigraphy: Detection of abnormal gallbladder motor function in patients with chronic acalculous gallbladder disease. J Nucl Med 1991;32:1695–1699
38. Zech ER, Simmons LB, Kendrick RR, et al. Cholecystokinin enhanced hepatobiliary scanning with ejection fraction calculation as an indicator of disease of the gallbladder. Surg Gynecol Obstet 1991;172:21–24
39. Misra DC, Blossom GB, Fink-Bennet D, et al. Results of surgical therapy for biliary dyskinesia. Arch Surg 1991;126:957–960
40. Halverson JD, Garner BA, Siegel BA, et al. The use of hepatobiliary scintigraphy in patients with acalculous biliary disease. Arch Intern Med 1992;152:1305–1309
41. Sorenson MK, Francher S, Lang NP, Eidt JF, Broadwater JR. Abnormal gallbladder nuclear ejection fraction predicts success of cholecystectomy in patients with biliary dyskinesia. Am J Surg 1993;166:672–675
42. Kleiger PS, O'Mara RE. The clinical utility of quantitative cholescintigraphy: the significance of gallbladder dysfunction. Clin Nucl Med 1998;23:278–282
43. Black NA, Thompson E, Sanderson CFB, ECHSS group. Symptoms and health status before and 6 weeks after open cholecystectomy: a European cohort study. Gut 1994;35:1301–1305
44. Desautels SG, Slivka A, Hutson WR, Chun A, Mitrani C, DiLorenzo C, Wald A. Postcholecystectomy pain syndrome: pathophysiology of abdominal pain in sphincter of Oddi type III. Gastroenterology 1999;116:900–905
45. Rubini G, Dmonte M. Postcholecystectomy syndrome. Evaluation by biliary cholescintigraphy and MR cholangiopancreatography. Clin Nucl Med 1999;24:784–789
46. Krishnamurthy GT, Bobba VR, Kingston E: Optimization of octapeptide of cholecystokinin (OP-CCK) dose for gallbladder emptying. In: Raynaud C, ed. Proceedings of the Third World Congress of Nuclear Medicine and Biology. Paris, France: Pergamon Press; 1982, pp 2224–2247
47. Toftdahl DB, Hojgaard L, Winkler K: Dynamic cholescintigraphy: Induction and description of gallbladder emptying. J Nucl Med 1996;37:261–266
48. Ziessman HA, Fahey FH, Hixon DJ. Calculation of a gallbladder ejection fraction: advantage of continuous Sincalide infusion over the 3-minute infusion method. J Nucl Med 1992;33:537–541
49. Krishnamurthy S, Krishnamurthy GT. Gallbladder ejection fraction: a decade of progress and future promise (editorial). J Nucl Med 1992;32;542–544

Pediatric Nuclear Hepatology

The liver and biliary system develop from a bilobed (cephalic and caudal) endodermal bud that sprouts along the ventral surface of the distal end of the foregut at its junction with the midgut. The cephalic bud divides into two branches which later form the right and left lobes of the liver. The caudal bud gives rise to the biliary tract and the gallbladder (Fig. 1.1.1, Chap. 1). The biliary tract starts first as a patent tubular structure but turns into a solid core during early intrauterine life due to proliferation of epithelial cells. After recanalization of the solid core by 12–14 weeks, bile secretion begins and flows into the small intestine. Most of the congenital abnormalities of the biliary tract are due to either failure of re-canalization of ducts (biliary atresia) or faulty re-canalization with cystic dilatation of intrahepatic (Caroli's disease) and extrahepatic ducts (choledochal cyst).

Physiologic jaundice usually clears within 2 weeks after birth. Therefore the jaundice which persists beyond 2 weeks in a neonate raises several possibilities (Table 11.1.1), some requiring immediate intervention while others may be managed by careful follow-up without a specific therapy. Neonatal hepatitis and congenital biliary atresia are two of the diseases that account for the great majority of persistent jaundice beyond 2 weeks after birth

Table 11.1.1. Causes of persistent jaundice beyond 2 weeks after birth

1. Neonatal hepatitis
   - Viral
     - Cytomegalovirus
     - Hepatitis B
     - Rubella
     - Herpes
     - Coxsackie
   - Bacterial
     - *E. coli*
     - *Klebsiella*
     - *Pseudomonas*
     - *Proteus*
     - *Bacteroides*
     - *Streptococcus*
     - *Treponema pallidum*
   - Parasitic
     - *Toxoplasma gondii*
2. Biliary atresia
   - Extrahepatic ducts (congenital biliary atresia)
   - Intrahepatic ducts.
     - Congenital rubella
     - Trisomy 17
     - Trisomy 18
     - Alagille's syndrome (arteriohepatic dysplasia)
3. Genetic or metabolic
   - Alpha$_1$-antitrypsin
   - Galactosemia
   - Hereditary fructosemia
   - Hypothyroidism

11.1 Congenital Biliary Atresia vs Neonatal Hepatitis

Congenital biliary atresia (CBA) is a progressive, sclerosing, inflammatory disease, primarily affecting the extrahepatic bile duct from the region of the porta hepatis to its termination in the duodenum. It is estimated to affect 1 in 12,000 live births [1]. Untreated, the disease progresses relentlessly leading to biliary cirrhosis and death. Hepatoportoenterostomy (Kasai procedure) is the definitive therapy in the early stages. The rate of success of establishing an adequate bile flow by the Kasai procedure depends very much on the duct size at birth and the time interval between birth and hepatoportoenterostomy (HPE). Effective bile flow is established in 77–82% of infants when HPE is performed within 60 days after birth. The success rate decreases to 45–59% when HPE is delayed for 60–90 days, and decreases further to 10–28% when HPE is delayed for 3–4 months. The success rate increases to 92% when the duct lumen is greater than 150 μm in size [2]. Early diagnosis, therefore, plays a critical role in determining the outcome of therapy (Table 11.1.2).

Table 11.1.2. Effect of timing and duct size on rate of success of hepatoportoenterostomy (HPE) for congenital biliary atresia [2]

Factor	Success rate
Age at HPE	
<60 days	77–82%
61–90 days	45–59%
90–120 days	10–28%
Duct size	
>151 μm	92%
50–150 μm	81%
No patent ducts	18%

Etiology

The exact etiology of CBA is unknown. Two theories have been proposed; one theory is that of metaplasia of the hepatocytes and the other is that of faulty metaplasia combined with ingrowth from extrahepatic ducts [3, 4]. Ischemia, toxins, and duct injury are well recognized risk factors. Recent studies suggest that atresia may be due to a failure of remodeling at the hepatic hilum with a continuation of the fetal type bile leak due to poor mesenchymal support. Bile leak through ducts initiates an intense inflammatory reaction with a subsequent obliteration of the bile duct lumen. The characteristic findings on liver biopsy include ductal proliferation, canalicular and cellular bile stasis, periportal edema, and fibrosis. The title "atresia" is reserved for patients with complete obliteration of the duct lumen. Hypoplasia is a transition phase before complete obliteration of the duct lumen [5].

Congenital biliary atresia is divided into two clinical forms: the fetal and perinatal forms. The perinatal form is the most common and is characterized by late onset neonatal jaundice, with a jaundice-free time interval after birth. There are no other accompanying congenital abnormalities. Remnants of bile duct are found within the hepatoduodenal ligament [2]. The fetal form is less frequent, and accounts for less than 25% of cases. It is characterized by an early onset of neonatal jaundice, with no clearance of physiologic jaundice (no jaundice-free time interval). It is frequently associated with other congenital anomalies including polysplenia, asplenia, cardiovascular defects, or abdominal situs inversus. No bile duct remnants are found in the hepatoduodenal ligament.

Clinical Presentation

Infants with CBA are usually born at full term with a normal birth weight and show a normal growth pattern in the immediate neonatal period. It is more common in girls than boys. Jaundice usually starts 2 weeks after birth with acholic stool. Serum shows non-specific elevation of direct bilirubin, alanine aminotransferase (ALT) and gamma-glutamyl transferase (GGT). About 90% of infants show serum conjugated bilirubin (direct bilirubin) levels greater than 4 mg/dl [6, 7]. Aspiration of bile through a nasoduodenal tube (after instillation of 25% magnesium sulfate into the duodenum to stimulate gallbladder contraction and bile emptying) establishes patency of the bile ducts and thus excludes the diagnosis of congenital biliary atresia and confirms the diagnosis of neonatal hepatitis. Bile is aspirated from the duodenum in more than 80% of infants with neonatal hepatitis but not from infants with biliary atresia [8]. Intubation and duodenal bile aspiration are relatively invasive in a newborn and a negative test (no bile aspiration) is not always specific for congenital biliary atresia.

Hepatomegaly is unusual at birth, and begins to develop 6–8 weeks later. Cholestasis, fibrosis, and cirrhosis develop as the infant grows. The incidence of biliary atresia is higher among Chinese and Filipinos (2–3/10,000 population) than in Japanese and Caucasians [9]. Serial liver function tests provide an indication of the severity of the disease. Serum values of total bilirubin, direct bilirubin, GGT, and alkaline phosphatase, and the alkaline phosphatase/GGT ratio, do not reliably distinguish congenital biliary atresia from neonatal hepatitis [10]. Laparoscopy has no diagnostic role as it cannot assess the patency of the bile ducts. Cholangiography is invasive and technically difficult to do due to the small size of the ducts.

Cholescintigraphy

The indication for cholescintigraphy in a neonate is persistent jaundice beyond the 2nd week of life or new jaundice that develops 3 weeks after birth. An ideal patient preparation includes treatment with 5 mg/kg/day phenobarbital, in two equally divided doses, for 5–7 days prior to cholescintigraphy. Phenobarbital stimulates bile production [11] and increases the secretion of the radiotracer into bile, enabling better delineation of bile ducts and duodenum in infants with neonatal hepatitis, but not in those with CBA [12–14]. Cholestyramine or ursodeoxycholic acid also promote bile secretion. The infant should not be fed for 1 h before and 1 h after injection of the radiotracer. The duration of fasting prior to cholescintigraphy should be increased in older children, in proportion to their age.

Data Collection. The agent of choice in neonatal cholestasis is ^{99m}Tc-mebrofenin, because it competes with serum bilirubin for hepatocyte uptake much more effectively than ^{99m}Tc-disofenin or any other ^{99m}Tc-HIDA agent [15]. A dose of 100 μCi/kg (1 mCi or 37 MBq minimum) of ^{99m}Tc-mebrofenin is injected intravenously. A gamma camera, preferably a small field of view, fitted with a low energy, parallel hole, all purpose collimator is positioned anteriorly over the upper abdomen. The computer data are collected on 64×64 word mode matrix at one frame per minute for 60 min (Fig. 11.1.1). Delayed images are obtained at 2–4 h and 20–24 h, when intestinal activity is not seen in early images.

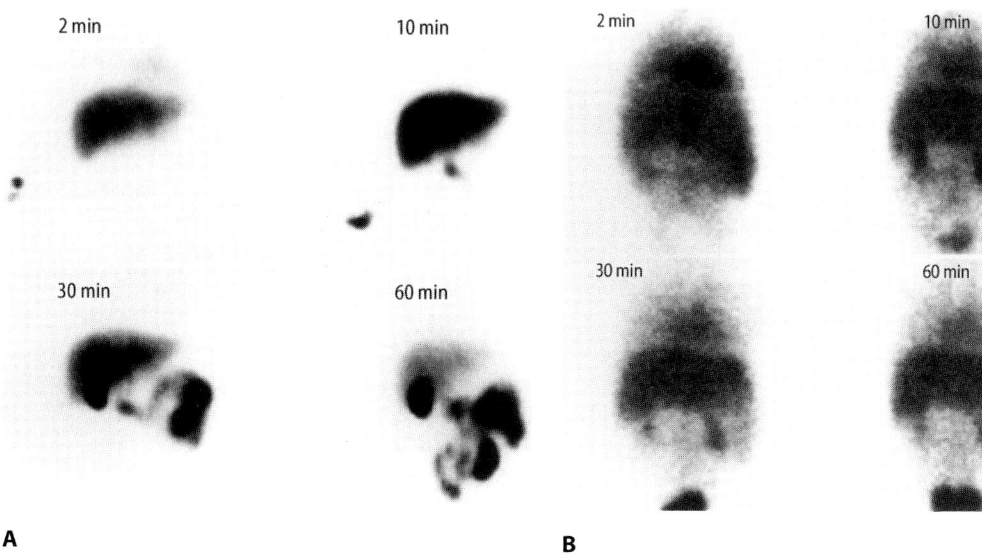

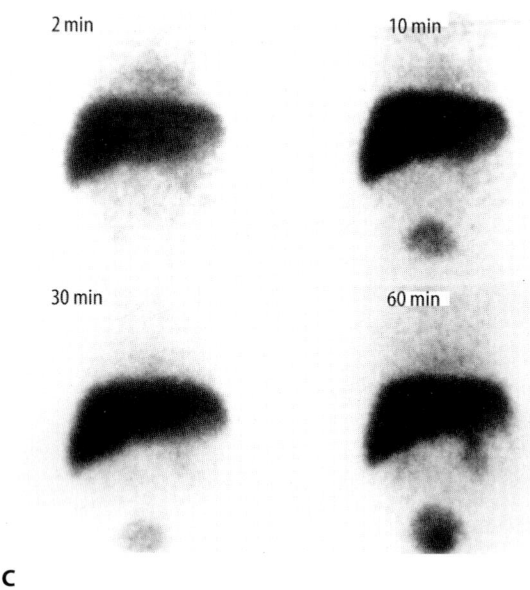

Fig. 11.1.1. Cholescintigraphy in the neonate. There is normal extraction and excretion of ^{99m}Tc-HIDA in a normal neonate **(A)**. The extraction is good but there is no excretion in congenital biliary atresia **(C)**. Both extraction and excretion are decreased and delayed, respectively, in neonatal hepatitis **(B)** [17]

Data Analysis. The normal neonate shows rapid liver uptake and excretion compared to the infant with CBA or hepatitis (Fig. 11.1.1). For quantification, three regions of interest are drawn and time/activity curves are generated separately over: (1) heart, (2) right upper lobe of the liver, and (3) spleen. The spleen ROI is used for blood background. Because both the hepatic and splenic arteries arise from the same celiac artery, the spleen serves as an ideal organ to represent the liver blood background. Hepatic extraction fraction and excretion half-times are obtained by subjecting data to the deconvolutional analysis, very similar to in adults (Fig. 11.1.2). Measurement of hepatic extraction fraction by deconvolutional analysis is equivalent to measuring first pass extraction by injecting the tracer directly into the hepatic artery or portal vein. Hepatic extraction fraction provides an objective criterion for separating biliary atresia from neonatal hepatitis in early cases of CBA [16, 17]. Liver extraction fraction and excretion half-time provide a measure of the severity of hepatobiliary disease. For a comparable level of serum bilirubin, infants with congenital biliary atresia show a relatively higher hepatic extraction fraction than infants with neonatal hepatitis [17, 18]. Obstruction over a longer period of time ultimately compromises hepatocyte function and the hepatic extraction fraction begins to decrease and loses its power to differentiate biliary from hepatocyte decrease. The diagnosis of congenital biliary atresia or neonatal hepatitis is also made by assessing both the images and the shape and direction of the curves (Fig. 11.1.3).

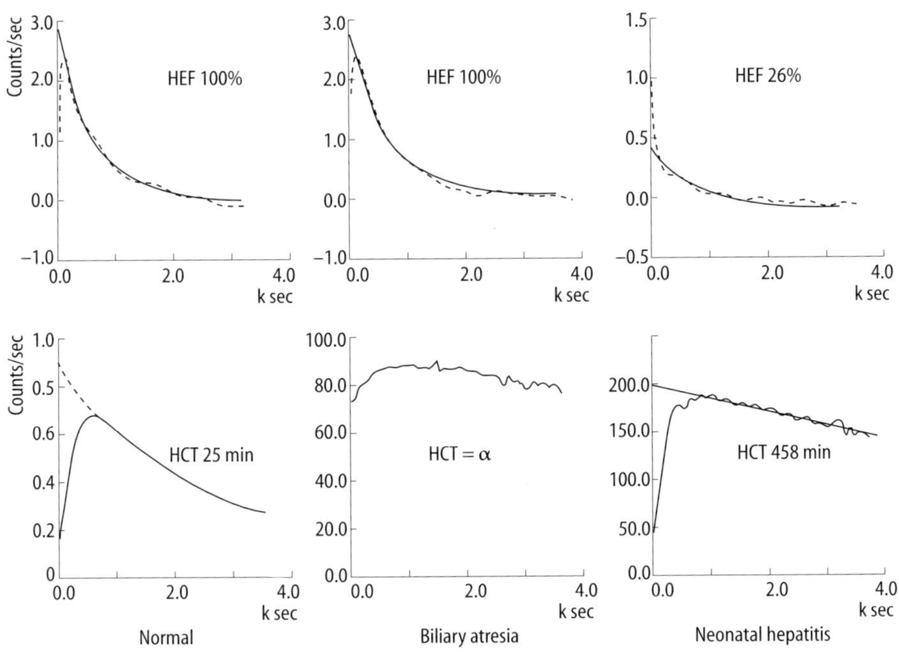

Fig. 11.1.2. Quantitative biliary dynamic studies in pediatrics. Hepatic extraction fraction (*HEF*) and excretion half-time (*HCT*) in a normal neonate, and a neonate with congenital biliary atresia or neonatal hepatitis. HEF remains relatively normal in biliary atresia, whereas both HEF and HCT are abnormal in neonatal hepatitis (modified from [17])

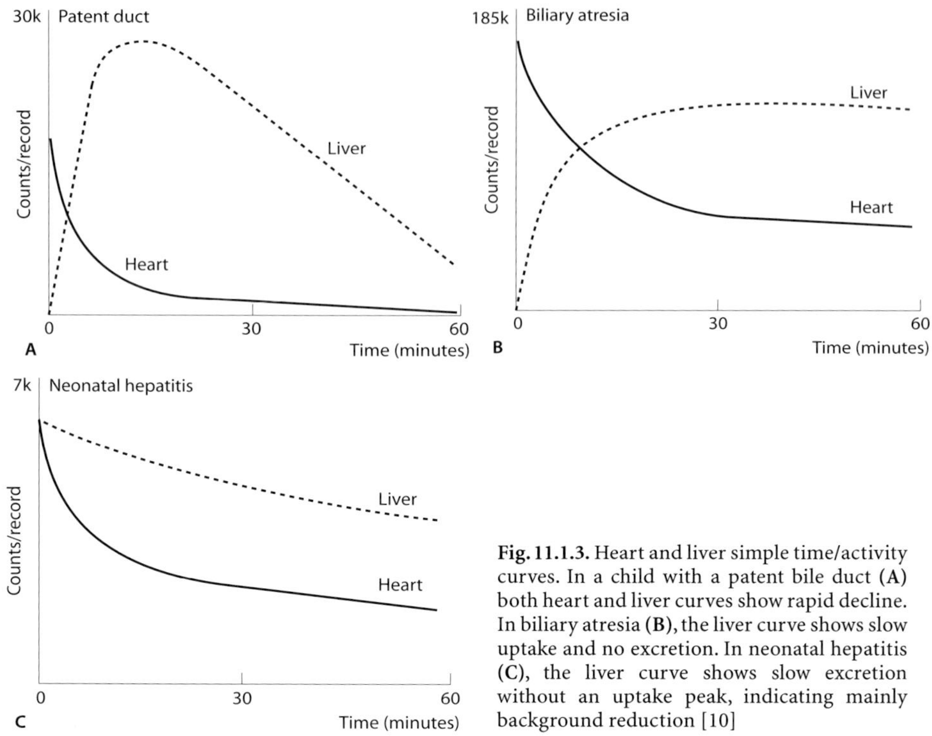

Fig. 11.1.3. Heart and liver simple time/activity curves. In a child with a patent bile duct (**A**) both heart and liver curves show rapid decline. In biliary atresia (**B**), the liver curve shows slow uptake and no excretion. In neonatal hepatitis (**C**), the liver curve shows slow excretion without an uptake peak, indicating mainly background reduction [10]

Normal Neonate. Cholescintigraphy in a normal neonate is characterized by rapid hepatocyte uptake and secretion of ^{99m}Tc-HIDA. Peak hepatic uptake occurs within 5 min, the gallbladder appears within 10 min, and intestinal activity is seen between 20 and 30 min. Unlike in adults and older children, the common hepatic duct, common bile duct, and cystic ducts are not seen in a neonate [13]. After reaching the peak within 5 min, the liver shows a rapid decline. Peak cardiac counts occur in the first frame (1 min) followed by a rapid decline, reaching a background activity level within 5 min. Both liver and heart curves converge towards the end [10]. A subjective analysis of the shape of the curves helps to separate normal infant from congenital biliary atresia or neonatal hepatitis (Fig. 11.1.3). Calculation of the hepatic extraction fraction and excretion half-time provide better and more powerful objective functional parameters than a simple subjective analysis of the curves (Fig. 11.1.2).

In a normal neonate, the hepatic extraction fraction value ranges between 87% and 100%, with an average of 99.0±3.6% (Table 11.1.3). A value below 92% (mean–2 SD) is considered abnormal. Mean excretion half-time with ^{99m}Tc-disofenin is 23.6±7.7 min; a value above 40 min is considered abnormal. An artifact in the calculation of hepatic extraction fraction due to an abrupt truncation of data collection is avoided by adding an appendage at the end of the curve [19].

Congenital Biliary Atresia. Neonates with congenital biliary atresia maintain relatively a high extraction of ^{99m}Tc-HIDA with clear delineation of the hepatic morphology with well defined borders and contour. Major abnormalities are confined to bile secretion. Despite a good extraction by the hepatocytes, there is total lack of secretion of ^{99m}Tc-HIDA into bile, resulting in non-visualization of the entire biliary tree. The liver image appears much like a radiocolloid scan, without the spleen. Delayed images at 24 h do not show any evidence of bile entry into small intestine [13, 14]. The liver time/activity curve shows good uptake but no excretion. Excretion half-time values often indicate infinity (Fig. 11.1.2). The hepatic extraction fraction value is maintained at a high level despite high serum bilirubin, especially when cholescintigraphy is obtained within 45 days after birth. When the extraction fraction value begins to decline in patients with CBA, however, it indicates functional compromise due to persistent bile duct obstruction over a longer period of time [18]. Diagnosis of congenital biliary atresia is a high probability in a neonate with conjugated (direct) hyperbilirubinemia, a relatively high hepatic extraction fraction in association with non-visualization of the entire biliary tree and the small intestine. Cholescintigraphy is unable to differentiate intrahepatic (Alagille's syndrome) from extrahepatic (congenital biliary atresia) ductal obstruction is the neonate.

The incidence of persistent jaundice beyond 2 weeks after birth, in general, is estimated to be 1 in 5000 live births; neonatal hepatitis occurs in 1 in 8000 and biliary atresia in 1 in 10,000–15,000 live births. Pure intrahepatic biliary atresia or hypoplasia is rare and occurs in 1 in 70,000 births [20]. The extrahepatic bile ducts are patent in most patients with intrahepatic biliary atresia. Intrahepatic biliary atresia is commonly associated with intrauterine infection and genetic abnormalities as listed in Table 10.1.1. Alagille's syndrome is a form of intrahepatic biliary hypoplasia or atresia in association with pulmonary stenosis, vertebral body abnormalities, sexual and mental underdevelopment, and typical facial features [21].

Table 11.1.3. Hepatic extraction fraction and excretion half-time (means ± SD) in normal subjects and children with congenital biliary atresia, hepatitis, and miscellaneous hepatobiliary diseases [17]

Parameter	Normal	CBA	Hepatitis	Miscellaneous
Number	12	9	16	8
Hepatic extraction fraction (%)	99.0±3.6	79.3±25.5	51.5±20.6	87.8±13.3
Hepatic excretion half-time (min)	23.6±7.7	183.1±201.1	101.9±77.0	44.8±35.7

Table 11.1.4. Efficacy of cholescintigraphy, ultrasonography, and liver biopsy in the differential diagnosis of congenital biliary atresia from neonatal hepatitis [22]

Parameter	Cholescintigraphy	Ultrasonography	Liver biopsy
Sensitivity (%)	100	70	95
Specificity (%)	80	70	100
Accuracy (%)	93	70	97
Positive predictive value	91	82	100
Negative predictive value	100	5491	

Neonatal Hepatitis. Neonatal hepatitis is usually caused by viral, fungal, or bacterial infection (Table 10.1.1). Jaundice persists beyond 2 weeks after birth and the liver function tests show non-specific elevation of enzymes with conjugated hyperbilirubinemia [9]. Cholescintigraphic features depend upon the severity of hepatocellular disease at the time of imaging. Uptake of ^{99m}Tc-HIDA by the hepatocyte is delayed and decreased. Both time to peak hepatic uptake and excretion half-time are increased. Intestinal and gallbladder visualization time may be either normal or markedly delayed. Due to a marked reduction in hepatocyte extraction of ^{99m}Tc-HIDA, the liver morphology is poorly defined with indistinct borders and contour. Heart and liver time/activity curves run in parallel, indicating mostly background reduction (Fig. 11.1.3). Hepatic extraction fraction value shows an inverse relationship with serum bilirubin level. Extraction fraction values as low as 30% are common [17]. Intestinal activity is seen by 24 h. An apparent appearance of good uptake by the liver is merely a reflection of hepatic blood pool radioactivity, and not due to true uptake by the hepatocytes as reflected by low hepatic extraction fraction value.

The success of cholescintigraphy is variable depending upon the time interval between birth and imaging (Table 11.1.4). A sensitivity of 100%, specificity of 80%, and accuracy of 93% have been reported from some centers with ^{99m}Tc-mebrofenin [22]. High accuracy is attributed partly to the agent's ability to compete effectively with serum bilirubin for uptake by the hepatocytes [15]. One cannot always separate congenital biliary atresia from neonatal hepatitis solely on the basis of HEF value, emphasizing the importance of combining quantification with image pattern to increase diagnostic accuracy [18].

Management of Neonatal Cholestasis

Neonatal hepatitis is treated medically with good nutrition, antiviral, antibacterial, or antiparasitic agents, depending upon its etiology. Most patients recover uneventfully (Fig. 11.1.4A). The Kasai procedure is the treatment of choice for congenital biliary atresia [23, 24]. The neonate is prepared for surgery with preoperative antibiotic prophylaxis, optimal hydration, and good nutrition. The abdomen is explored through a high transverse incision and a fine catheter is inserted into the gallbladder by piercing the fundus. Fibrosis of the wall with no bile within the gallbladder and obliteration of the common bile duct lumen confirms biliary atresia. The presence of bile inside the gallbladder with patency of the common bile duct, on the other hand, indicates neonatal hepatitis. A cholangiogram is obtained by injecting the radiocontrast through the catheter.

In the original Kasai procedure, the jejunum is cut beyond the ligament of Treitz and a portoenterostomy is established (Fig. 11.1.5). The proximal part of the jejunum is anastomosed to the side wall of the Roux-en-Y limb, below the portoenterostomy. The most common complication of portoenterostomy is acute ascending cholangitis, due to reflux of the intestinal contents into the bile ducts. Several modifications to the original portoenterostomy were made mainly with the hope of preventing acute ascending cholangitis. The temporary jejunostomy stoma created for decompression is usually closed at 3 months after confirming adequacy of bile flow. Most pediatric surgeons now seem to prefer the original Kasai procedure (Kasai 1) and avoid creating

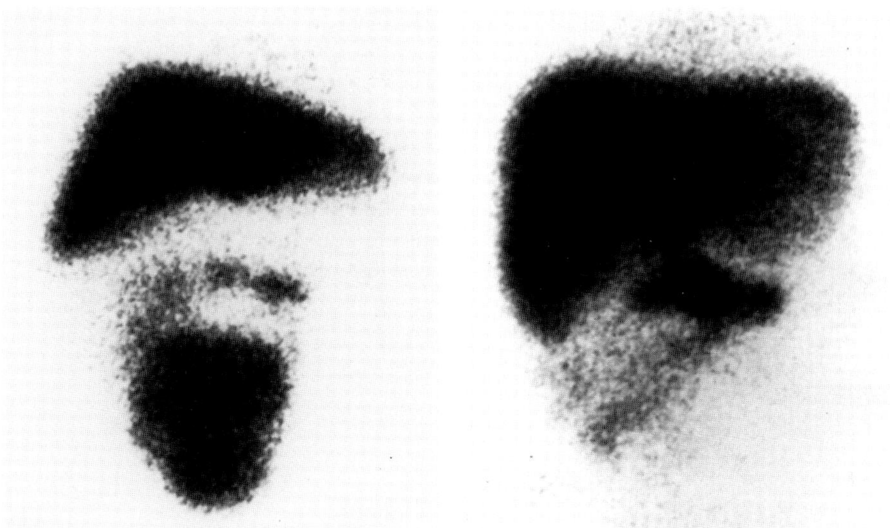

A B

Fig. 11.1.4. Response to therapy in neonatal cholestasis. An infant with giant cell neonatal hepatitis responds to medical therapy and shows bile secretion into intestine (**A**). An infant with congenital biliary atresia (**B**) shows bile secretion into intestine after a Kasai procedure. (Courtesy of Dr. V. Tolia, Detroit, MI [18])

an external fistula. Administration of appropriate antibiotics reduces the incidence of acute or recurrent cholangitis. A successful Kasai procedure establishes free bile flow into small intestine (Fig. 11.1.4B).

The rate of success of portoenterostomy for congenital biliary atresia depends primarily upon the time interval between birth and surgery and also upon the size of the duct lumen at birth (Table 11.1.2). Poor results are generally attributed to delayed portoenterostomy. A success rate of 89% and a 10-year survival rate of 33–74% are obtained when the neonate with congenital biliary atresia receives portoenterostomy within 60 days after birth (Table 11.1.5).

Liver transplantation is the ultimate therapy when HPE fails. The usual cause for HPE failure is continued fibrosis secondary to recurrent cholangitis. Approximately 65% of infants who receive HPE for biliary atresia ultimately require liver transplantation [26]. Biliary atresia is the most common indication and accounts for 54% of all liver transplantation in children. Other indications include metabolic diseases (14%), acute hepatic necrosis (11%), autoimmune and other cirrhosis (7%), malignancy, and other miscellaneous conditions [27]. Split liver and living donor liver transplantations have helped to overcome, to some extent, the shortages of donor livers in the pediatric populations [28, 29]. The high cost and limited availability of donors still remain two major factors limiting liver transplantation in children (see Chap. 12). The Kasai operation remains the first choice of treatment and its application early at experienced centers reduces the need for liver transplantation [30]. Non-invasive functional imaging with quantification is ideal for children, for evaluation of both native or transplant livers. Congenital biliary atresia, metabolic diseases, and acute hepatic necrosis alto-

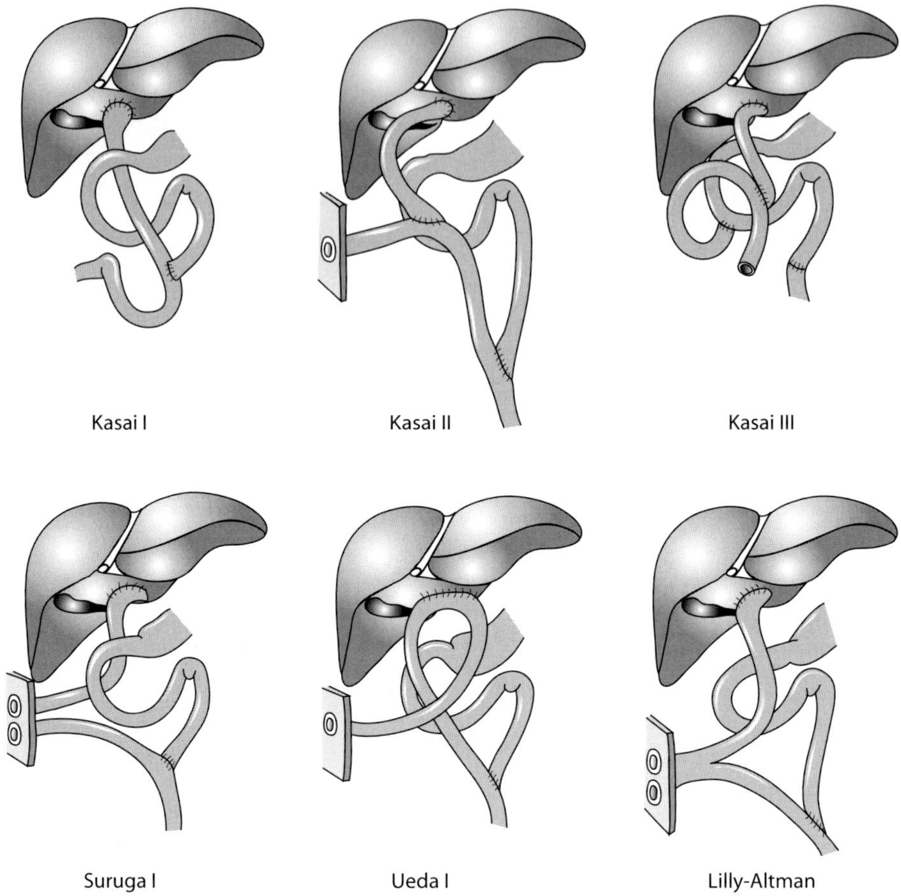

Fig. 11.1.5. Portoenterostomy for congenital biliary atresia. In Kasai I, an open end of a loop of the jejunum is attached directly to the undersurface of the liver to serve as a bile conduit. In Kasai II and Kasai III, a temporary external fistula is created. Other types of anastomoses include Segura I, Ueda I, and Lilly-Altman (modified from [9])

Table 11.1.5. Clinical outcome after the Kasai procedure for congenital biliary atresia [2]

Parameter	Success rate
Effective bile excretion	89%
Clearance of jaundice	62%
Jaundice free survival	53–62%
Ten-year survival	33–74%
Onset of esophageal varices	29–73%

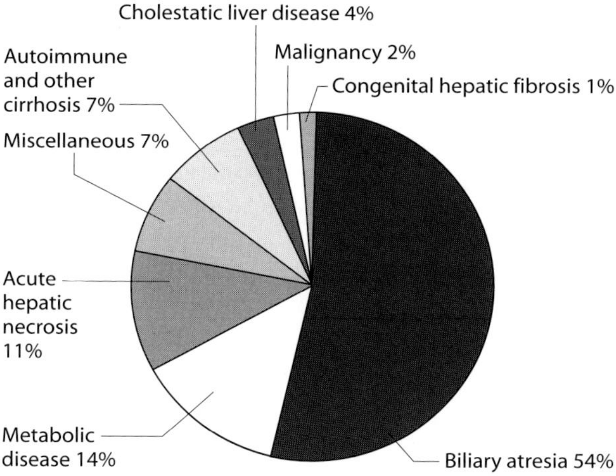

Fig. 11.1.6. Indications for liver transplantation in children. Congenital biliary atresia is the most common indication, followed by metabolic diseases, acute hepatic necrosis, and others [31]

gether account for nearly 80% of all transplants in children (Fig. 11.1.6). In the case of congenital biliary atresia, cholescintigraphy is suitable not only for diagnosis but for assessing the function after the Kasai procedure or transplant liver function when the Kasai procedure fails [31].

References

1. Balistreri WF. Neonatal cholestasis. J Pediatr 1985;106:171–184
2. Balistreri WF, Grand R, Hoofnagle JH, Suchy FJ, Ryckman FC, Perlmutter DH, Sokol RJ. Biliary atresia: current concepts and research directions. Summary of a symposium. Hepatology 1996;23:1682–1692
3. Cocjin J, Rosenthal P, Buslon V, Luk L Jr, Barajas L, Geller SA, Ruebner B, French S. Bile ductule formation in fetal, neonatal, and infant livers compared with extrahepatic biliary atresia. Hepatology 1996;24:568–574
4. Desmet VJ. Congenital diseases of intrahepatic bile ducts: variations on the theme "ductal plate malformation". Hepatology 1992;16:1069–1083
5. Tan CEL, Davenport M, Driver M, Howard ER. Does the morphology of the extrahepatic biliary remnant in biliary atresia influence survival? A review of 205 cases. J Pediatr Surg 1994;29:1459–1464
6. Mieli-Vergani G, Howard ER, Portman B, Mowat AP. Late referral for biliary atresia-missed opportunities for effective surgery. Lancet 1989;1:421–423
7. Mowat AP, Davidson LL, Dick MC. Earlier identification of biliary atresia and hepatobiliary disease: selective screening in the third week. Arch Dis Child 1995;72:90–92
8. Greene HL, Helinek GL, Moran R, O'Neill J. A diagnostic approach to prolonged obstructive jaundice by 24-hour collection of duodenal fluid. J Pediatr 1979;95:412–414
9. De Lorimier AA, Harrison MR. Congenital biliary atresia. In: Way LW, Pelligrini CA (eds). Surgery of the gallbladder and bile ducts. WB Saunders, Philadelphia 1987, pp 581–607
10. Leonard JC, Hitch DC, Manion CV. The use of diethyl-IDA Tc-99m clearance curves in the differentiation of biliary atresia from other forms of neonatal jaundice. Radiology 1982;142;773–776
11. Jaffe SJ, Jachau MR. Perinatal pharmacology. Ann Rev Pharmacology 1974;14:219–238
12. Thaler MM. Effect of phenobarbital on hepatic transport and excretion of 131I-rose bengal in children with cholestasis. Pediatric Res 1972;6:100–110

13. Majd M, Reba RC, Altman RP. Effect of phenobarbital on 99mTc-IDA scintigraphy in the evaluation of neonatal jaundice. Semin Nucl Med 1981;11:194–204
14. Majd M, Reba RC, Altman RP. Hepatobiliary scintigraphy with 99mTc-PIPIDA in the evaluation of neonatal jaundice. Pediatrics 1981;67:140–145
15. Krishnamurthy S, Krishnamurthy GT. Technetium-99m-iminodiacetic acid organic anions: review of biokinetics and clinical application in hepatology. Hepatology 1989;9:139–153
16. Brown PH, Juni JE, Lieberman DA, Krishnamurthy GT. Hepatocyte versus biliary disease: a distinction by deconvolutional analysis of Technetium-99m IDA time-activity curves. J Nucl Med 1988;29:623–630
17. Howman-Giles R, Moase A, Gaskin K, Uren R. Hepatobiliary scintigraphy in a pediatrc population: determination of hepatic extraction fraction by deconvolution analysis. J Nucl Med 1993;34:214–221
18. Tolia V, Kottamasu SR, Tabassum D, Simpson P. The use of hepatocyte extraction fraction to evaluate neonatal cholestasis. Clin Nucl Med 1999;24:655–659
19. Juni JE, Thrall JH, Froelich JW, Wiggins RC, Campbell DA Jr, Tuscan M. The appended curve for deconvolutional analysis – method and validation. Eur J Nucl Med 1988;14:403–407
20. Shim WKT, Kasai M, Spence MA: Racial influence on the incidence of biliary atresia. In: Bill MA, Kasai M (eds). Progress in pediatric surgery, Urban, Scharzenberg 1979
21. Alagille D, Odievre M, Gautier M, Dommergues JP. Hepatic ductular hypoplasia associated with characteristic facies, vertebral malformation, retarded physical, mental, and sexual development, and cardiac murmur. J Pediatr 1975;56:63–71
22. Maini A, Khanduri A, Gambhir S, Yacha SK, Das BK. Role of Tc-99m-mebrofenin in evaluation of neonatal cholestasis syndrome. Indian J Nucl Med 1997;12:84–87
23. Kasai M, Kimura S, Asakura Y. Surgical treatment of biliary atresia. J Pediatr Surg 1968;3:665–668
24. Kasai M, Suzuki H, Ohashi F, Ohi R, Chiba T, Okamoto A. Technique and results of operative management of biliary atresia. World J Surg 1978;2:571–579
25. Otte JB, deVille de Goyet J, Reding R, Hausleithner V, Sokal E, Chardot C, Debande B. Sequential treatment of biliary atresia with Kasai portoenterostomy and liver transplantation: a review. Hepatology 1994;20 (suppl):41S–48S
26. Ryckman F, Fisher R, Pedersen S, Dittrich V, Heubi J, Farrell M, Balistreri W, Ziegler M. Improved survival in biliary atresia patients in the present era of liver transplantation. J Pediatr Surg 1993;28:382–385
27. Reyes J, Mazariegos GV. Pediatric transplantation. Surgical Clinic of North America 1999;79:163–189
28. Egawa H, Uemoto S, Inomata Y, Shapiro J, Asonuma K, Kiuchi T, Okajima H, Itou K, Tanaka K. Biliary complications in pediatric living related liver transplantation. Surgery 1998;124:901–910
29. Reding R, Goyet J, Delbeke I, Sokal E, Jamart J, Janssen M, Otte J. Pediatric liver transplantation with cadaveric or living related donors: comparative results in 90 elective recipients of primary grafts. J Pediatr 1999;134:280–286
30. Chardot C, Carton M, Spire-Bendelac, Pommelet CL, Golmard J, Auvert B. Prognosis of biliary atresia in the era of liver transplantation: French national study from 1986 to 1996. Hepatology 1999;30:606–611
31. Reyes J, Mazariegos GV. Pediatric transplantation. Surgical Clinic of North America 1999;79:163–189

11.2 Cystic Diseases of the Hepatobiliary System

Cysts are abnormal spaces within the liver parenchyma or along the biliary tract (choledochal cysts). They vary in size and location and contain mostly clear liquid. Choledochal cysts are rare, 1 in 100,000–150,000 live births. About 80% of choledochal cysts become symptomatic early and are diagnosed before the age of 10 years. Cysts are classified in many ways and the classification provided in Table 11.2.1 is primarily for diagnostic purposes using various imaging techniques including ultrasound, CT, MRCP, and cholescintigraphy. Cystic diseases due to parasites (hydatid cyst) and bacte-

Table 11.2.1. Classification of congenital cystic diseases of the hepatobiliary system

a) Intrahepatic
  i) Solitary or multiple intrahepatic cysts with no communication with the bile ducts (adult polycystic liver disease)
  ii) Mixed variety where few cysts communicate with the bile ducts.
  iii) Diffuse or segmental cystic dilatation of the bile ducts (Caroli's disease)
b) Extrahepatic
  i) Choledochal cyst
    a) Cystic
    b) Fusiform
    g) Cylindrical
    d) Rosary (multiple cysts)
    e) Diverticular
    z) Choledochocele

ria (abscess) are covered separately under space occupying lesions of the liver in Chap. 4. This section deals primarily with those congenital cysts that have direct communication with the bile ducts and hence fill in with radiolabeled bile. The diagnosis of a non-communicating cyst is inferred when radioactive bile does not enter the cyst.

Cysts are either solitary or multiple. Solitary cysts are rare, are found at all ages, and most remain asymptomatic [1]. The cysts occur mostly along the hepatobiliary tract, starting at the smallest intralobular duct to the termination of the common bile duct into the duodenum. Most of the cysts are congenital. Few of the acquired cysts usually follow an infection, trauma, or obstruction of a duct. The cyst may be entirely extrahepatic or intrahepatic in location. The occurrence of both intrahepatic and extrahepatic cysts in a patient is rare but is well recognized [2].

Etiology

The exact cause of cystic dilatation of the bile ducts is unknown. Various hypotheses have been proposed including weakness of the duct wall, angulation of the duct, presence of a valve-like structure within the lumen, inflammation, or sphincter dysfunction, all of which increase in intraductal pressure with impedance to bile flow [3]. The dilatation is initiated by an irregular and unequal proliferation of duct cells during recanalization of solid core during early intrauterine life. Cysts are relatively more common in the Japanese and other Asians than people elsewhere in the western hemisphere. An incidence of 1 in 13,000 hospital admissions has been reported in Japanese children [4]. The cyst wall ranges in thickness from 1 to 10 mm and consists mostly of fibrous tissue lined with cuboidal cells, or often with no lining cells at all. The cyst wall lacks mucous glands and muscle layer. The cyst volume varies from a few milliliters to several liters [3].

Classification of Choledochal Cysts

Cysts are classified mainly into the intrahepatic and extrahepatic variety. Kami et al. and Todani et al. recommend classification based upon the shape, size, extent, and location of the cyst [5, 6]. The cystic type is the most common variety and accounts for

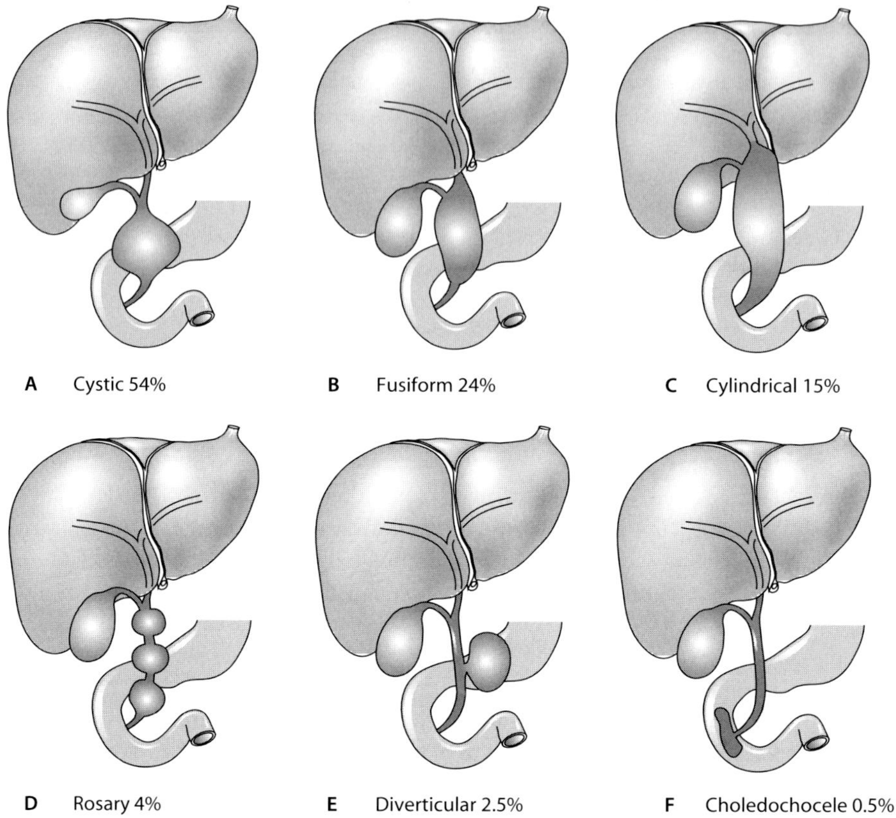

Fig. 11.2.1A–F. Classification of extrahepatic bile duct cysts. The cystic type is the most common (54%), followed by the fusiform (24%), cylindrical (15%), rosary (4%), and diverticular forms (2.5%). Choledochocele is a cystic dilatation of the intraduodenal part of the common bile duct before its entrance into the duodenum

54% of all choledochal cysts (Fig. 11.2.1). Fusiform is the next most common (24%), followed by the cylindrical (15%) and rosary types (4%). Together, these four account for nearly 97% of all cystic lesions. The diverticular type arises from one side of the duct wall, consists of a narrow opening and may compress the adjoining structures, manifesting clinical symptoms of obstruction. A cyst at the distal end of the common bile duct, situated within the duodenal wall close to the ampulla of Vater, is called a choledochocele, and is the rarest type (0.5%). The gallbladder remains normal in size and gallstones are relatively rare in patients with choledochal cysts [3].

Intrahepatic Cystic Dilatation (Caroli's Disease)

Caroli et al. in 1958 first described an entity of pure intrahepatic cystic dilatation [2]. Numerous authors have since described frequent association of intrahepatic cysts with cysts of the extrahepatic ducts. Studies from Japan report as many as 28–42% of

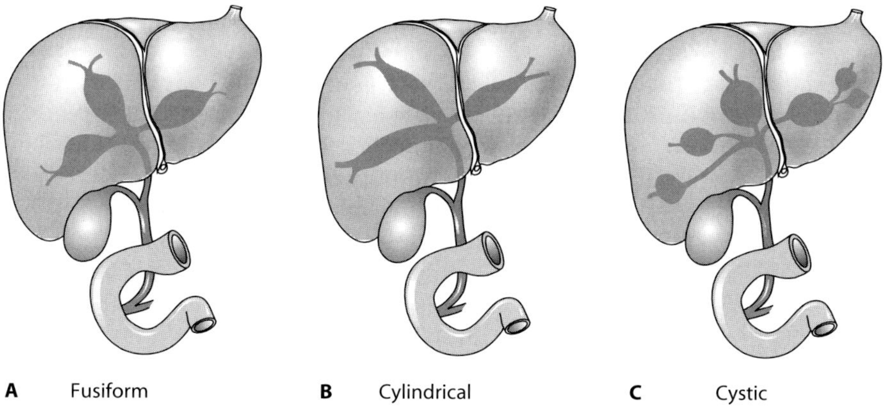

Fig. 11.2.2A–C. Classification of intrahepatic bile duct cysts. The fusiform and cylindrical types are typical examples of Caroli's disease. The cystic type may affect both the intrahepatic and extrahepatic ducts. Simultaneous involvement of both intrahepatic and extrahepatic ducts is found in 28–42% of patients

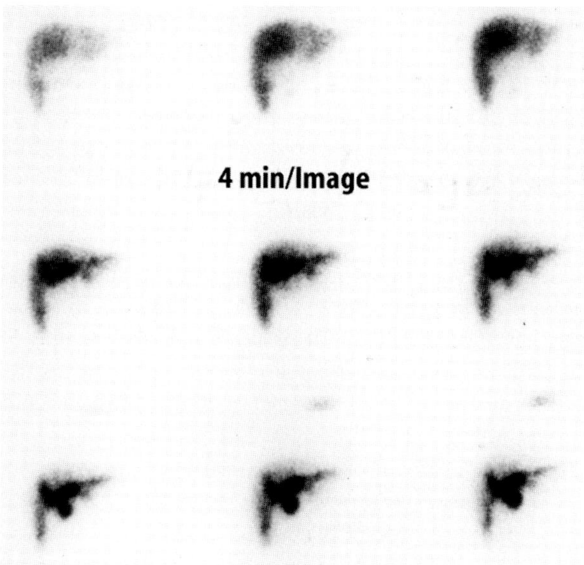

Fig. 11.2.3. Cholescintigraphic features of a choledochal cyst. A choledochal cyst fills in with radiolabeled bile and appears as a round structure in the middle of the common duct. The gallbladder is not seen

patients with extrahepatic cysts having simultaneous intrahepatic cysts [3, 5, 7]. The fusiform and cylindrical type are more common in patients with intrahepatic cysts (Fig. 11.2.2).

Diagnosis

Choledochal cysts are three times more common in women than men, and are more common in Asia and the Orient than in the western hemisphere [3]. Cysts remain asymptomatic for many years. When symptoms occur, more than one-half of patients present with a triad of abdominal pain, abdominal mass, and jaundice. Pain is usually localized to the right upper quadrant. The onset of symptoms usually coincides with the enlargement of the cyst and the symptoms subside when the cyst decreases in size or drains spontaneously into the duodenum. Liver function tests show mild non-specific elevation. Ultrasonography or CT is the initial diagnostic procedure of choice. Once a cyst is identified with one of the imaging modalities, cholescintigraphy confirms the diagnosis. A cyst by ultrasound or CT in the vicinity of the biliary tract that fills with radiolabeled bile is specific for a choledochal cyst (Fig. 11.2.3). Choledochal cysts must be differentiated from cysts in other nearby organs including cystic lesions of the kidney (renal cyst, hydronephrosis, Wilms' tumor), pancreas (pseudocyst), or duodenum (diverticulum). The malignant potential of a choledochal cyst is about 2.4% [6].

Cholescintigraphy

The imaging study is obtained 4–6 h after fasting. Usually there is no need for pretreatment with phenobarbital, unless the child is severely jaundiced. Any one of the ^{99m}Tc-HIDA agents may be chosen when serum bilirubin is within normal range. Routinely one minute per frame images are obtained for 60 min (Fig. 11.2.3). Delayed images are obtained at 4 and 24 h when necessary.

The most common cholescintigraphic feature of a choledochal cyst is that of an early defect (90%) in the vicinity of the common hepatic or common bile duct that fills with radioactive bile at 4 or 24 h (Table 11.2.2). Intrahepatic ductal prominence or bile pooling is seen in 22% [8]. The gallbladder usually appears late. Only about 25% of gallbladders are seen within 60 min, and as many as 25% remain non-visualized even at 24 h [8–10].

Delayed filling or non-filling of the native gallbladder in a patient with choledochal cyst suggests that the cyst may act as low pressure reservoir for bile. Gallbladder histopathological changes indicative of acute cholecystitis are found in 7%, and of chronic cholecystitis in 59% of patients with choledochal cysts [8]. This raises the possibility that the presenting symptoms may be due to onset of cholecystitis and not

Table 11.2.2. Cholescintigraphic features of choledochal cyst

Parameter	Frequency
1. Prolonged intrahepatic ductal prominence	22%
2. Visualization of the gallbladder within 1 h	25%
3. Non-visualization of the gallbladder by 2–4 h	71%
4. Non-visualization of the gallbladder by 24 h	25%
5. Filling defect in the region of the cyst in early images	90%
6. Filling of the defect with the radiolabel in late images	89%

to the choledochal cyst itself. Large cysts (one measured 400 ml) may compress adjoining structures and present clinically as an acute emergency [11]. Combined application of ultrasound and ^{99m}Tc-HIDA cholescintigraphy is the most cost-effective approach in the diagnosis of choledochal cyst [12].

Management of Choledochal Cyst

Surgical excision of the cyst is the treatment of choice [13]. The cyst is excised with the hepatic duct Roux-en-Y jejunal anastomosis. This approach results in the most favorable postsurgical outcome, with a low incidence of ascending cholangitis. Total excision of the cyst is recommended because of its high malignant potential, which is 20 times higher than in the general population [3]. Surgical management of pure intrahepatic cysts (Caroli's disease) remains controversial. Lobectomy is advocated when cysts involve only one lobe of the liver. In the severe form of Caroli's disease, recurrent ascending cholangitis often leads to fibrosis and portal hypertension. About 20% of choledochal cysts which are diagnosed in adults are treated much like in children with total surgical excision [14].

Cystic Disease of the Liver Parenchyma

Liver cysts can be either solitary or multiple. Solitary cysts are uncommon, non-hereditary, and not associated with cysts in other organs. The Mayo Clinic reported only 38 solitary asymptomatic liver cysts during a follow-up period of 47 years [15]. Frequent use of abdominal ultrasound examination may now detect many more asymptomatic liver cysts than before. Symptomatic solitary liver cysts are four times more common in women than in men and are found more frequently in the anterior-inferior area of the right lobe [16]. The cyst surface is usually smooth with wall thickness less than 1 cm. The cyst size varies from a few milliliters to several liters. One reported cyst contained 17 l fluid [17]. Most of the cysts contain clear fluid. Some cysts may contain blood, mucin, proteins, and cholesterol. Bile is rarely found in a solitary cyst, indicating its non-communication with the bile ducts. A solitary cyst on ultrasound or CT that does not fill with radiolabeled bile indicates a non-communicating simple liver cyst (Fig. 11.2.4A).

Polycystic Liver Disease

Polycystic liver disease is classified into two main categories, non-communicating and communicating. Non-communicating cysts are usually multiple, are common in adults (adult polycystic liver disease), and show an autosomal dominant pattern of inheritance. They are associated with cysts in other organs, especially of the kidneys [18]. Cysts become symptomatic when they rupture or become infected. ^{99m}Tc-HIDA cholescintigraphy can establish reliably whether or not the abdominal pain is due to rupture of the liver cyst [19]. In patients with polycystic liver disease on CT or ultrasound, non-filling with radiolabeled bile indicates a non-rupture (Fig. 11.2.4B,C).

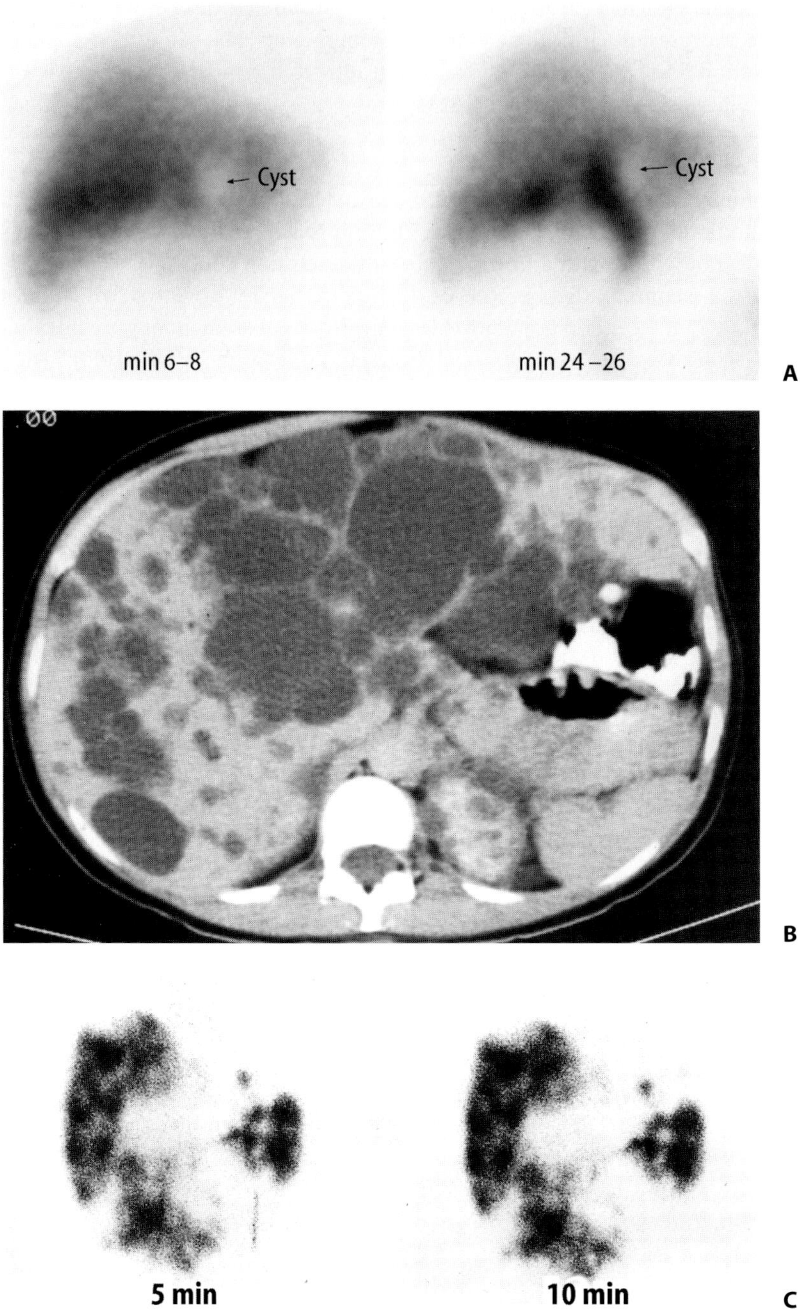

Fig. 11.2.4. Liver cyst. A simple liver cyst appears as a round defect early and does not fill in with radiolabeled bile later (**A**). A polycystic liver shows multiple small and large liver cysts on CT (**B**). Cholescintigraphy shows functioning liver tissue along the margins of the right and left lobes (**C**). No filling of the cysts occurs later indicating no wall rupture [19].

References

1. Witzleben C. Cystic disease of the liver. In: Zakim D, Boyer TD (eds). Hepatology. A textbook of liver disease. WB Saunders, Philadelphia 1996, Volume II, pp 1630–1649
2. Caroli J, Soupault R, Kossakowski J et al. La dilatation polycystic congenitale des voies biliares intrahepatiques. Sem Hop Paris 1958;34:488–491
3. Fonkalsrud E. Biliary cystic disease in children and adults. In: Way LW, Pelligrini CA. (eds). Surgery of the gallbladder and bile ducts. WB Saunders, Philadelphia, 1987, pp 609–629
4. Kimura K, Tsugawa C, Ogawa K, Matsumoto Y, Yamamoto T, Kubo M, Asada S, Nishiyama S, Ito H. Choledochal cysts. Etiological considerations and surgical management in 22 cases. Arch Surg 1978;113:159
5. Komi N, Udaka H, Ikeda N, Kashiwagi Y. Congenital dilatation of the biliary tract; new classification and study with particular reference to anomalous arrangement of the pancreaticobiliary ducts. Gastroenterol JPN 1977;12:293–304
6. Todani T, Watanabe Y, Narusue M, Tabuchi K, Okajima K. Congenital bile duct cysts: classification, operative procedure, and review of thirty-seven cases including cancer arising from choledochal cyst. Am J Surg 1977;134:263–269
7. Saito S. Surgical treatment and long term followup results of congenital dilatation of the biliary duct. Presented at international symposium on cholestasis in infancy – its pathogenesis, diagnosis, and treatment. Sendai, Japan 1978, June 7–9
8. Kao PF, Huang MJ, Tzen KY, You DL, Liaw YF. The clinical significance of gall-bladder non-visualization in cholescintigraphy of patients with choledochal cysts. Eur J Nucl Med 1996;23:1468–1472
9. Camponovo E, Buck JL, Drane WE. Scintigraphic features of choledochal cyst. J Nucl Med 1989;30:622–628
10. Padhy AK, Gopinath PG, Basu AK, Upadhyay P. Hepatobiliary scintigraphy in congenital cystic dilatation of biliary tract. Clin Nucl Med 1985;10:703–707
11. Williams LE, Fisher JH, Courtney RA, Darling DB. Preoperative diagnosis of choledochal cyst by hepatoscintigraphy. N Engl J Med 1970;283:85–86
12. Gates GF, Miller JH. Combined radionuclide and ultrasonic assessment of upper abdominal masses in children. Am J Roentgenol 1977;128:773–780
13. Tsardakas E, Rdonett AH. Congenital cystic dilatation of the common bile duct. Arch Surg 1956;72;311–315
14. Weyant MJ, Maluccio MA, Bertagnolli MM, Daly JM. Choledochal cysts in adults. A report of two cases and review of the literature. Am J Gastroenterol 1998;93:2580–2583
15. Henson SW Jr, Gray HK, Dockery MB. Benign tumors of the liver III. Solitary cysts. Surg Gynecol Obstet 1956;103:607–609
16. Caplan LH, Simon M. Nonparasitic cysts of the liver. Am J Roentgenol Radium Ther Nucl Med 1966;96:421–428
17. Flagg RS, Robinson DW. Solitary nonparasitic hepatic cysts. Report of oldest known case and review of the literature. Arch Surg 1967;95:964–973
18. Gabow PA, Ikle DW, Holmes JH. Polycystic kidney disease: prospective analysis of nonazotemic patients and family members. Ann Intern Med 1984;101:238–247
19. Salam M, Keeffe EB. Liver cysts associated with polycystic kidney disease: role of Tc-99m hepatobiliary imaging. Clin Nucl Med 1989;14:803–807

Liver Transplantation

After many years of experiments and clinical experience, liver transplantation is now considered an optimal therapy for various types of end stage liver disease [1]. The first liver transplantation was performed by Welch in 1955 in a dog and the first human liver transplantation was performed by Starzl et al. in 1963 [2, 3]. Early clinical results were disappointing. The advent of modern immunosuppressive agents has improved survival rates in both children and adults. The survival rates at 1, 3, 5, and 10 years in children are 82%, 80%, 78%, and 76%, respectively [4]. The indications for liver transplantation for varieties of end stage liver diseases are shown in Table 12.1.1.

Types of Liver Transplantation

There are essentially three types of liver transplantation: (1) cadaver liver, (2) living-donor liver, and (3) auxiliary liver. During cadaver liver transplantation, the recipient entire liver is removed and replaced in its place (orthotopic) by a donor liver usually from a cadaver (Fig. 12.1.1). In the case of a living donor transplantation, either the lateral segment or the entire left lobe from the donor liver replaces the entire native liver of the recipient. In the case of an auxiliary liver transplantation (for patients with fulminant hepatic failure), the donor liver, which acts as a transient bridge until the native liver recovers, is placed either adjacent to the native liver or it replaces the left lobe of the native liver [5–8]. The transplantation procedure usually involves four stages: (1) hepatectomy of the native liver, (2) anhepatic stage, the time interval during

Table 12.1.1. Indications for liver transplantation

Parenchymal diseases	Cholestatic diseases
Postnecrotic cirrhosis	Biliary atresia
Primary biliary cirrhosis	Cystic fibrosis
Primary sclerosing cholangitis	Biliary cirrhosis
Alcoholic liver failure	Sclerosing cholangitis
Viral hepatitis	Familial cholestasis
Inborn errors of metabolism	Graft-vs-host disease
Fulminant hepatic failure	Chronic hepatic rejection
Autoimmune hepatitis	
Cystic fibrosis	Tumors
Neonatal hepatitis	Hepatoma
	Hepatoblastoma
	Apudomas
	Miscellaneous
	Budd-Chiari syndrome
	Trauma

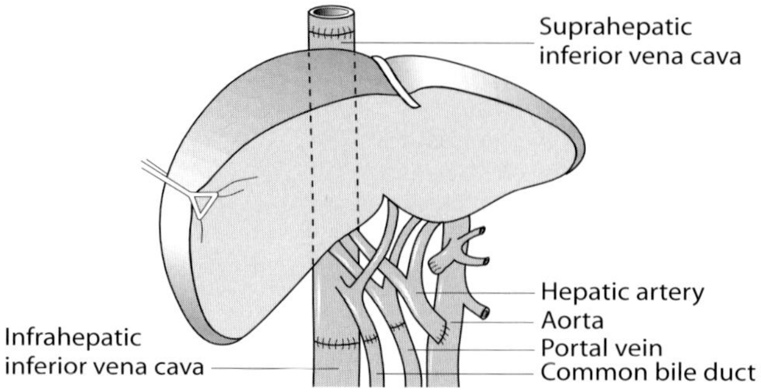

Orthotopic liver transplant

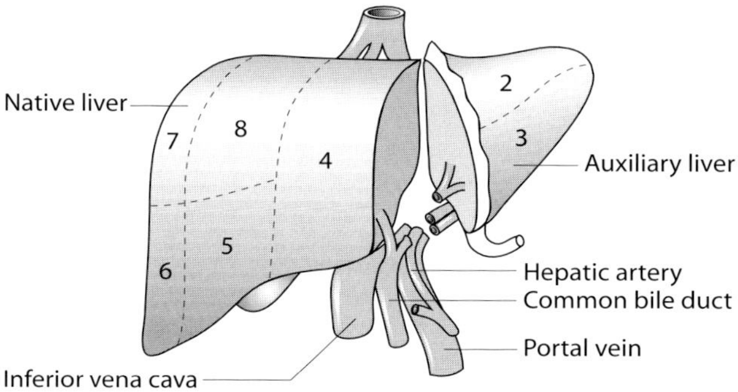

Auxiliary orthotopic liver transplant

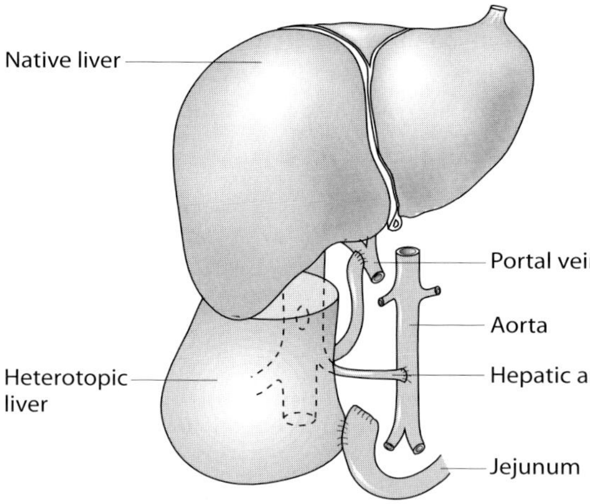

Auxiliary heterotopic liver transplant

Fig. 12.1.1. Liver transplantation. Orthotopic liver transplant with end-to-end anastomosis is the most common type. In auxiliary transplantation, the donor liver is placed in either the orthotopic or the heterotopic position which the native liver is removed and the blood flow through the vena cava, portal vein, and hepatic artery is interrupted, (3) reperfusion stage when the donor liver is being revascularized in the recipient, and (4) biliary reconstruction stage where a choledochocholedochostomy (adults) or a choledochojejunostomy [in children less than 35 lb (16 kg)] is performed.

Nuclear medicine procedures are used for the evaluation of liver function in the recipient, both in the pre- and post-transplant period. In the case of a living donor liver transplantation, both the donor and the recipient may undergo pretransplant evaluation, which generally includes assessment of the functional reserve of the donor liver and determination of the ideal time for transplantation in the recipient [9]. Since no single test is found to be adequate either for the determination of end-stage liver disease or for predicting the ideal time for transplantation, assessment of liver function generally involves application of serial imaging and non-imaging diagnostic procedures over many months or years. Just prior to transplantation, multiple gated blood pool (MUGA) and myocardial perfusion studies are obtained in the recipient to exclude significant heart disease. After the transplantation, nuclear studies are used to detect immediate and late postoperative complications (Table 12.1.2) and also for the assessment of functional recovery of the donor liver. Cholescintigraphy is used for detection of bile leak and to assess functional recovery, and blood pool studies are obtained to identify vascular complications, such as bleeding or thrombosis [9–11]. Post-transplant chronic ischemia causes diffuse bile duct stenosis, manifesting a vanishing bile duct syndrome in some patients [12].

Normal Functioning Liver Transplant

A normal functioning liver transplant functions much like a normal native liver and maintains its normal shape and size. The gallbladder is absent due to cholecystectomy performed as an integral part of transplantation to prevent future complications due to gallstones. Hepatic extraction fraction and excretion half-time values are maintained within the normal range for normal native liver. Common hepatic and common bile ducts show normal features. Duodenogastric bile reflux is rare (Fig. 12.1.2, Table 12.1.3).

Complications

Liver transplant complications occur both in the immediate and delayed postoperative period:

Table 12.1.2. Complications of liver transplantation [10]

Complication	Frequency (%)
Infections	30.0–60.0
Biliary obstruction	15.0–25.0
Rejection	10.0–15.0
Bile leak	7.5–10.0
Bleeding	5.5–6.5
Renal failure (requiring dialysis)	5.0
Arterial thrombosis	3.0–5.0
Lymphoproliferative disorder	2.0–2.5
Portal vein thrombosis	1.0–2.0

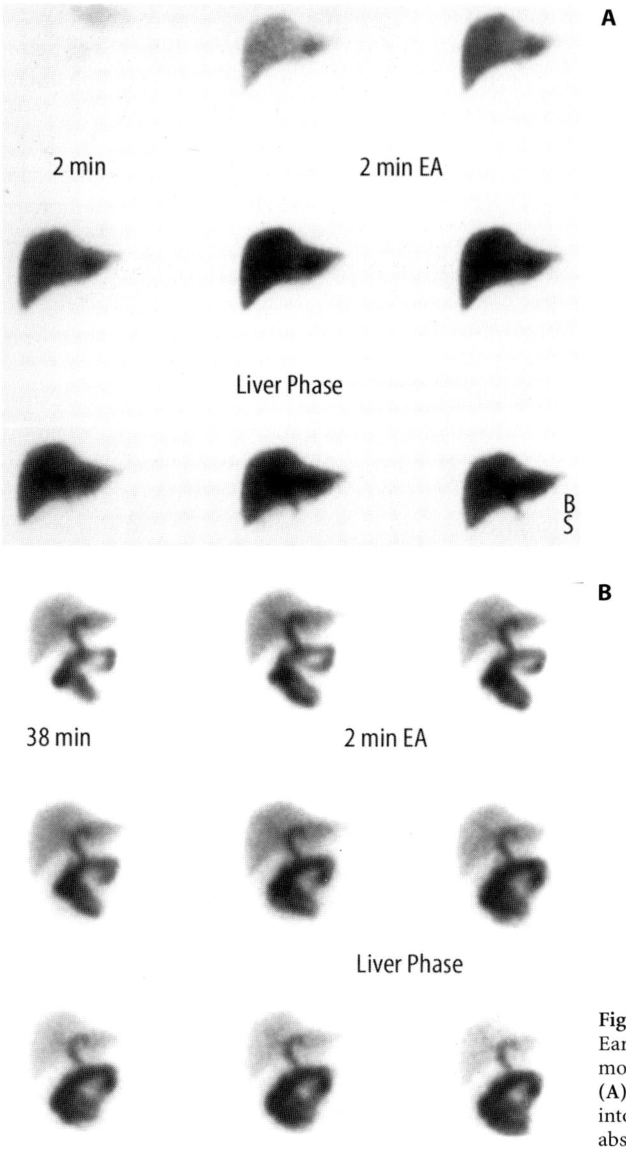

Fig. 12.1.2. Normal liver transplant. Early images show normal morphology and bile formation **(A)**. Late images show free bile flow into intestine. Gallbladder is absent due to cholecystectomy **(B)**.

Table 12.1.3. Hepatic extraction fraction and excretion half-time of a normal liver transplant.

	Hepatic extraction fraction (92–100%)	Hepatic excretion, $T_{1/2}$ (11–31 min)	Hepatic uptake, $T_{1/2}$ (1.1–9.0 min)
RU lobe	100%	10.5 min	7.2 min
RL lobe	100%	11.1 min	8.2 min
LT lobe	100%	12.1 min	9.0 min

Immediate complications include bile leak, arterial or venous thrombosis infection bleeding, etc., and delayed complications are immunological in nature.

Bile Leak. Leak is inferred when bile enters an unanticipated region or an anticipated region at an unanticipated time [13]. Bile leak at the anastomotic site is relatively common and accounts for 10% of all complications. Bile may leak into the liver parenchyma (abscess) or into the subhepatic space, forming a biloma, or it may leak into the peritoneal space, causing bile peritonitis. Space occupying lesions due to biloma or other benign or malignant conditions produce a filling defect within the liver in early images. Biloma fills with ^{99m}Tc-HIDA radiolabeled bile in late images, whereas a benign or malignant space-occupying lesion remains as a "cold" defect throughout. Bile may enter an abscess cavity when the abscess penetrates into a bile duct. Healing of the abscess cavity can be demonstrated with serial imaging (Fig. 12.1.3). Bile leak at the duct anastomotic site (choledochocholedochal) is usually small and closes spontaneously. Bile leak at the choledochoduodenal junction, on the other hand, tends to be large in volume and carries a much higher morbidity and mortality due to simultaneous leakage of intestinal contents into the peritoneal space. In the supine position, leaked bile gravitates to the right or the left paracolic gutter and later enters the pelvic cavity. Opioids prescribed for pain control increase volume of bile leak due to their constrictive effect on the native sphincter of Oddi.

Bile Duct Stricture. Stricture is a late complication and accounts for 15–25% of the total complications of liver transplantation. Stricture is attributed to bile duct ischemia caused by arterial stenosis or thrombosis. Cholescintigraphy shows bile pooling in ducts proximal to the stricture. Segmental and area ducts are seen with unusual prominence [14]. Denervation during transplant surgery alters sympathetic-parasympathetic-hormonal interaction on the ducts and sphincter of Oddi. Nervous and hormonal imbalance may cause biliary dyskinesia. A distinction between anatomic stricture and biliary dyskinesia is made with the use of amyl nitrite or calcium channel blockers (nifedipine), very similar to studies in non-transplant patients [15, 16].

Primary Non-Function vs Rejection. Primary non-function is non-recovery of donor liver function despite good surgical technique establishing adequate portal vein and hepatic artery blood flow. Clinically it presents as liver failure in association with encephalopathy, persistent acidosis, and severe coagulopathy and requires therapy which is different from that of acute or chronic transplant rejection. Acute rejection occurs within 3 months of transplantation and chronic rejection follows later. Unlike the kidneys, the liver does not manifest an hyperacute rejection. Rejection is a microvascular phenomenon where fibrin, immune, and inflammatory cells deposit within and around the capillaries manifesting an obliterative angiopathy and chronic ischemia. Chronic ischemia leads to obliteration of bile ducts (vanishing bile duct syndrome) and intrahepatic cholestasis. Rejection and intrahepatic cholestasis due to other causes manifest similar cholescintigraphic findings and are hence unable to be used to separate one from the other [18]. Rejection is managed by a combination of several immunosuppressive agents [19].

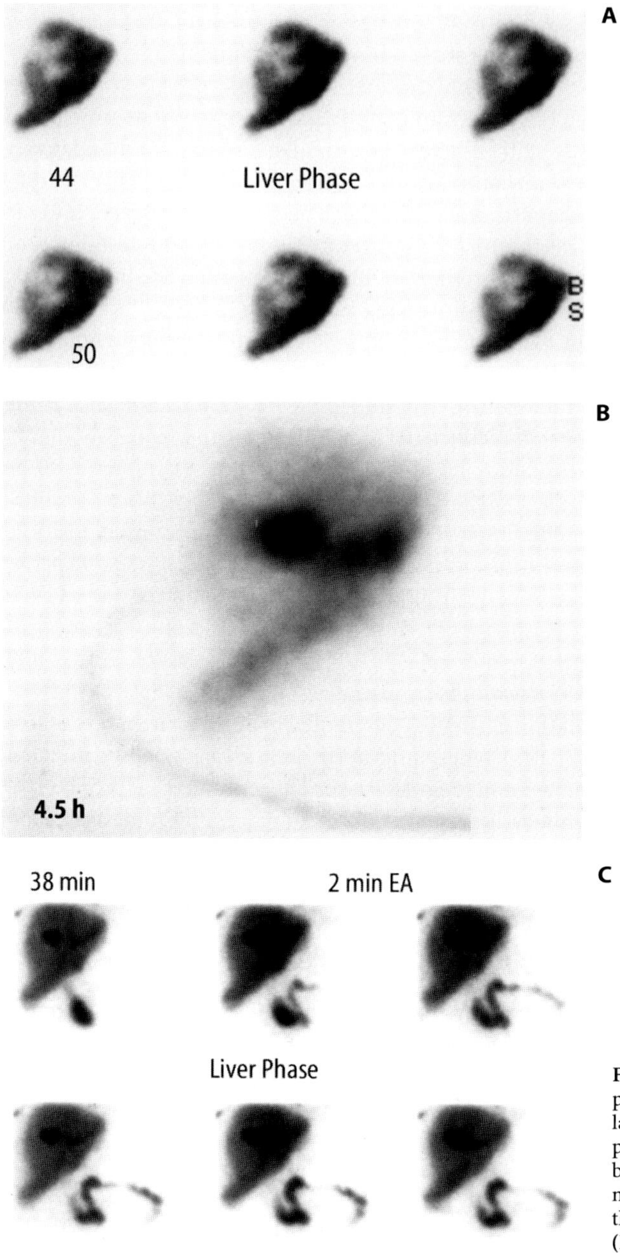

Fig. 12.1.3. Abscess in a transplant liver. An abscess causes a large filling defect within liver parenchyma (**A**) and fills with bile at 4.5 h (**B**). A repeat study 3 months later shows shrinkage of the abscess, but fistula persists (**B**).

Cholescintigraphy

The data are collected with a large field of view gamma camera fitted with a low energy, all purpose, parallel hole collimator, using 3–8 mCi ^{99m}Tc-HIDA. ^{99m}Tc-mebrofenin is preferred in jaundiced patients. Liver perfusion images are obtained at 2 s/frame during the first 1 min, followed by functional images at 1 min/frame for 59 min, for a total of 1 h, and recorded on a 64×64 word mode matrix. A short imaging interval is essential for location of the exact site of the bile leak. The first place of unexpected bile radioactivity usually indicates the site of origin of the leak. Once there is collection of a large volume of bile, it becomes difficult to identify the exact site of the bile leak.

Auxiliary Liver Transplantation

In an auxiliary transplant, the donor liver is placed in a heterotopic position adjacent to the native liver or in the space created by partial hepatectomy of the native liver (Fig. 12.1.4). Auxiliary liver transplantation is restricted mostly to patients with fulminant hepatic failure, where the native liver has the potential for full functional recovery, if the patient survives the acute episode. Fulminant hepatic failure consists of liver failure and encephalopathy occurring within a 2- to 8-week period in a previously healthy person. Fulminant hepatic failure is relatively rare, and accounts for 6% of all adult liver transplants and 11% of all pediatric liver transplants in a year in the United States [20]. Mortality is 100% in untreated patients. Spontaneous full functional recovery is attributed to regeneration capacity of the native liver in those patients who can withstand an acute insult.

Fulminant hepatic failure heals slowly over several months to attain full functional recovery (Table 12.1.4). When serum liver function tests show either an improvement or a deterioration in a patient with auxiliary liver transplantation, it is not clear from the serum levels whether the changes reflect the function of the native or the donor liver. The immunosuppressive dose needs to be increased when there is rejection of the donor liver. An improvement of the native liver function, on the other hand, calls for either a reduction in dosage or total discontinuation of immunosuppressive agents. The donor liver undergoes spontaneous regression and atrophy when the native liver recovers its full function, and steroids are withdrawn safely at this time. The donor liver is surgically removed if it does not undergo spontaneous atrophy and interferes with the function of the native liver [21, 22].

Differentiation of Native vs Donor Liver Function

Cholescintigraphy is able to measure the total liver function as well as the individual function of the donor and native liver. The differential liver function information helps in adjusting the dose of immunosuppressive agents.

Table 12.1.4. Differentiation of native from donor liver function following auxiliary liver transplantation for fulminant hepatic failure in a patient shown in Fig 12.1.4. (Courtesy of Dr. Muriel Buxton-Thomas, Kings College Hospital, London, UK)

Study no.	Time post-transplant	Native liver function			Auxiliary liver function		
		HEF (%)	Ex. *T*1/2 (min)	Function (%)	HEF (%)	Ex. *T*1/2 (min)	Function (%)
1	10 days	37	27	15	73	21	85
2	7 months	51	18	44	54	17	56
3	8.5 months	78	16	64	50	53	36
4	11.5 months	100	8	>99	–	–	<1

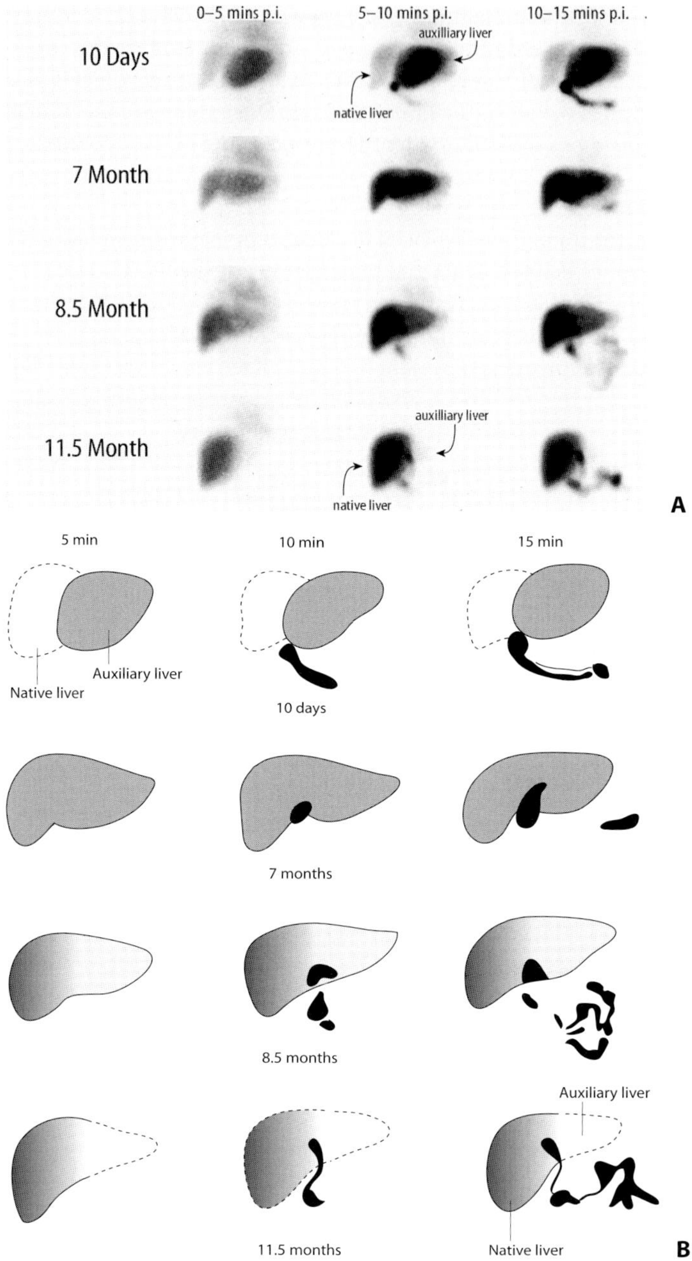

Fig. 12.1.4A,B. Pattern of recovery of native liver function following auxiliary liver transplantation. Cholescintigram (**A**) and a corresponding schematic diagram (**B**) are shown in a 2-year-old child with auxiliary liver transplant for fulminant hepatic failure. At 10 days, the native liver shows poor uptake and the auxiliary liver has good uptake of ^{99m}Tc-HIDA. Function appears equal by 7 months. Function of the auxiliary liver begins to decrease by 8.5 months, and disappears completely at 11.5 months. The native liver recovers its function completely with 100% extraction fraction. (Courtesy of Dr. Muriel Buxton-Thomas, Kings College Hospital, London, UK)

Cholescintigraphy is obtained in adults with a large field of view and in children with a standard or even a small field of view gamma camera, fitted with a low energy, general-purpose, parallel-hole collimator. With the patient in the supine position, the camera is positioned anteriorly to cover the entire native and donor liver. A dynamic 60 frame images at minute intervals are obtained with 4–6 mCi ^{99m}Tc-HIDA, and recorded on a 64×64 computer matrix. The preferred imaging agent in jaundiced patients is ^{99m}Tc-mebrofenin, which has superior biokinetic behavior in patients with hyperbilirubinemia [23]. Some obtain a liver scan with ^{99m}Tc-S-colloid to outline the liver borders, but this is not essential since early ^{99m}Tc-HIDA images, obtained within the first 5–6 min, provide similar morphologic information (Fig. 12.1.2).

Quantification. Many different methods have been used for quantification of transplant function. Deconvolutional analysis (Chap. 5) is applied to measure the extraction fraction of the native and auxiliary liver separately, by choosing heart for the input and liver for the output function. Excretion half-time is measured with a monoexponential fit. Some express the function as uptake of the injected dose by the native vs donor liver. Four regions of interest (ROIs) are drawn: two ROIs over the liver (one over the entire native liver and the other over the entire donor liver) and two ROIs for background just lateral to each liver. Background counts (from ^{99m}Tc-S-colloid when a preliminary scan is obtained) are subtracted from the liver counts and the net liver counts and curve are displayed. From the net liver curve, three functional parameters are generated [24]:

1. T_{max} = time to maximum liver counts
2. $T_{1/2}$ = clearance half-time using a monoexponential fit to the data points from peak counts
3. Relative uptake (RU) by the liver. RU is obtained by noting the area under the time-activity curves of the native and graft livers between 2 and 10 min

$$\text{RU by native liver} = \frac{\text{Native liver area between 2–10 minutes} \times 100}{\text{Native liver area between 2–10 min} + \text{donor liver area between 2–10 min}}$$

$$\text{RU by graft liver} = \frac{\text{Graft liver area between 2–10 minutes} \times 100}{\text{Graft liver area between 2–10 min} + \text{native liver area between 2–10 min.}}$$

The authors of one study followed patient recovery for up to 30 months and calculated the percentage uptake by the native liver by using the area under the curve between the 2nd and 10th min and showed the value of the scintigraphic method in management of the patient with auxiliary liver transplantation [24].

Deconvolutional analysis is applied when the software is available. In children, where the liver physiology is much faster than in adults, the data are collected at a much shorter interval, 30 s per frame for 30 min. The hepatic extraction fraction calculation uses only the first 30 frames (15 min) and the excretion $T_{1/2}$ is calculated using all 60 frames. Native and donor liver HEF and excretion half-times are measured separately for both. The contribution of each liver to the total function is calculated and expressed as a percentage (Table 12.1.4).

Recovery Pattern in Auxiliary Liver Transplantation

Immediately after the transplant, the function of the native liver remains depressed, with a median uptake value of 27% (range 4%–36%) during the first 4 weeks. The median uptake value raises gradually, increasing to twice the baseline value within 6–12 months after transplantation. When serum liver function tests show a stable normal value, the relative uptake by the native liver rises above 90%. The native liver T_{max} value may normalize within a month but the excretion $T_{1/2}$ value remains elevated for a much longer period of time. The dose of immunosuppressive agents may be decreased when the relative uptake value rises above 30% and the drug may be withdrawn completely when the uptake value rises above 90% [24]. The pattern of recovery of native liver function following an auxiliary liver transplantation in a 2-year-old child is shown in Table 12.1.4. Hepatic extraction fraction and excretion half-time of the native liver and auxiliary liver are measured separately for each liver (Fig. 12.1.4). As the function of the native liver improves gradually and recovers fully, the auxiliary liver function deteriorates with regresses of functional liver volume.

Living Donor Liver Transplantation

Although the liver is one solid organ, its distinct and separate segmental and lobar anatomy and physiology allow resection into smaller portions for transplantation [25]. Resection of the donor liver is performed along the physiological planes (Fig. 1.3, Chap. 1). The lateral segment of the left lobe (areas 2 and 3) or the entire left lobe (areas 2, 3, 4A, and 4B) is resected from the donor for transplantation in the recipient (Fig. 12.1.1). The first living donor liver transplantation was performed by Raia et al. in Brazil in 1989 [26]. The left lobe of the liver from a mother was transplanted successfully into her son in Australia in 1989 [27]. After addressing the ethical issues, numerous other centers around the world have started performing living donor liver transplantations [28–30]. The major advantages of living donor liver transplantation are: (1) reduction in waiting time, (2) high quality of donor liver, and (3) immunological similarity in haploidentical donors.

Complications

Postoperative complications are a major concern both in the donor and the recipient. Among the first 100 living-donor liver donor transplantations performed at the University of Chicago, 91 donors had resection of the lateral segment of the left lobe (areas 2 and 3) and the remaining 9 had resection of the entire left lobe (areas 2, 3, 4A, and 4B). Thirteen of the 100 donors had complications, which included bile leaks, infection, and injury to bile ducts and spleen [31]. Bile leak, bleeding, thrombosis, or infection may occur in either the recipient or the donor or both. Rejection is an additional complication in the recipient. The living donor liver transplantation procedure is found to be safe both for the donor and the recipient. Donor survival is 100% and the recipient survival ranges from 80% to 94% in centers that have done at least 15 or more living donor transplantations [21]. Common complications occurring within 30 days after transplantation include bleeding, extrinsic obstruction, hemobilia, and bile leak around the T-tube or at the anastomotic site. Bile leak around the T-tube usually close spontaneously and those that continue to leak may require sphincterotomy or insertion of a biliary stent. Common complications occurring after 30 days include stricture at or proximal to the site of anastomosis [32]. Viral, bacterial, and fungal infections are always a concern in an immunocompromised liver transplant patient [33].

Future Directions

The major advantage of functional hepatobiliary imaging is the opportunity to detect disease early before irreversible morphological changes take place. Simultaneous quantification of function provides a measure of the severity of disease and enables the clinician to determine the appropriate time to intervene with therapy and also to test later whether or not the chosen therapy has achieved the intended goals. Following a thorough clinical evaluation and analysis of liver function tests, ^{99m}Tc-HIDA cholescintigraphy is an appropriate initial imaging procedure for detection of most pathophysiologic changes associated with bile formation and flow [34]. Cholescintigraphic results can guide the clinician in developing a management strategy and also aid in determining the need as well as the type of imaging or non-imaging procedure that will lead to ultimate diagnosis. Liver biopsy is the most appropriate next step for patients with intrahepatic cholestasis. For extrahepatic cholestasis, the clinician may choose percutaneous transhepatic cholangiography for obstruction at or proximal to the union of the right hepatic and left hepatic ducts. ERCP is preferred for obstructions in the common hepatic or common bile duct [23]. Magnetic resonance cholangiopancreatography is being developed as an alternative to ERCP and early results appear very optimistic [35]. Receptor based imaging may enable the selection of receptor specific therapy. Asialoglycoprotein receptor quantitative imaging with ^{99m}Tc-DTPA galactosyl human serum albumin enables the prediction of residual liver function after resection of hepatocellular cancer and cholangiocarcinoma and the forecast of prognosis of liver cirrhosis [36–38]. A somatostatin receptor positive liver metastatic gastrinoma may respond to therapy with octreotide. Current FDA-approved radiotracers meet the clinical need for functional imaging in nuclear hepatology and their full potential is gradually being harnessed [39].

References

1. National Institute of Health consensus development conference statement, Liver transplantation. June 20–23, 1983, Hepatology 1983;3: Suppl 107S–110S
2. Welch CS. A note on transplantation of whole liver in dogs. Transplant Bull 1955,2:54
3. Starzl TE, Marchioro TL, Von Kaulla KN, Hermann G, Brittain RS, Waddell UR. Homotransplantation of the liver in humans. Surg Gynecol Obstet 1963;117:659–676
4. Goss JA, Shackleton CR, McDiarmid SV, Maggard M, Swenson K, Seu P, Vargas J, Martin M, Ament M, Brill J, Harrison R, Busuttil RW. Long-term results of pediatric liver transplantation. An analysis of 569 transplants. Ann Surg 1998;228:411–420

5. Starzl TE, Demetris AJ, Van Thiel D. Liver transplantation (1). N Engl J Med 1989;321:1014–1022
6. Kawasaki S, Makuuchi M, Matsunami H, Hashihura Y, Ikegami T, Nakazawa Y, Chisuwa H, Terada M, Miyagawa S. Living related liver transplantation in adults. Ann Surg 1998;227:269–274
7. Terpstra OT, Schalm SW, Weimar W, Willemse PJ, Baumartner D, Groenland TH, ten Kate FW, Porte RJ, de Rave S, Reuvers CB et al. Auxiliary partial liver transplantation for end-stage chronic liver disease. N Engl J Med 1988;319:1507–1511
8. Sudan DL, Shaw BW Jr, Fox IJ, Langnas AN. Long-term followup of auxiliary orthotopic liver transplantation for the treatment of fulminant hepatic failure. Surgery 1997;122:771–778
9. Shah AN, Dodson F, Fung J. Role of nuclear medicine in liver transplantation. Semin Nucl Med 1995;25:36–48
10. Stieber AC, Gordon RD, Galloway JR. Orthotopic liver transplantation. In: Zakim D, Boyer TD. (eds). Hepatology. A text book of liver disease. WB Saunders, Philadelphia, 1996, pp 1759–1780
11. Brown RK, Memsic LD, Busuttil RW, Pusey E, Ray RA, Kangarloo H, Hawkins RA. Accurate demonstration of hepatic infarction in liver transplant recipients. J Nucl Med 1986;27:1428–1431
12. Sanchez-Urdazpal L, Gores GJ, Ward EM, Maus TP, Wahlstrom HE, Moore SB, Wiesner RH, Krom RA. Ischemic-type biliary complication after orthotopic liver transplantation. Hepatology 1992;16:49–53
13. Von Moll LK, Juni JE, Merion RM. Scintigraphic demonstration of accessory hepatic duct leak following liver transplantation. J Nucl Med 1988;29:259–262
14. Lantsberg S, Lanchbury EE, Drolc ZA. Evaluation of bile duct complications after orthotopic liver transplantation by hepatobiliary scanning. Nucl Med Commun 1990;11:761–769
15. Madacsy L, Velosy B, Lonovics J, Csernay L. Differentiation between organic stenosis and functional dyskinesia of the sphincter of Oddi with amyl nitrite-augmented quantitative hepatobiliary scintigraphy. Eur J Nucl Med 1994;21:203–208
16. Bhatnagar A. Nifedipine interventional cholescintigraphy. A new method for assessing sphincter of Oddi? Indian J Nucl Med 1997;12:93–96
17. Krishnamurthy S, Krishnamurthy GT. Biliary dyskinesia: role of the sphincter of Oddi, gallbladder and cholecystokinin. J Nucl Med 1997;38:1824–1830
18. Hawkins RA, Hall T, Gambhir SS, Busuttil RW, Huang SC, Glickman S, Marciano D, Brown RK, Phelps ME. Radionuclide evaluation of liver transplant. Semin Nucl Med 1988;18:199–212
19. Jain A, Khanna A, Molmenti EP, Rishi N, Fung JJ. Immunosuppressive therapy Surgical Clinic of North America 1999;79:59–76
20. Shakil AO, Mazariegos GV, Kramer DJ. Fulminant hepatic failure. Surgical Clinic of North America 1999;79;77–108
21. Boudjema K, Cherqui D, Jaeck D, Chenard-Neu MP, Steib A, Freis G, Becmeur F, Brunot B, Simeoni U, Bellocq JP, et al. Auxiliary liver transplantation for fulminant and subfulminant hepatic failure. Transplantation 1995;59:218–223
22. Metselaar HJ, Hesselink EJ, de Rave S, ten Kate FJ, Lameris JS, Groenland TH, Reuvers CB, Weimar W, Terpstra OT, Schalm SW. Recovery of failing liver after auxiliary heterotopic transplantation. Lancet 1990;335:1156–1157
23. Krishnamurthy S, Krishnamurthy GT. Technetium-99m-iminodiacetic acid organic anions: review of biokinetics and clinical application in hepatology. Hepatology 1989;9:139–153
24. Buyck D, Bonnin F, Bernuau J, Belghiti J, Bok B. Auxiliary liver transplantation in patients with fulminant hepatic failure: hepatobiliary scintigraphy followup. Eur J Nucl Med 1997;24:138–142
25. Bismuth H, Houssin D. Reduced-size orthotopic liver graft in hepatic transplantation in children. Surgery 1984;95:367–372
26. Raia S, Nery JR, Mies S. Liver transplantation from live donors. Lancet 1989;2:497
27. Strong RW, Lynch SV, Ong TH, et al. Successful liver transplantation from a living donor to her son. N Eng J Med 1990;322:1505–1507
28. Emond JC. Clinical application of living-related liver transplantation. Gastroenterol Clin North Am 1993;22:301–315
29. Donovan J. Nonsurgical management of biliary tract disease after liver transplantation. Gastroenterol Clin North Am 1993;22:317–336
30. Reding R, Goyet JV, Delbeke I, Sokal E, Jamart J, Janssen M, Otte J. Pediatric liver transplantation with cadaveric or living related donors: comparative results in 90 elective recipients of primary grafts. J Pediatr 1999;134:280–286
31. Grewal HP, Thistlethwaite JR Jr., Loss GE, Fisher JS, Cronin DC, Siegel CT, Newell KA, Bruce DS, Woodle ES, Brady L, Kelly S, Boone P, Oswald K, Millis JM. Complications in 100 living-liver donors. Ann Surg 1998;228:214–219

32. Stratta RJ, Wood RP, Langnas AN, Hollins RR, Bruder KJ, Donovan JP, Burnett DA, Lieberman RP, Lund GB, PillenTJ et al. Diagnosis and treatment of biliary tract complications after orthotopic liver transplantation. Surgery 1989;106:675–684
33. Mazariegos GV, Molmenti EP, Kramer DJ. Early complications after orthotopic liver transplantation. Surgical Clinic of North America 1999;79:109–129
34. Krishnamurthy S, Krishnamurthy GT. Nuclear hepatology: where is it heading now? J Nucl Med 1988;29:1144–1149
35. Fulcher AS, Turner MA, Capps GW, Zfass AM, Baker KM. Half-Fourier RARE MR cholangiopancreatography: experience in 300 subjects. Radiology 1998;207:21–32
36. Sasaki N, Shiomi S, Iwata Y, Nishiguchi S, Kuroki T, Kawabw J, Ochi H. Clinical usefulness of scintigraphy with Tc-99m galactosyl-human serum albumin for prognosis of cirrhosis of the liver. J Nucl Med 1999;40:1652–1656
37. Hwang E, Taki J, Shuke N, Nakajima K, Kinuya S, Konoshi S, Michigishi T, Aburano T, Tonami N. Preoperative assessment of residual hepatic functional reserve using Tc-99m-DTPA-galactosyl-human serum albumin dynamic SPECT. J Nucl Med 1999;40:1644–1651
38. Uetake M, Koizumi K, Yagawa A, Nogata H, Tezuka T, Kono H, Ozawa T, Kusano T, Miyabukuro M, Hosaka M. Use of Tc-99m DTPA galactosyl human serum albumin to predict postoperative residual liver function. Clin Nucl Med 1999;24:428–434
39. Krishnamurthy S, Krishnamurthy GT. Functional imaging in nuclear hepatology. Indian J Nucl Med 1997;12:216–232

Subject Index

Printing (Computer to Film): Saladruck, Berlin
Binding: Stürtz AG, Würzburg